W9-BER-184

THE
pregnancy
BIBLE

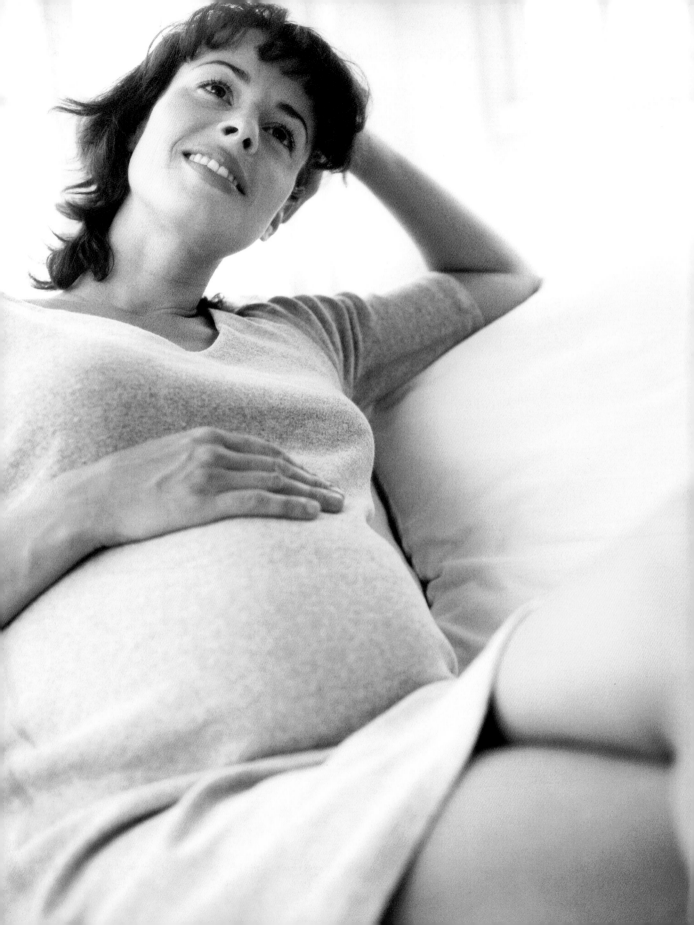

THE
pregnancy
BIBLE

*Your Complete Guide to Pregnancy
and Early Parenthood*

CONSULTING EDITORS

Joanne Stone, MD
Keith Eddleman, MD

FIREFLY BOOKS

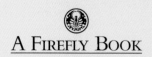

A FIREFLY BOOK

Published by Firefly Books Ltd., 2003

Copyright © 2003 Carroll & Brown

All rights reserved. No part of this publication may be reproduced, stored in a retrieval system or transmitted in any form or by any means, electronic, mechanical, photocopying, recording, or otherwise, without the prior written permission of the Publisher.

Fourth printing 2005

Publisher Cataloging-in-Publication Data (U.S.)
The pregnancy bible : your complete guide to pregnancy and early parenthood / consulting editors Joanne Stone and Keith Eddleman.—1st ed.
[392] p. ; col. photos. : cm.
Includes index.
Summary: A comprehensive guide for expecting mothers and fathers.
ISBN 1-55297-848-6
ISBN 1-55297-796-X (pbk.)
1. Pregnancy—Popular works. 2. Childbirth--Popular works.
3. Infants--Care. 4. Parenthood—Popular works. I. Stone, Joanne. II. Eddleman, Keith. III. Title.
618.2/ 4 21   RG525.P74 2003

National Library of Canada Cataloguing in Publication
The pregnancy bible : your complete guide to pregnancy and early parenthood / consulting editors, Joanne Stone, Keith Eddleman. --1st ed.
Includes index.
ISBN 1-55297-848-6 (bound).--ISBN 1-55297-796-X (pbk.)
1. Pregnancy--Popular works. 2. Childbirth--Popular works.
I. Stone, Joanne II. Eddleman, Keith
RG551.S64 2003   618.2'4   C2003-900394-9

Published in the United States by
Firefly Books (U.S.) Inc.
P.O. Box 1338, Ellicot Station
Buffalo, New York 14205

Published in Canada by
Firefly Books Ltd.
66 Leek Crescent
Richmond Hill, Ontario L4B 1H1

Created and produced by
Carroll & Brown Limited
20 Lonsdale Road, Queen's Park
London NW6 6RD

Project Editors: Kirsten Chapman, Alison Mackonochie and Debbie Musselwhite
Managing Art Editor: Emily Cook
Photography: Jules Selmes

Reproduced by Colourscan, Singapore
Printed by SNP Leefung, China

The contributors and publisher specifically disclaim any responsibility for any liability, loss, or risk (personal, financial, or otherwise) that may be claimed or incurred as a consequence—directly or indirectly—of the use and/or application of any of the contents of this publication.

CONTENTS

CONSULTANTS AND CONTRIBUTORS

Joanne Stone, MD
Associate Professor of Obstetrics, Gynecology, and Reproductive Science, and Director of Perinatal Ultrasound at Mount Sinai School of Medicine, New York, NY.

Keith Eddleman, MD
Associate Professor of Obstetrics, Gynecology, and Reproductive Science and Director of the Division of Maternal-Fetal Medicine at Mount Sinai School of Medicine, New York, NY.

Eve R Colson, MD
Assistant Professor of Pediatrics, Yale University School of Medicine, Director, Well Newborn Nursery, Yale-New Haven Hospital, CT.

Marilyn Graham, PhD, MD
Associate Professor of Clinical OB/Gyn, Indiana University, Indianapolis, IND.

David K James, MA, MD, FRCOG, DCH
Professor, Division of Feto-Maternal Medicine, Academic Division of Obstetrics & Gynecology, The University of Nottingham, Nottingham, UK.

James J Walker, MD, FRCP, FRCOG
Professor, Department of Obstetrics & Gynecology, St James University, Leeds, UK.

Michelle F Mottola, PhD
Associate Professor and Director, R Samuel McLaughlin Foundation—Exercise and Pregnancy Lab., School of Kinesiology, University of Western Ontario, Canada.

Richard Woolfson, PhD, FBPS
Writer, journalist, and child psychologist, with experience of working with children and families.

Peter Hepper, PhD, FBPsS, CPsychol
Professor of Psychology, Head of School of Psychology, and Director of the Fetal Behavior Research Center, Queen's University, Belfast, UK.

Wendy Doyle, SRD, PhD
Dietitian, London Metropolitan University, London, UK.

Kathleen Capitulo, DNSc, RN, FACCE
Director of the Maternal-Child Health Care Center and Associate Hospital Director at The Mount Sinai Hospital in New York, NY.

Patricia M Barnes, PNNP, MS, CNM
Certified Nurse-Midwife at Nativiti Women's Health and Birth Center, Houston, TX.

Jane Butler, RN, CNM, BS, MPH
Certified Nurse-Midwife at Maggee Women's Hospital, Pittsburgh, PA.

Christine Obremski, CNM, MS, RN
Director of Midwifery at The Mount Sinai Hospital in New York, NY.

Gayla Vanden Bosche, MA
Writer and Assistant Director, Magee Women's Hospital National Center of Excellence in Women's Health, Pittsburgh, PA.

June Thompson, RGN, RM, RHV
Health Visitor and freelance health writer.

Jeanne Langford, PGCE
Prenatal teacher and tutor with The National Childbirth Trust, London, UK.

Mary Nolan, PhD, MA, RGN
Prenatal teacher at The National Childbirth Trust, London, UK.

Lenore Abramsky
Genetic Associate, North Thames Perinatal Public Health Unit, Northwick Park Hospital, London, UK.

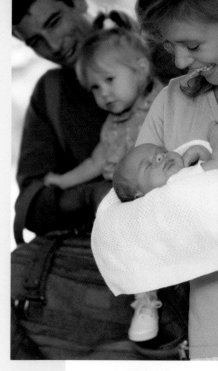

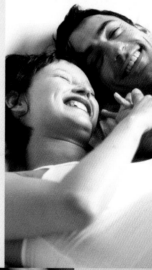

INTRODUCTION

Pregnancy is a unique experience and one that you will want to enjoy while doing what's best for your baby. Until recently, however, pregnancy did not always result in a healthy infant and mother. But today, great progress has been made—not only in understanding the risks to a baby's normal development, but also in knowing what a woman needs to do to successfully meet the challenges of pregnancy, labor, and delivery. All the information that is now available, particularly relating to situations that may be, evenly remotely, out of the ordinary, is rarely known in total to a single physician, no matter how well trained and experienced he or she is. That is why, to create a thoroughly researched book, we worked with a team of experts in every related field including genetics, midwifery, gynecology and obstetrics, pregnancy nutrition and exercise, psychology, fetology, and pediatrics. Additionally, we consulted teachers in natural childbirth techniques, breastfeeding, and baby care.

The Pregnancy Bible is the result. It covers every aspect of pregnancy, birth, and new parenthood. Although it cannot replace the care and attention that you'll receive from your healthcare providers, who'll know you as an individual, it can supplement that advice, explain procedures, give handy hints, and answer many questions that you may not have thought of asking.

It also contains many special features such as life-size illustrations, color photography, and the very latest 3-D images, which allow you to see how your baby develops week by week. Special gatefold pages give you an at-a-glance guide to what you can expect in each of the three trimesters.

Comprehensive sections on nutrition, exercise, and what you should do to maintain good health will help you achieve a healthy pregnancy and prepare for the birth that you want. There is also advice on the the emotional aspects of pregnancy for both you and your partner. Once your baby is born, further chapters contain information on how to take care of yourself and how to respond to, bond with, and feed, bath, change, dress, and carry your newborn.

Two reference sections form an in-depth guide to the tests and procedures that may be used during your pregnancy and to the treatment of the medical complaints and problems that can affect you or your newborn.

Most importantly, *The Pregnancy Bible* has been designed to help you achieve a positive attitude, which has been shown to be one of the most significant factors in a rewarding birth experience. With knowledge and understanding, you can take on pregnancy and parenthood with confidence.

Joanne Stone, MD and *Keith Eddleman*, MD

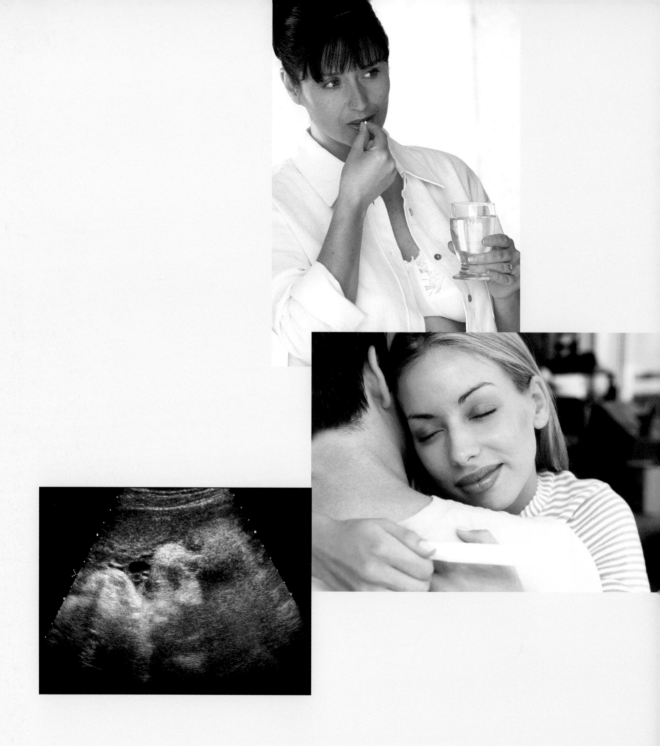

PART I   MIRACULOUS BEGINNINGS

THE STORY OF PREGNANCY

When a woman conceives, it's just the beginning of an amazing process. This chapter tells the story of how the fertilized egg reaches the uterus, how your baby inherits your characteristics, and how he or she develops week by week. It also outlines the major external changes to your body and the important milestones of the following nine months.

SPERM MEETS EGG

The beginning of life occurs at a microscopic level, when an egg no larger than a speck unites with a single sperm, the sole winner of a race with several million competitors.

To meet, egg and sperm undergo amazing, arduous journeys that are both fraught with failure. However, if they succeed, their meeting leads to the creation of a single cell containing genetic information from each partner. It's this unique blueprint that forms the basis of a new life.

Conception takes place in three basic stages: ovulation, fertilization, and the division of the fertilized egg, which then implants in the uterus—it's not until this is successful that pregnancy begins.

THE EGG COMES FIRST

A woman is born with her lifetime's supply of approximately 2 million eggs. From the moment of birth the eggs begin to die off, and by the time a girl reaches puberty only an estimated 400,000 eggs will remain. Of these, some 400 to 500 will mature over her lifetime and be released during ovulation.

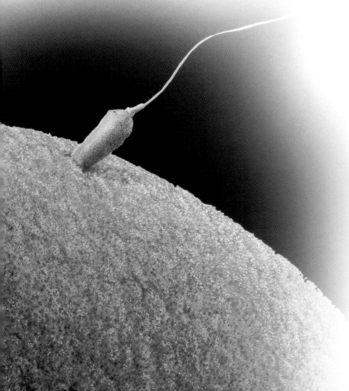

In most women ovulation happens every month in response to a hormone released by the pituitary gland. Each month around 100 to 150 ova (eggs) begin to ripen inside protective, fluid-filled sacs called follicles. Usually only one of these eggs reaches maturity, and as this happens, the hormone estrogen is released into the bloodstream, effectively stopping the ripening of other eggs. This hormone also triggers the lining of the uterus to thicken, forming a blood-rich cushion in preparation for the possible development of an embryo.

HOW OVULATION HAPPENS

At ovulation, which occurs about midway through the menstrual cycle, the follicle that has outgrown the others finally ruptures, and the egg bursts out. The site of the release is called the stigma, and the ruptured follicle goes on to form the corpus luteum. Translated as "yellow body," the corpus luteum produces a hormone, progesterone, which sustains the growing baby until the placenta takes over the role. At this stage the egg is no more than a dot, barely visible to the naked eye.

As the egg is released from the ovary it's moved along the fallopian tube toward the uterus by tiny, hairlike projections called cilia. If conception takes place, it normally happens toward the outer end of the tube, near the ovary.

If the egg isn't fertilized within 12 hours of being released, the egg dies, the follicle dries up, the lining of the uterus is shed, and a menstrual period occurs. This is all due to a drop in the level of the hormone progesterone. However, if the egg is fertilized, then progesterone levels will increase and the uterus lining continues to thicken.

Signs of ovulation

Although most women are completely unaware of ovulation, around 25 percent experience lower abdominal pain, usually on the side near the ovary that's ovulating. The pain is called mittelschmerz

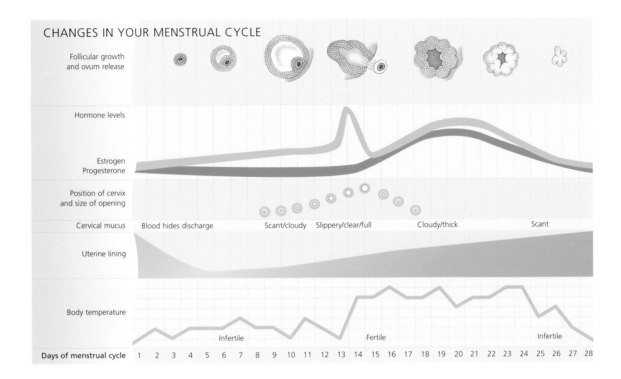

CHANGES IN YOUR MENSTRUAL CYCLE

Follicular growth and ovum release

Hormone levels

Estrogen
Progesterone

Position of cervix and size of opening

Cervical mucus | Blood hides discharge | Scant/cloudy | Slippery/clear/full | Cloudy/thick | Scant

Uterine lining

Body temperature | Infertile | Fertile | Infertile

Days of menstrual cycle | 1 2 3 4 5 6 7 8 9 10 11 12 13 14 15 16 17 18 19 20 21 22 23 24 25 26 27 28

(literally, "middle pain") and is thought to be caused by irritation from fluid or blood from the follicle when it ruptures. However, this pain is not considered a reliable sign of ovulation, as it doesn't occur with every cycle.

A more concrete sign of ovulation is a change in the mucus secreted by the cervix (the neck of the uterus). Just after menstruation the mucus is scant, thick, and sticky, making it impenetrable to sperm. As ovulation approaches, the mucus becomes thinner and wetter, allowing healthy sperm to travel through it at speed. After ovulation, the mucus reverts back to its usual, more inhospitable consistency. Another sign of ovulation is body temperature. Progesterone causes a small but distinct rise in body temperature from 97.5 to 98°F (36.4 to 36.7°C). When a man and woman make love during the woman's fertile period—that is, when ovulation has just happened or is imminent—this is the optimum time for conception.

THE GREAT SPERM RACE

When the man ejaculates into the vagina he releases hundreds of millions of sperm at a speed of around 10 miles (16 km) an hour. The sperm are mixed with a sugar-containing fluid that gives them energy for the testing journey ahead. The fastest will reach the egg in 45 minutes, the slowest take around 12 hours. However, most don't even make the journey—they either trickle out of the vagina or are lost or destroyed along the way. Only a few hundred of the strongest swimmers will eventually arrive at the fallopian tubes where fertilization can take place.

Obstacles and advantages

Sperm have to traverse the vagina, the cervix, and uterus, and swim out into the fallopian tubes before they reach the egg. It's a distance of only some 6 to 7 inches (15 to 18 cm), but is the equivalent of a human swimming over 100 lengths of an olympic-sized swimming pool.

The odds are stacked against sperm ever reaching their destination. When they enter the vagina they aren't fully active and are incapable of fertilization. It's only as they travel through the mucus in the vagina that they become activated and capable of fusing with an egg. Millions get lost in the numerous crevices of the vagina or arrive at the wrong fallopian tube. Others, mainly weak or damaged sperm, are destroyed by the deadly acidic environment in the vagina. Interestingly, it seems that female sperm, which contain an X chromosome

MORE **ABOUT**   sperm

Sperm development begins in puberty when a clutch of hormones, including testosterone, kickstart production. Sperm continues to be made throughout adulthood, though the quantity and quality begin to decrease from about the age of 40. The average healthy young man produces 2 to 6 ml of semen per ejaculation, with each milliliter containing 50 to 150 million sperm. Each sperm looks like a tadpole and measures approximately 0.05 mm in length. A sperm has a long tail that helps it swim along the vagina and up the fallopian tube, and an oval-shaped head that contains genetic information.

(see page 18), are more comfortable with the acidic conditions in the vagina than male sperm, which contain a Y chromosome. Millions more sperm are pushed back by microscopic hairs inside the uterus.

However, other factors give the sperm a helping hand. If a woman orgasms during intercourse, it's thought that wavelike contractions in her vagina draw the sperm in toward the cervix—although you don't have to have an orgasm to become pregnant. During a woman's fertile period (see diagram, page 11), the mucus that usually forms a barrier to the cervix becomes slippery and thin, so helping the sperm's progression into the uterus. The opening of the cervix also becomes wider in readiness for receiving sperm. It's estimated that some 40 million healthy sperm travel through the cervix and across the uterus, a journey that takes around 45 minutes.

The fallopian tubes also release an alkaline mucus, which nourishes the sperm as it waits for the egg to be released.

A matter of timing
The moment of conception is wholly dependent on timing. A woman must have a ripe egg ready as a healthy sperm arrives in the fallopian tube. Sperm can survive for up to four days in the female body, but any longer than this and they'll die before the egg arrives. This means that if a woman has intercourse two to three days before ovulation, she can still conceive. If sperm arrive after ovulation they never have the chance to meet the egg in the fallopian tube.

And the winner is…
Only around 200 sperm make it to the site of fertilization, but the race isn't yet over. The egg is surrounded by thousands of cells that nourish it. The sperm fight their way through these cells, flipping them out of the way with their tails. When they reach the wall of the egg, a sticky substance on the surface helps them attach. The objective now is to burrow through the outer layer of the egg, called the corona radiata, and through a further layer, the zona pellucida. Several sperm may break through the outer layer, but usually only one reaches the nucleus. When this happens, the head of the sperm fuses with the nucleus of the egg, and the egg immediately throws up a chemical barrier around it to stop other sperm from penetrating.

The beginning of life
As the egg and sperm fuse together, the sperm loses its tail and its head enlarges. The egg and sperm form a single cell containing 46 chromosomes of genetic information—23 from each parent. The inside of the cell swirls around, forcing chromosomes to mingle. In a matter of hours this

single cell will duplicate material known as deoxyribonucleic acid (DNA) and split into two. The building blocks of life are now forming.

YOUR CHANCES OF CONCEIVING

Fertility varies widely, so it can take longer for some couples to conceive than others. On average, among couples having regular intercourse, 25 percent of women will conceive within one month, 60 percent within six months, 80 percent within a year, and 90 percent within 18 months.

However, certain factors on both the male and female side can mean that it may take longer to conceive. For example, smoking, drinking alcohol, certain medications, obesity, and exposure to heat and chemicals can all affect sperm quantity and quality. Insufficient and poor quality sperm won't survive the journey to the egg. Even if they meet, damaged sperm or eggs may not be able to fuse successfully or they may produce a fertilized egg that can't survive the early stages of growth. In women, the quality of eggs deteriorates with age, and, after the age of 35, you may not ovulate every month, even though you still have regular periods. Smoking and abusing drugs or alcohol can also damage your

eggs. In some women a fallopian tube may be blocked or scarred, hindering the progress of a ripe egg. You can improve your chances of conceiving with the following:

- *Regular exercise* It not only improves your physical well-being, but helps reduce stress, promotes relaxation, and encourages good sleep.
- *A general health check* Visit your doctor to find out if you are in peak physical condition.
- *Tracking your ovulation* You can do this by keeping a menstrual calendar—ovulation usually occurs 14 days before menstruation—checking for raised body temperature, and using ovulation detection kits. Make love at least every other day during your fertile period.
- *Avoiding smoking* It not only has a damaging affect on overall health but can affect your partner's sperm count.
- *A balanced diet* Make sure that you receive adequate amounts of vitamin B12, which is found in meat, fish, eggs, and milk. More importantly, take a folic acid supplement.

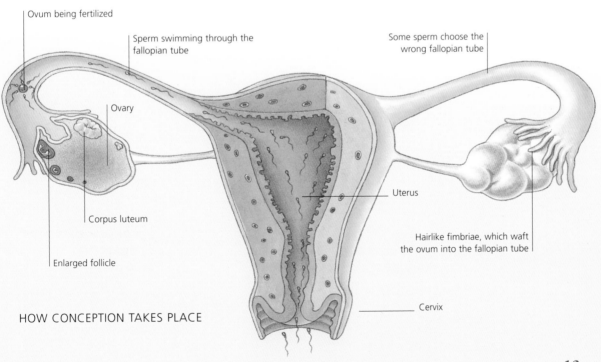

Ovum being fertilized

Sperm swimming through the fallopian tube

Some sperm choose the wrong fallopian tube

Ovary

Corpus luteum

Enlarged follicle

Uterus

Hairlike fimbriae, which waft the ovum into the fallopian tube

Cervix

HOW CONCEPTION TAKES PLACE

THE JOURNEY TO THE UTERUS

Between 12 and 20 hours after the egg is fertilized, the cell that is formed begins to divide in two, replicating its DNA as it does so. This division continues rapidly, and all the while this bundle of cells is heading toward the uterus, where the fetus will eventually grow.

It takes the fertilized egg around seven days to reach the uterus after leaving the ovary. This journey along the fallopian tube is helped along by the cilia (hairlike feelers) that line the tube. The fallopian tube also nourishes the developing cells and removes waste products produced by the cells as they divide. During this time the fertilized egg goes through several stages of development.

FROM EGG TO BLASTOCYST
The fertilized egg is called a zygote, and this divides and subdivides until it forms a solid ball the size of a pinhead. Consisting of 16 to 32 cells, this is now called a morula. The morula continues dividing at 15-hour intervals so that by the time it reaches the uterus, some 90 or so hours later, it has approximately 64 cells. Of these, only a few cells will actually develop into the embryo; the rest will go to form the placenta and the membranes that surround the baby in the uterus.

The morula gradually goes from being solid to being a fluid-filled ball of cells, and at this stage it is called a blastocyst. The surface of the blastocyst consists of a single layer of large, flat cells called trophoblast cells. These later develop into the placenta. Inside the ball is a small cluster of inner cells that will become the embryo.

In the early stages of development, when the zygote is no bigger than a few cells, each one of these has the potential to become a human being. If the zygote splits, identical twins are formed.

IMPLANTATION TAKES PLACE
About five to seven days after ovulation occurs, progesterone production is at its height, stimulating the growth of the rich blood vessels that supply the endometrium (the lining of the uterus). This coincides with the arrival of the blastocyst in the uterus ready for implantation. At this stage, the blastocyst is less than one hundredth of an inch (0.23 mm) across. It floats freely in the uterus for a few days as it continues to develop and grow. Approximately nine days after fertilization, the blastocyst attaches itself to the uterine wall by means of spongelike projections of trophoblast cells which burrow into the endometrium. These cells grow into the chorionic villi (see page 140), which will later develop into the placenta. Occasionally, implantation causes a small amount of bleeding, known as spotting.

If the blastocyst doesn't implant, it will be swept out with the next menstrual period, and the woman won't even be aware that she had conceived.

THE DEVELOPING EMBRYO

Zygote

Morula

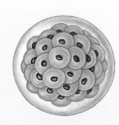

Blastocyst

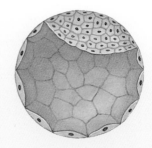

Cross-section of blastocyst

Finding nourishment

By the time it implants, the blastocyst is made up of hundreds of cells. It releases enzymes that penetrate the lining of the uterus and cause tissue to break down. This provides a nourishing mix of blood and cells on which it can feed. Occasionally, the lining of the uterus doesn't supply a rich enough source of food for the blastocyst. In this case, a miscarriage occurs, rather like a late, heavy period.

It's also after implantation that the placenta begins to develop and the embryo begins to produce the pregnancy hormone human chorionic gonadotrophin (HCG). It's this hormone that can be detected by pregnancy testing kits.

What happens next

It takes around 13 days for the embryo to implant firmly. Miscarriage is still a possibility but is much less likely now. The embryo begins to produce progesterone of its own, encouraging the endometrium to develop. It's also at this stage that the embryo's first organs start to form, beginning with the nervous system and, later, the heart. Thirteen days is the latest date that an embryo can split into two to become twins. If the split occurs later, conjoined (Siamese) twins are formed.

CONCEIVING TWINS

Over the past 20 years, largely because of the increase in fertility treatments, the chances of conceiving twins—and more—have increased. In Canada, twins accounted for around 2.9 percent of all births in 2000. While in the United States, the rate of twin births increased from 28.1 per 1000 live births in 1998 to 28.9 in 1999. This rate has risen more than 25 percent since 1990. Interestingly in 2000, the rate of triplet and other higher-order multiple births declined for the second consecutive year, after increasing more than fivefold between 1980 and 1998. This may be due to changes in infertility treatments.

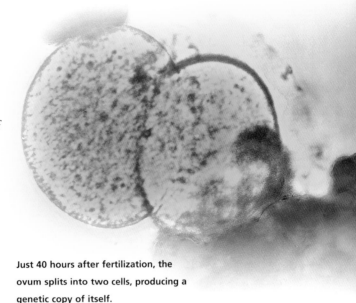

Just 40 hours after fertilization, the ovum splits into two cells, producing a genetic copy of itself.

Many more twins are conceived than are actually born. Known as the "vanishing twin" syndrome, this occurs when one of the fetuses spontaneously aborts, usually during the first trimester, and the fetal tissue is absorbed by the other twin, the placenta, or the mother, making it seem that the twin has vanished.

DID YOU KNOW...

Implantation can often fail Attaching to the endometrium is a risky business. It's estimated that around 40 percent of blastocysts entering the uterus never implant. Instead they die and are swept out with the next menstruation. It appears that timing plays a part, with an early or late arrival impacting negatively on the blastocyst's success in implanting.

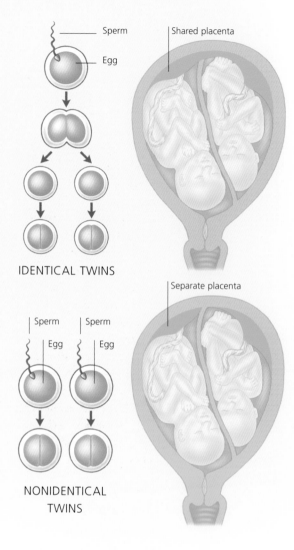

Sperm

Egg

Shared placenta

IDENTICAL TWINS

Separate placenta

Sperm   Sperm

Egg   Egg

NONIDENTICAL
TWINS

Identical or nonidentical twins

About one third of twins are identical—technically monozygotic—and two thirds are nonidentical—technically dizygotic—twins. Identical twins develop when, as in a normal conception, an egg is fertilized by a single sperm. The fertilized egg then splits into two, causing two separate embryos to develop—if it splits into three, triplets result, and so on. Identical twins may or may not share a placenta and amniotic sac, but each twin has its own umbilical cord. These babies will have the same identical genetic makeup and will be the same sex. They will also have the same hair, eye color, and blood type.

Nonidentical twins—also called fraternal twins—are produced when a woman releases more than one egg when she ovulates. This could be two eggs from one ovary, or one from each. Each egg is fertilized by a different sperm and two genetically different babies are conceived. They can be the same sex or boy and girl, and will look as much alike or different as any other siblings.

In the case of triplets, quads and more, there can be any combination of identical and nonidentical children. For example, three—or four or more—eggs can be fertilized creating nonidentical triplets. Or, one fertilized egg can split into identical twins with another fertilized egg making it a triplet pregnancy with two identical babies and one nonidentical. Or a single egg can divide into three, thereby creating identical triplets.

The hereditary factor

One factor influencing the conception of twins is your age. After the age of 35, the chances of conceiving identical twins rises. However, the chances of conceiving nonidentical twins rises until about the age of 35 and then drops off. This may be due to the fact that as you age you naturally produce more ovulation-stimulating hormones, which could trigger your ovaries to release more eggs each month.

Your chances of having twins also increase with each subsequent pregnancy, and it seems that larger, taller women are 25 to 30 percent more likely to have them. Nonidentical twins also may run in families, on the mother's side. Finally, there seems to be an ethnic predisposition: Twins are more common in women of African origin and occur least frequently in women of Asian origin.

YOUR BABY'S INHERITANCE

Your baby's genetic endowment is determined at the moment of conception. Half of that will have come from the egg and half from the sperm. So, no matter who the baby looks like, both you and your partner have contributed equally in terms of her inherited makeup.

The process whereby you pass on characteristics to your children is amazingly intricate, but the natural rules that govern it can be easily understood. To understand more about how you and your partner influence your baby's characteristics, you first have to be clear about some basic genetics.

GENES AND CHROMOSOMES

Your body is made up of millions of cells, all of which are copies of the fertilized egg from which you developed, and the nucleus (center) of each of these cells contains a copy of all your genes. Genes

Your child may resemble you more than your partner because of the way the genes you gave her have mixed.

are the blueprints that instructed your body how to form when you were an embryo and determine how it functions now. These blueprints are encoded in miniscule units of deoxyribonucleic acid (DNA).

DNA influences how your baby will look. The color and efficiency of her eyes, the texture of her hair, the shape of her nose, her blood type, her bone structure, and many more of her characteristics are determined by her genes, which she inherits from you—and you inherited from your parents. There are about 30,000 genes in each of the body's millions of cells, so it takes little imagination to realize that they're extremely small—too small to be seen even under a very powerful microscope. All these genes combine to make you unique.

Genes don't float around loose inside the body's cells; they're packaged systematically onto structures called chromosomes. Normally, in each cell, your baby has 46 chromosomes that exist in matching pairs. One chromosome in each pair came from you and the matching one from your partner. Each chromosome carries thousands of genes and is large enough to be seen under a powerful microscope.

YOUR GENETIC MAKE UP

Who are you most like—your mother or your father? You have one pair of genes for each characteristic: one from your mother and one from your father. For some characteristics, both your parents may have given you the same version of a gene, and for others they may have given you different versions. Sometimes, one version of a gene dominates over another; in other cases, both influence the outcome equally. It's the total effect of the combination of all your genes that determines your hereditary makeup.

Variety is the spice of life

Many genes exist in a variety of different forms, just as there are many possible recipes for chocolate cake. If this weren't the case, people would all look exactly alike and the world would be a very boring place. Since there are many versions of the thousands of genes you inherit from your parents, you are genetically unique, unless, that is, you have an identical twin. Even your brothers and sisters will be genetically different, because their genetic inheritance all depends on the unique combination of genes in a particular egg and a particular sperm. This idea carries through for your baby and any children you have in the future.

Some genes do not form correctly. If both genes of the pair are abnormal, this can result in problems such as cystic fibrosis or sickle-cell disease (see page 240). These disorders are said to be inherited recessively (see below). Other abnormal genes cause problems even if only one gene of the pair is abnormal, for example in Huntington's disease (see page 240). Some abnormal genes that are carried on the X chromosome cause problems only for boys. These so-called X-linked disorders include Duchenne muscular dystrophy and hemophilia (see page 240). For information on genetic counseling, see the Prenatal Reference section.

Who will your baby look like?

If you and your partner both passed on your full complement of 46 chromosomes in the egg and sperm, your baby would have 92 chromosomes in her cells, and the numbers would continue to double with every generation. This system wouldn't work. Instead, in the formation of eggs and sperm, the cells go through a specialized division, in which they halve the number of chromosomes within each—so each egg and sperm contains only 23 chromosomes. Therefore, for any given chromosome you will give your baby either the one you received from your mother or the one your received from your father; your partner does the same.

Your baby will receive some chromosomes that you inherited from both your parents, so she could have, for example, your father's build and hair color but your mother's eye color. If you plan to expand your family in the future, your next child will inherit a slightly different combination, so will be another unique addition to your family.

Silent genes

Your baby can inherit genes from you that you didn't know you had. For example, your baby may turn out to have red hair, even though neither you or your partner do. This is because some genes are dominant and others are recessive, and, in the pairs of chromosomes that are formed, the dominant genes override the information coded on the recessive genes. So you and your partner may carry both the gene for black hair, which is dominant, and the gene for red hair, which is recessive. In each of you, the black hair gene dominates. However, if you both pass on the red hair gene to your baby, there is no dominant gene to override the recessive gene, so your baby will have red hair.

How chromosomes determine the sex of a child

Just like physical characteristics, your baby's sex is also decided at the moment of conception. Of the 23 pairs of chromosomes, only one pair determines whether your baby is a boy or a girl. This crucial pair are the sex chromosomes: X and Y. Girls have two X-chromosomes, boys have one X and one Y chromosome. Because of the way that eggs and sperm are produced, all eggs contain a single X chromosome. Half the sperm contain an X and half contain a Y chromosome. At fertilization, when the sperm and egg pool their chromosomes, if the sperm carries an X the baby will be a girl and if it carries a Y he will be a boy. It's ironic that historically women have borne the blame for failing to produce boys, when the sex of the baby is determined entirely by which of the father's sperm fertilized the egg.

THE FIRST SIGNS OF PREGNANCY

Some women just intuitively know when they're pregnant and are even able to pinpoint the exact moment that they conceived. For other women, it might not be so obvious.

You don't have to "feel" pregnant to actually be pregnant and while there are certain telltale symptoms of pregnancy, you might not necessarily experience them all.

EARLY INDICATIONS

You may experience one or two, or all, of the following symptoms of pregnancy. Morning sickness is the classic giveaway sign, but you may be one of the lucky ones and hardly have it at all. Likewise, while missing a period is another classic symptom, if your periods have always been irregular, it can be difficult to tell if you're late because you're pregnant or late because of the irregularities in your cycle.

Missing a period
This is one of the clearest indications of pregnancy. However, there are other reasons why menstruation may be delayed. Stress, illness, extreme fluctuations in weight—excessive gain or anorexia—or coming off the oral contraceptive pill can all stop periods for a while. Irregular periods are a common symptom with polycystic ovary syndrome, a condition in which periods can occur several months apart.

Breast tenderness
Changes in the size and feel of your breasts are one of the earliest signs of pregnancy. As early as a few days after conception your breasts will begin to enlarge in readiness for breastfeeding, and you'll probably experience heaviness and soreness. Many women report that their breasts are very sensitive and experience a sharp, tingling sensation, too, although this often disappears a few weeks later. These breast changes may be less dramatic with subsequent pregnancies.

Nausea and vomiting
Feeling sick is the most common complaint in early pregnancy and is experienced by most women from around 5 to 6 weeks of pregnancy, but it can also begin as early as two weeks after conception. Although termed "morning sickness," the nausea can occur at any time of day and can vary from an occasional, faint sensation to being an overwhelming nausea and vomiting (see page 67). By and large, these symptoms tend to disappear by around 14 to 16 weeks of pregnancy.

Tiredness
Many women report feelings of extreme tiredness during pregnancy, especially at the beginning. Typically, after getting in from work in the evening all you want to do is go to bed, or you may be

Carried out correctly, home pregnancy testing kits are 98 to 99 percent accurate, so you can trust the results.

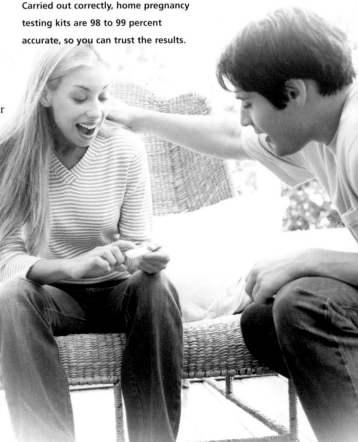

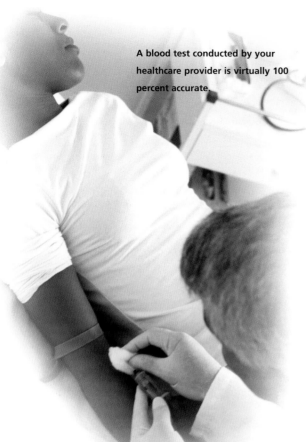

A blood test conducted by your healthcare provider is virtually 100 percent accurate.

desperate for a mid-afternoon nap. When you reach week 14 of your pregnancy, your energy levels should start to pick up.

Frequent urination

As early as two to three weeks after conception you will find yourself wanting to urinate more frequently. This is due to the pressure of the enlarging uterus on the bladder, literally reducing the capacity of your bladder. At about 14 weeks the uterus rises up into the abdomen, which often relieves this annoying symptom until the last few weeks of pregnancy when the baby's head engages (drops down in the uterus), again causing pressure on your bladder. Rising levels of the pregnancy hormone progesterone also stimulate the bladder muscle so that you feel your bladder is full even when there's not much urine in there. In addition to this, your kidneys are working harder in response to being pregnant and an extra 13 to 15 pints (6 to 7 liters) will be added to your circulation to increase the blood flow around your body.

Changes in taste and smell

Don't be surprised if certain foods suddenly make you feel queasy or if you start to crave particular foods (see page 99) or even certain smells. You also may have a strange metallic taste in your mouth.

Constipation

A common early symptom of pregnancy, this is caused by high levels of progesterone, which relaxes the bowel and slows your digestion (see page 72).

Mood swings

High levels of pregnancy hormones flood your body in early pregnancy, making you extra emotional and sometimes weepy (see page 151).

CONFIRMING YOUR PREGNANCY

Two weeks after conception your baby is just a ball of cells, not much bigger than a pinhead, starting to develop in the lining of the uterus. Already the placenta is forming and starting to produce a hormone called human chorionic gonadotrophin (HCG), which passes into your bloodstream and urine from the day of your first missed period.

Home pregnancy tests

These tests, which you can buy from most drug stores, confirm pregnancy by detecting HCG in the urine. They are very accurate, so don't be surprised if your healthcare provider relies on your own home test for confirmation of your pregnancy. Normally

DID YOU KNOW...

You can have "a period" when you're pregnant
Some women experience light bleeding around nine days after the egg was fertilized. This bleeding is usually lighter than a proper period and is thought to be caused when implantation occurs as the ovum first attaches to the uterine wall.

doctors only repeat the test if complications arise, such as a concern about miscarriage. However, if you receive a positive result, you should make an appointment to see your healthcare provider for proper medical follow-up.

Office urine test

A urine test carried out in your healthcare provider's office works in the same way as a home pregnancy test—detecting the presence of HCG in the urine to confirm pregnancy. It's almost 100 percent accurate, and doesn't require a urine sample at the start of the day. As it's carried out by a professional, you can have more confidence in the result.

Pregnancy blood tests

Your healthcare provider may also use a blood test to help detect and date a pregnancy. The test your healthcare provider uses may simply give you a positive or negative result or it may test levels of HCG in your blood, depending on your symptoms and medical history or simply what your healthcare provider prefers. The more sophisticated blood tests are virtually 100 percent accurate and can detect a pregnancy from as early as the first week after conception. If the exact amounts of HCG are measured, these can help date the pregnancy, as the values of this hormone change as pregnancy progresses. However, an ultrasound scan is still the best way to date pregnancy, and you may be offered one at your first prenatal visit (see page 87).

Pregnancy blood tests are useful if there are any concerns about miscarriage or if your healthcare provider suspects an ectopic pregnancy (see page 274). In these situations HCG blood levels don't usually rise as fast and may even fall, indicating that the pregnancy has failed.

Internal exam

Four to six weeks after conception, your healthcare provider can receive definite proof of pregnancy by examining you internally. He or she will be looking

HOW TO use a pregnancy testing kit

You can perform a home pregnancy test from the first day that you've missed your period and onward. There are several different home kits on the market, so always read the manufacturer's instructions carefully.

It is best to use the first urine passed when you get up in the morning; this will be the most concentrated, so even tiny amounts of HCG can be picked up by the test. Later in the day your urine tends to get more dilute because of what you've been drinking and eating, so early pregnancy hormone levels may be too low for a home kit to detect.

Some tests ask you to hold a stick in your urine flow **1**, others require that urine is passed first into a clean container and then a few drops squeezed from the dropper provided **2** onto a window on an oblong stick.

Usually the result appears within minutes and can be read by looking for a colored line in a window on the stick. Often there is also a line indicating that the test has been carried out correctly. If the test is negative, but you still feel that you may be pregnant, repeat the test in five to seven days. It may be that the pregnancy is too early to detect and you became pregnant later than you thought. This is most likely if you have irregular periods.

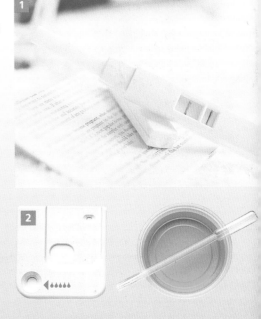

How to calculate your due date

Once your pregnancy's been confirmed, one of the first things you'll want to know is when your baby will be born. Your pregnancy, which is described as being 40 weeks long—according to Naegele's rule of dating (see box, right)—is dated from the first day of your last menstrual period (LMP).

If you have a regular 28-day cycle and know the date of the first day of your LMP, you can use Naegele's rule to work out your baby's due date by counting on nine months plus seven days—or 280 days—after the first day of your LMP. You can adjust the date according to the length of your cycle. If you have a 26-day cycle, count on nine months plus five days from your LMP—or 278 days. If you have a

32-day cycle, count on nine months plus 11 days from your LMP—or 284 days—and so on.

Alternatively, use the chart below to find out your estimated date of delivery (EDD). First, find the date that your last menstrual period was due by looking at the numbers in bold. Then look at the number in the line directly below it, which represents your EDD. If, for instance, your LMP was 12 April, your baby will be due on 17 January the following year. Remember, however, that this is just a general guide—only about 5 percent of babies are born on their estimated birth date.

DATING PREGNANCY

In the 1800s, a German obstetrician called Naegele fixed the length of pregnancy at ten lunar months—nine calendar months—or 280 days, and now all pregnancies are dated according to "Naegele's Rule." He based his calculations on the first day of the woman's LMP, but as conception usually occurs two weeks later, a pregnancy is actually 38 weeks long—or 266 days—not 40 weeks. So, two weeks after you conceived, you're described as being in week 4 of your pregnancy.

January	1	2	3	4	5	6	7	8	9	10	11	12	13	14	15	16	17	18	19	20	21	22	23	24	25	26	27	28	29	30	31
Oct/Nov	8	9	10	11	12	13	14	15	16	17	18	19	20	21	22	23	24	25	26	27	28	29	30	31	1	2	3	4	5	6	7
February	1	2	3	4	5	6	7	8	9	10	11	12	13	14	15	16	17	18	19	20	21	22	23	24	25	26	27	28			
Nov/Dec	8	9	10	11	12	13	14	15	16	17	18	19	20	21	22	23	24	25	26	27	28	29	30	1	2	3	4	5			
March	1	2	3	4	5	6	7	8	9	10	11	12	13	14	15	16	17	18	19	20	21	22	23	24	25	26	27	28	29	30	31
Dec/Jan	6	7	8	9	10	11	12	13	14	15	16	17	18	19	20	21	22	23	24	25	26	27	28	29	30	31	1	2	3	4	5
April	1	2	3	4	5	6	7	8	9	10	11	12	13	14	15	16	17	18	19	20	21	22	23	24	25	26	27	28	29	30	
Jan/Feb	6	7	8	9	10	11	12	13	14	15	16	17	18	19	20	21	22	23	24	25	26	27	28	29	30	31	1	2	3	4	
May	1	2	3	4	5	6	7	8	9	10	11	12	13	14	15	16	17	18	19	20	21	22	23	24	25	26	27	28	29	30	31
Feb/Mar	5	6	7	8	9	10	11	12	13	14	15	16	17	18	19	20	21	22	23	24	25	26	27	28	1	2	3	4	5	6	7
June	1	2	3	4	5	6	7	8	9	10	11	12	13	14	15	16	17	18	19	20	21	22	23	24	25	26	27	28	29	30	
Mar/Apr	8	9	10	11	12	13	14	15	16	17	18	19	20	21	22	23	24	25	26	27	28	29	30	31	1	2	3	4	5	6	
July	1	2	3	4	5	6	7	8	9	10	11	12	13	14	15	16	17	18	19	20	21	22	23	24	25	26	27	28	29	30	31
Apr/May	7	8	9	10	11	12	13	14	15	16	17	18	19	20	21	22	23	24	25	26	27	28	29	30	1	2	3	4	5	6	7
August	1	2	3	4	5	6	7	8	9	10	11	12	13	14	15	16	17	18	19	20	21	22	23	24	25	26	27	28	29	30	31
May/Jun	8	9	10	11	12	13	14	15	16	17	18	19	20	21	22	23	24	25	26	27	28	29	30	31	1	2	3	4	5	6	7
September	1	2	3	4	5	6	7	8	9	10	11	12	13	14	15	16	17	18	19	20	21	22	23	24	25	26	27	28	29	30	
Jun/Jul	8	9	10	11	12	13	14	15	16	17	18	19	20	21	22	23	24	25	26	27	28	29	30	1	2	3	4	5	6	7	
October	1	2	3	4	5	6	7	8	9	10	11	12	13	14	15	16	17	18	19	20	21	22	23	24	25	26	27	28	29	30	31
Jul/Aug	8	9	10	11	12	13	14	15	16	17	18	19	20	21	22	23	24	25	26	27	28	29	30	31	1	2	3	4	5	6	7
November	1	2	3	4	5	6	7	8	9	10	11	12	13	14	15	16	17	18	19	20	21	22	23	24	25	26	27	28	29	30	
Aug/Sept	8	9	10	11	12	13	14	15	16	17	18	19	20	21	22	23	24	25	26	27	28	29	30	31	1	2	3	4	5	6	
December	1	2	3	4	5	6	7	8	9	10	11	12	13	14	15	16	17	18	19	20	21	22	23	24	25	26	27	28	29	30	31
Sept/Oct	7	8	9	10	11	12	13	14	15	16	17	18	19	20	21	22	23	24	25	26	27	28	29	30	1	2	3	4	5	6	7

for telltale signs such as the uterus softening and an alteration in the texture of the cervix. The vaginal tissues thicken and produce more secretions, resulting in a heavier discharge. The uterus grows so quickly—it's already about the size of a small orange by 8 weeks—that an internal exam can accurately date a pregnancy.

LETTING PEOPLE KNOW

You may be so excited when you discover the good news that you want to tell everyone you meet in the street. However, you may decide to wait a while. There are some people that you'll want to tell as soon as possible, such as your partner and your healthcare provider, and others that you might want tell at a later stage, once you're sure that your pregnancy is progressing well.

Healthcare provider

If you've found out that you're pregnant with a home testing kit, one of the first things you should do is make an appointment to confirm the pregnancy, either with your family doctor or a midwife. Once you know, you'll need to make an appointment for your first prenatal check-up (see page 87)—in some cases you may be able to have this at the same time.

Friends and family

When to tell your friends and family is very much a personal decision. You might choose to tell only your nearest and dearest at first, such as your partner and close relatives and friends, and then start to spread the news as your pregnancy becomes more obvious. Alternatively, you might choose to postpone making your pregnancy common knowledge until after the third month, once the risk of miscarriage has reduced—women who have suffered a previous miscarriage often choose to do this.

Your employer and colleagues

The question of how to break the news at work sometimes causes concern for moms-to-be. But you can make it easier on yourself if you plan what you're going to say. Find out about maternity law and company policies before you talk to your boss.

One of the major issues is deciding when to tell your employers and work colleagues, and this depends on a number of factors. If you're putting on weight and suffering from morning sickness and tiredness, you may want to tell others soon, before they draw their own conclusions. However, if you have a review coming up, you may want to hold off until you've heard that you're going to get that promotion or pay raise. If you work in an environment that you think may be harmful for your baby, it's best to talk to your employer as soon as possible to find out about the possibility of changing duties. For more information about working safely, see page 79.

MORE **ABOUT** | trimesters

The nine-and-a-bit months of pregnancy are divided into three trimesters, which mark the major milestones in your and your baby's progress. The trimesters are of slightly uneven length. The first trimester represents the first 13 weeks, and is the period during which your baby's major systems and organs are formed. The beginning of the second trimester, at 14 weeks, is a turning point for both you and your baby: You will probably feel some relief from any early pregnancy symptoms, and your pregnancy may start to show, while your baby is now fully formed and will start to grow. The third trimester, starting at week 28, is the home stretch, as your body prepares for birth and your baby continues to grow in weight and length.

1 YOUR PREGNANT BODY

Weeks

| 1 | 2 | 3 | 4 |

Although you're unlikely to put on much weight or look significantly pregnant during the first 13 weeks of pregnancy, momentous changes are happening inside you. Emotionally, you're adjusting to the idea of being pregnant and beginning to take on board the incredible changes this will make to your life. Expect to put on 2 to 4 lbs (0.9 to 1.8 kg) this trimester, of which just 1¾ oz (650 g) will be due to your baby.

1
Your healthcare provider will date your pregnancy from the first day of your last menstrual period, which will be written as LMP in your prenatal records. Pregnancy usually lasts about 280 days or 40 weeks.

2
Your ovaries have begun to ripen an egg, which will be released into the fallopian tube in a process known as ovulation. This usually happens 12 to 16 days before the start of your next period.

You may notice that your vaginal secretions are wetter and more transparent at this time, and some women even feel slight pain with ovulation.

If you haven't already been taking a folic acid supplement, then start as soon as possible and continue for the rest of the first trimester.

3
Conception has taken place. Your egg has fused with a single sperm to create the unique cell destined to become your baby.

4
Your uterus is beginning to enlarge and soften, and the texture of your cervix is changing.

You may experience some breakthrough bleeding as the fertilized egg embeds in the lining of the uterus.

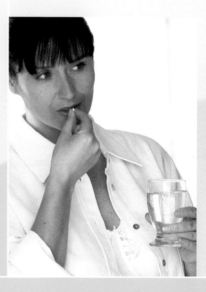

1-4

- You won't look any different, but your baby is starting to develop, and his brain and spinal cord are beginning to form.
- Some women "feel" they are pregnant soon after conception even before they have missed their next period.

10

You may find yourself becoming upset or irritable over things that wouldn't normally bother you. This is due to hormonal changes, but can be exacerbated by natural anxieties about pregnancy and motherhood.

11

You may notice that your hands and feet feel warmer, due to the increase in blood volume. You may also find yourself feeling thirstier than usual, as your body signals that it needs extra fluids.

It's normal to have gained around 2¼ lbs (1 kg) in weight by this stage, although some women actually lose weight in the first trimester if they suffer from nausea.

12

You may be offered the nuchal translucency test for Down syndrome, which involves the use of ultrasound (see page 238).

If you suffered from morning sickness you should start to feel better now.

13

This marks the end of the first trimester, when the development of your baby's vital organs and structures is complete.

The risk of miscarriage is reduced by around 65 percent.

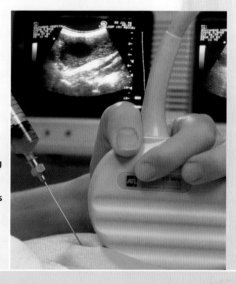

Chorionic villus sampling (CVS) can be carried out at around 11 weeks. This tests for chromosomal abnormalities and inherited disorders.

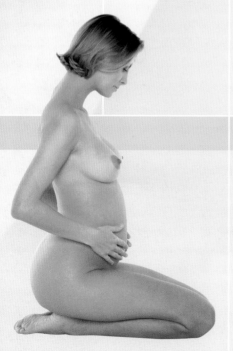

10–13

- ◆ You'll feel the urge to pass water more frequently.
- ◆ Changes in blood pressure make faintness or dizziness common, especially with changes in position, such as getting up from a chair quickly.
- ◆ Blood vessels are often visible on the breasts and small nodules, called Montgomery's tubercles, may appear around the nipples.
- ◆ Hormonal changes may lead to a breakout in pimples.

2 YOUR PREGNANT BODY

Weeks

14	15	16	17

During this trimester many of the discomforts of early pregnancy will have passed, and you may begin to appear and feel incredibly well. At long last you look pregnant. Expect to gain about 12 lbs (5.4 kg) this trimester, 2 lbs (900 g) of which will be due to your baby.

You may find that you're suffering from constipation due to increasing levels of progesterone, which cause the muscles of the intestine to slow. The pressure of your growing uterus also affects the bowel and inhibits its normal function. The simplest solution is to drink more water and eat fiber-rich fruit and vegetables.

By now, you may have noticed that you have trouble fastening your trousers, so it may be time to start thinking about maternity clothes. For advice on what to wear, see page 135.

Your next prenatal visit will likely take place between now and week 20. You will be offered an ultrasound scan to check your baby's anatomy (see page 92).

If you've had a previous pregnancy, you may feel your baby's first movements.

The urge to urinate frequently should have passed by now.

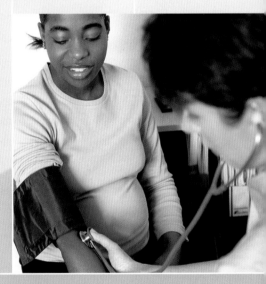

Your blood pressure will be tested at each prenatal visit. After week 20, this will be to check for signs of pre-eclampsia (see page 254).

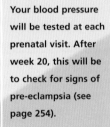

14-17

- Your placenta is fully formed and takes over the task of hormone production from you.
- Morning sickness has usually passed completely by now, and you begin to feel like your old self again.
- Changes in hormone levels are likely to affect the texture of your skin and hair.
- You may experience cravings for certain foods.

18	**19**	**20**	**21**	**22**

At this stage, your energy levels are probably back to normal, and you may experience an increase in your libido. The extra estrogen in your body boosts blood flow to the pelvic area, making sexual arousal more frequent and faster than before. Gentle lovemaking is perfectly safe during pregnancy, but if you have any concerns, speak to your healthcare provider.

Your increased metabolism and blood supply has a positive effect on your nails.

High estrogen levels mean that a few women develop chloasma, dark patches of skin on the face.

Your next prenatal check takes place around now.

If this is your first baby, you might feel her move at around 18 to 20 weeks.

You may notice that you are perspiring more than usual because of the effort of carrying around extra weight.

Your breasts may have started leaking colostrum, your baby's first food. Montgomery's tubercles (small nodules on the areolas) produce a moisturizing substance that will protect the nipples during breastfeeding.

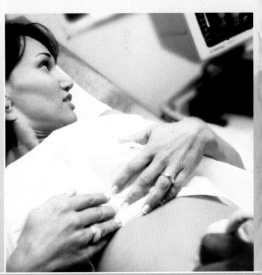

Ultrasound is used to check on the health of your baby. Your healthcare provider will measure your baby's length, check her heart, spinal cord, and limbs.

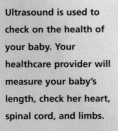

18-22

- Changes to skin tone are common, with pigmented areas—areolas, moles, freckles—becoming darker.
- Your hair may appear thicker, as the natural cycle of shedding hair comes to a halt and doesn't resume again till after the birth.
- Increased blood flow to the pelvic area coupled with highly sensitive breasts make achieving orgasm more likely.
- The top of your uterus can now be felt by pressing around 3 inches (7.5 cm) below your navel.

You've missed your period. An over-the-counter pregnancy test will confirm that you're pregnant.

Once confirmed, you should set up a visit with your healthcare provider.

You may notice a change in your breasts, due to hormonal stimulation of the milk-producing glands. Your breasts may feel full and tender, and your nipples may already be more prominent.

The areolas, the brownish circles of skin around the nipples, become darker, and bluish veins may be seen just under the skin as the blood supply to the breasts increases.

Your first prenatal visit is scheduled for between now and week 12. A physical exam, blood-pressure check, and routine tests will be carried out. You may be offered an ultrasound scan to confirm your due date (see page 22).

If you haven't already, you may start to experience the nausea and vomiting of "morning sickness," and you're likely to feel extremely tired.

Your heart rate rises steeply and your metabolic rate increases up to 25 percent.

Your uterus has doubled in size since you conceived.

Although you won't look pregnant yet, you might notice that your waistband is starting to get tighter.

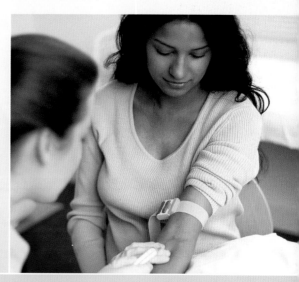

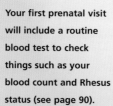

Your first prenatal visit will include a routine blood test to check things such as your blood count and Rhesus status (see page 90).

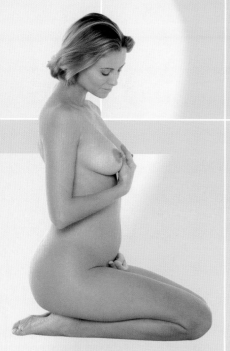

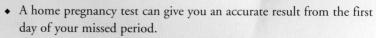

5-9

- A home pregnancy test can give you an accurate result from the first day of your missed period.
- The earliest physical signs of pregnancy, other than a missed period, include tiredness, changes in smell and taste, and your breasts becoming fuller and more tender.
- It's very common to go off foods that you previously enjoyed.
- Mood swings are common, and you may feel emotionally vulnerable.

23

As your abdomen grows, so does its impact on your digestive system. For some women this results in the discomforts of indigestion and heartburn.

To ease heartburn eat several small snacks, rather than two or three large meals, and, whenever possible, take a gentle walk after meals to aid digestion.

24

Your next prenatal checks may take place between now and week 28.

If you haven't already, start practicing Kegel exercises now (see page 122) to strengthen your pelvic-floor muscles.

25

As your abdomen gets bigger and heavier, you may experience backache, pressure in the pelvis, and cramps in the legs. Shortness of breath may also be a problem. Paying attention to your posture and getting plenty of rest will help.

Make sure you book your childbirth classes now. These will give you the opportunity to meet your healthcare providers and other moms-to-be.

26

You next prenatal check takes place between now and week 28.

If you're going to get stretch marks they'll appear around now, usually on your belly and breasts.

27

This is the end of the second trimester. Your abdomen is now quite prominent, although its size depends on your height, weight, and frame, whether or not you've been pregnant before, and the amount of amniotic fluid surrounding your baby.

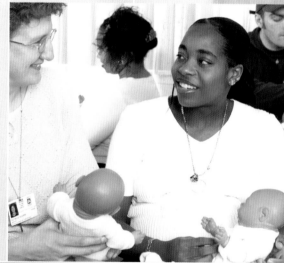

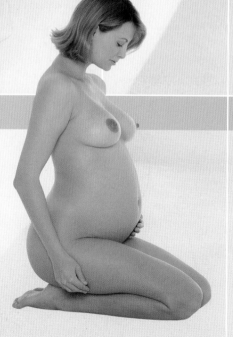

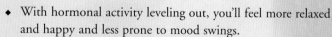

23-27

- With hormonal activity leveling out, you'll feel more relaxed and happy and less prone to mood swings.
- Pelvic-floor muscles are becoming stretched, which may result in stress incontinence (leaking urine when laughing or coughing).
- You'll be accumulating fat stores around your breasts and hips, and it's likely that your pre-pregnancy clothes won't fit anymore.
- Your heart and kidneys are working extra hard to maintain adequate blood circulation and process surplus fluids.

YOUR BABY WEEK BY WEEK

YOUR BABY'S SIZE

During the first trimester, babies follow a very predictable growth pattern, and measuring their body length, which can be done as early as 7 weeks, is the most accurate way of determining their age. It's easier to measure from crown to rump than from crown to heel, because the baby's legs are often bent. However, in later pregnancy, a baby's size can vary considerably, and crown-to-rump measurements are less accurate in determining the baby's age than the use of ultrasound.

The story of your unborn baby's development is an incredible one, beginning life as a fertilized egg and growing and maturing into a fully fledged human being, equipped with all the essential functions to survive in the outside world.

Conception usually occurs two weeks after a period. Most women, however, don't know exactly when they conceived, so it's easier for healthcare providers to date pregnancy from the first day of your last period. If, for example, your last period was ten weeks ago, you'll be considered in week 10 of your pregnancy, even though your baby will probably only be 8 weeks old. The descriptions below detail the development of your baby according to your weeks of pregnancy.

Pregnancy lasts for approximately 40 weeks. Babies born before 37 weeks are regarded as premature, while infants born after 42 weeks are regarded as postmature.

WEEK 4

...of your pregnancy.
Your baby is 2 weeks old.

Your baby measures between $\frac{1}{70}$ and $\frac{1}{25}$ inch (0.36 and 1 mm) from crown to rump.

This is a time of astounding development for your baby. At the end of the third week, the fertilized ovum (egg) is embedded in the lining of your uterus where it continues to multiply and grow. What was originally a simple sperm and egg cell has become a blastocyst (fluid-filled ball) of several hundred cells. This blastocyst now divides into two, one half inside the other. The half attached to the wall of the uterus becomes the placenta. Its outer layer forms the umbilical cord, the amniotic and yolk sacs, and the chorion (protective membranes in the uterus).

The inner half of the blastocyst will become your baby. This divides into three layers, known as germ layers, which grow to form different parts of your baby's body. The inner layer will form the liver, pancreas, bladder, thyroid gland, and the lining of the gastrointestinal tract. The middle layer develops into muscle, bone, cartilage, blood vessels, and kidneys, while the outer layer will become the brain and nervous system, skin, and hair.

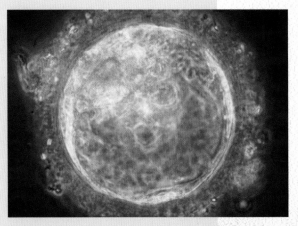

WEEK 5

...of your pregnancy.
Your baby is 3 weeks old.

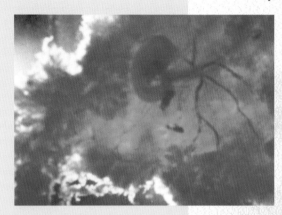

Your baby measures about ¹⁄₂₀ inch (1.25 mm) from crown to rump.

What was a round mass of cells has begun to elongate and a head and tail are now distinguishable. The central nervous system begins to develop, and your baby's brain and spinal cord start to form. Traces of the eyes and ears are discernible on the sides of her head, the liver and kidneys are beginning to develop, and muscle and bone are also in the early stages of development, although her bones will not ossify (harden) for a while yet. The walls of your baby's heart are now forming—her heart will begin to beat by the end of the week.

At this stage your baby derives most of her nourishment from nutrients stored in the uterine walls, but from as early as week 4 the placenta begins to provide nourishment.

WEEK 6

...of your pregnancy.
Your baby is 4 weeks old.

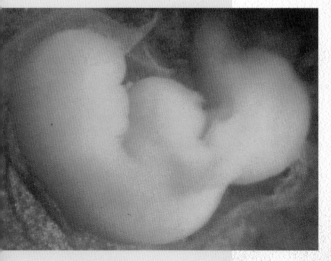

Your baby measures about ¹⁄₂ to ¹⁄₆ inch (2 to 4 mm) from crown to rump.

Growth is very rapid this week. Your baby might look like a tadpole, with his curved back and tail, but he now has a brain. His tiny heart is no bigger than a poppy seed, but it is beating on its own. Other major organs, including the kidneys and liver, continue to develop, and the neural tube, which connects the brain and spinal cord, closes. Your baby's head now begins to take shape.

A rudimentary digestive tract begins to form, together with the abdominal and chest cavities and the backbone. What will eventually become the testes or ovaries appear as a cluster of cells. Rudimentary arms and legs appear as tiny buds on the body. Your baby now has his own bloodstream, which has started to circulate blood.

WEEK 7

...of your pregnancy.
Your baby is 5 weeks old.

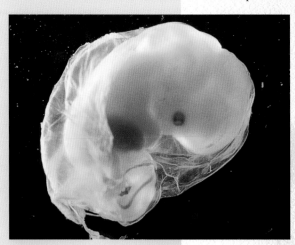

Your baby measures about ⅙ to ⅕ inch (4 to 5 mm) from crown to rump.

Your baby is beginning to look more human now, and her tail has almost vanished. However, her head is still bumpy and bent forward. Dark spots on the sides of her head will be her eyes, two holes represent the beginnings of nostrils, and her lips, tongue, and first tooth buds are visible. Her arms and legs have lengthened, and she has rudimentary hands and feet.

This is a vulnerable stage for your baby when all her major organs are forming, so you need to avoid any potential hazards, which could adversely affect this development. Her heart has divided into the right and left chambers and is beating about 150 beats a minute—about twice the rate of an adult. Her liver, kidneys, lungs, intestines, and internal sex organs are all nearing completion.

WEEK 8

...of your pregnancy.
Your baby is 6 weeks old.

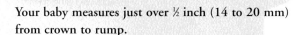

Your baby measures just over ½ inch (14 to 20 mm) from crown to rump.

Your baby's head is still larger than the rest of his body, and his facial features continue to develop. He now has a tongue and nostrils—you can even see the tip of his nose—while his jaw is fusing to shape his mouth. The next eight days are crucial for the development of his eyes and inner ears, responsible for balance and hearing.

Most of your baby's internal organs such as his heart, brain, liver, lungs, and kidneys have developed in their basic forms. His intestines are starting to develop in the umbilical cord. His heartbeat has normalized and the pumping capacity has increased. Under his paper-thin skin, you can see a network of blood vessels.

Up to now, your baby's framework has been made up of cartilage. Now bone cells begin to replace this. His leg and arm bones are hardening and lengthening, and his joints start to form. He begins to move around, although you can't feel him yet.

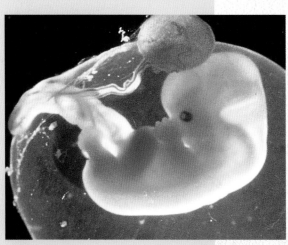

WEEK 9

...of your pregnancy.
Your baby is 7 weeks old.

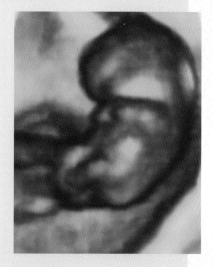

Your baby measures about 1 inch (22 to 30 mm) from crown to rump.

Your baby is now beginning to look like a proper baby. This three-dimensional (3D) ultrasound scan clearly shows her head bent forward onto her chest, and her developing limbs. Her hands, feet, and limbs are growing quite fast. Her fingers and toes are nearly complete, and touch pads form on the fingers. Her eyelids almost cover her eyes and her nose has taken shape.

   During the next few days your baby's diaphragm will develop; this is the muscle that will enable her to breathe after birth. Her intestines now begin to move out of the umbilical cord, where they started to form, and into her abdominal cavity where the space is increasing as her body gets bigger.

WEEK 10

...of your pregnancy.
Your baby is 8 weeks old.

Your baby measures about 1¼ to 1⅔ inches (31 to 42 mm) from crown to rump, and weighs about ⅕ oz (5 g).

Your baby switches from being an embryo to a fetus—which means "little one"—this week. His brain has grown so much by now that his head still looks too big for the rest of his body. His eyes and nose are clearly visible. Twenty tiny baby tooth buds are forming in his gums.

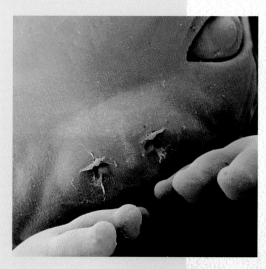

   Your baby's wrists and ankles have formed by now, and you can make out fingers and toes. Most of his joints are formed. Genitals have begun to form, but it's too early to distinguish the sex.

   Your baby's nervous system is responsive and many of his internal organs begin to function. His lungs continue to develop, and his stomach and intestines are developing in his abdomen. His kidneys are moving into their final positions in the upper abdomen, and his heart is almost completely developed.

WEEK 11

...of your pregnancy.
Your baby is 9 weeks old.

Your baby measures about 1¾ to 2¼ inches (44 to 60 mm) from crown to rump, and weighs about ⅓ oz (8 g).

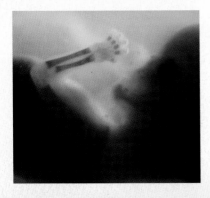

Your baby's development has passed its critical stage, and from now on she'll be at less risk of developing any sort of congenital abnormality or being affected by most infections and certain drugs.

By the end of the week her body will double in length, and her head will be almost half the length of her body. Underneath her fused eyelids, the irises start to develop, and these will later protect her eyes from too much light. However, her ears won't be fully developed for some time. Even this early on, your baby can yawn, suck, and swallow.

Your baby's vital organs—liver, kidneys, intestines, brain, and lungs—are fully formed and beginning to operate. For the rest of the pregnancy they just need to grow. Finishing touches, such as fingernails and downy hair, start to appear. Her heart carries on pumping blood to all her internal organs, including the umbilical cord, which transfers blood to the placenta.

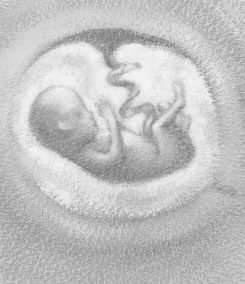

At week 12, your baby is fully formed. His face is rounder and he's looking more and more like a human baby.

WEEK 12

...of your pregnancy.
Your baby is 10 weeks old.

Your baby measures about 2½ inches (61 mm) from crown to rump, and weighs between ⅓ to ½ oz (8 to 14 g).

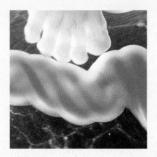

Your baby is fully formed from top to toe, although his organs continue to develop, particularly the brain. His fingers and toes have separated, and his hair and nails continue to grow. His bones continue to harden. The genitals begin to take on their gender characteristics. Your baby's vocal cords are forming and the pituitary gland at the base of the brain is beginning to make hormones.

It's astonishing what your baby can do at this stage: He can move his arms, fingers, and toes. He can smile, frown, and suck his thumb.

His digestive system is now capable of absorbing glucose (sugar). However, the umbilical cord is busy circulating blood between the placenta and your baby to provide nourishment and get rid of waste products produced by his rapid growth.

WEEK 13

...of your pregnancy.
Your baby is 11 weeks old.

Your baby measures 2⅗ to 3 inches (65 to 78 mm) from crown to rump and weighs between ½ to ⅔ oz (13 to 20 g).

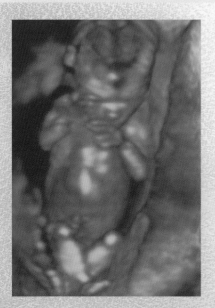

Although fully formed—as seen on this three-dimensional (3D) ultrasound scan—your baby wouldn't be able to survive outside the uterus yet, as her internal organs, particularly her lungs, haven't matured sufficiently. The intestines have moved farther into her body, while her liver begins to secrete bile, and her pancreas starts to produce insulin. The external genital organs continue to grow.

Your baby's neck is fully formed and can support head movements. Her eyes are moving into position on the front of her head, and her ears move to their normal position. Research suggests that your baby starts to sense sounds now. The ears aren't fully formed until around 24 weeks, but it's thought that babies "hear" sound through vibration receptors on their skin.

WEEK 14

...of your pregnancy.
Your baby is 12 weeks old.

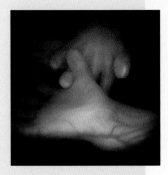

Your baby measures about 3¼ to 4 inches (80 to 93 mm) from crown to rump now and weighs almost 1 oz (25 g).

This week marks the beginning of the second trimester. Your baby's growth speeds up as his internal organs mature. The placenta is now his support system, producing hormones and supplying him with essential nutrients and oxygen.

Your baby's movements are now less jerky, and he can bend, flex, and twist his fingers, hands, wrists, legs, knees, and toes. His nervous system has begun to function. His eyelids, fingernails, and toenails continue to develop, and he has a sprinkling of hair on his head.

Your baby now "practices" the movements of breathing in and out, in readiness for life outside the uterus. He doesn't need to breathe in his watery world, as his oxygen comes straight from you, via the umbilical cord and the placenta.

WEEK 15

...of your pregnancy.
Your baby is 13 weeks old.

Your baby measures 4 to 4½ inches (104 to 114 mm) from crown to rump and weighs about 1¾ oz (50 g).

Your baby's ribs, blood vessels, and retinas—which appear as dark spots on her head—are clearly visible through her wafer-thin skin, but her skin now starts to be covered with lanugo, extra-fine hair that helps regulate her body temperature. This body hair follows the pattern of her skin, creating patterns that look like fingerprints all over her body. She also starts to develop eyebrows, and the hair on her head continues to grow, but this hair may change its color and texture after she's born.

The mechanisms enabling your baby to hear are developing. Very small bones in her middle ear have begun to harden, but as her brain's auditory centers haven't developed yet, she won't be able to make sense of the sounds she hears. The amniotic fluid she swims in acts as a sound conductor, so over time she'll begin to hear your voice and your heartbeat.

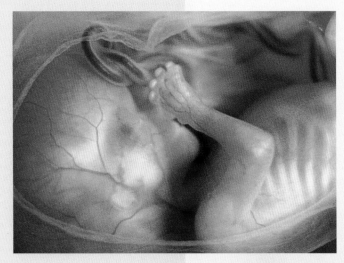

WEEK 16

...of your pregnancy.
Your baby is 14 weeks old.

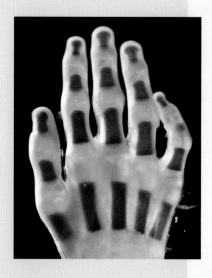

Your baby measures about 4⅓ to 4⅗ inches (108 to 116 mm) from crown to rump and weighs 2¾ oz (80 g).

Your baby's arms and legs are complete, and his joints are working. Bones that have already formed are getting harder and retaining calcium—a process known as ossifying. On the picture, left, hardened bone shows up as dark red.

Your baby's nervous system is operating and his muscles are responding to stimulation from his brain, so he can coordinate his movements. He continues to be very active in his private space, rolling over, doing somersaults, and kicking. However, you won't feel more than a fluttering sensation, as amniotic fluid cushions your baby's more vigorous movements. If this is your first baby, you won't usually recognize these as your baby's movements for another few weeks. You can now tell your baby's sex on an ultrasound scan.

WEEK 17

...of your pregnancy.
Your baby is 15 weeks old.

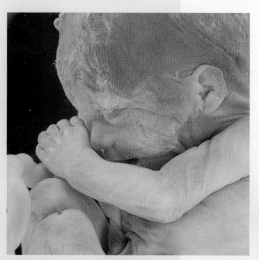

Your baby measures about 4½ to 5 inches (11 to 12 cm) from crown to rump and weighs about 3½ oz (100 g).

Your baby's head, while still big, is beginning to look in proportion to the rest of her body. Her eyes are still closed but are much larger, and her eyelashes and eyebrows have grown longer. This is a period of rapid growth, as fat starts to be laid down under your baby's skin, helping her keep warm and giving her energy. She's getting more hair on her head, eyebrows, and eyelashes, and she has fingernails and toenails in miniature. Her small heart can be pumping as much as 25 qt (24 liters) of blood a day.

Your baby can now hear sounds outside your body, and some might even make her jump. As she practices breathing, her chest rises and falls. Her lungs are beginning to exhale amniotic fluid.

Your baby measures 5 to 5¾ inches (12.5 to 14 cm) from crown to rump and weighs about 5¼ oz (150 g).

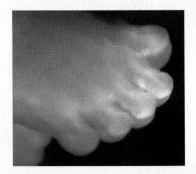

There's no stopping your baby now as he begins his most active phase. He's twisting, turning, wriggling, punching, and kicking, and generally giving his reflexes a good workout.

Inside his fast-growing lungs, tiny air sacs called alveoli begin to develop. Pads have formed on his fingertips and toes, and the unique swirls and whorls that are your baby's fingerprints begin to appear. His eyes have moved to their correct position. Meconium, which forms your baby's first bowel movement, is accumulating in his bowels. If your baby is a boy, his prostate gland is forming.

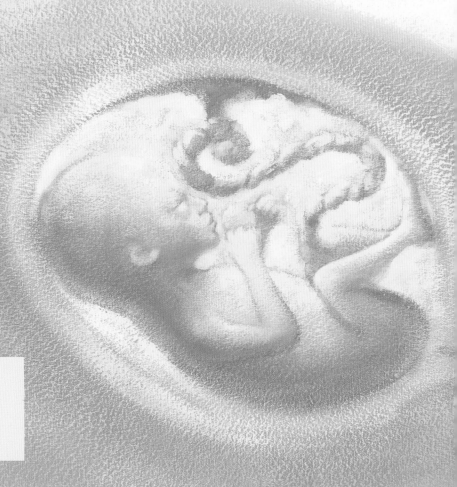

At week 20, your baby still has room to move freely. As he gets bigger, his movements will become more constrained.

WEEK 19

...of your pregnancy.
Your baby is 17 weeks old.

Your baby measures about 5¼ to 6 inches (13 to 15 cm) from crown to rump and weighs about 7 oz (200 g).

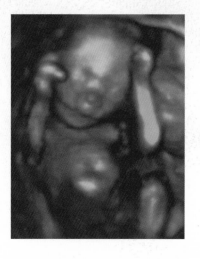

A thick, white greasy substance called vernix caseosa is being secreted by glands in your baby's skin. This acts as a waterproof barrier, to prevent her skin from getting waterlogged in the amniotic fluid.

Throughout your baby's body, nerves are being coated with a fatty substance called myelin, which insulates the nerves, allowing the smooth, rapid exchange of information necessary for coordinated, skillful movement. The poorly coordinated movements of newborns—and particularly premature infants—are for the most part due to their comparative lack of myelin.

Your baby's gut has begun to produce gastric juices that help absorb amniotic fluid and pass it to her kidneys where it's filtered and excreted back into the amniotic sac.

WEEK 20

...of your pregnancy.
Your baby is 18 weeks old.

Your baby measures about 5½ to 6½ inches (14 to 16 cm) from crown to rump and weighs about 9 oz (255 g).

Your baby has reached the halfway mark. She's still tiny but growing rapidly. This is a crucial stage for the development of her senses— taste, smell, hearing, seeing, and touch. Now your baby can finally hear and recognize your voice. The nerve cells serving each of the senses are now developing into their particular areas of the brain. The increase in the number of nerve cells is slowing, but the complex connections required for the development of memory and thinking functions are being formed.

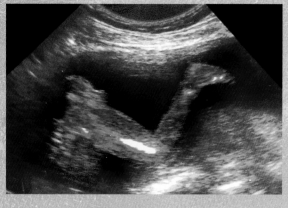

If your baby is a girl, she already has roughly 2 million eggs in her ovaries. However, by the time she's born, this number will have reduced to a mere million.

She can also enjoy a good stretch of her limbs—a tiny leg is colored blue on this ultrasound—as her nervous and muscular systems have developed sufficiently to allow this.

WEEK 21

...of your pregnancy.
Your baby is 19 weeks old.

Your baby measures about 7¼ inches (16 cm) from crown to rump and weighs about 10½ oz (300 g).

Your baby's digestive system is developed enough to absorb water from the amniotic fluid she swallows. At full term, your baby can swallow as much as 18 fl oz (500 ml) of amniotic fluid in a 24-hour period. In the early stages, amniotic fluid is produced by the placenta. Once the baby's kidneys start functioning, around the fourth month, they take over this production. Although your baby's kidneys remove some waste products from her blood and make urine, there isn't much urine in the amniotic fluid. Most waste products are conveyed through the placenta to your bloodstream and are then filtered by your kidneys. Your baby also secretes body chemicals into the amniotic fluid, and a sample taken via an amniocentesis or chorionic villus sampling can reveal important information about her health.

The senses your baby will use to learn about the world are developing daily. Taste buds have formed on her tongue, and the development of her brain and nerve endings are advanced enough to let her sense touch. She can be seen on ultrasound sucking her thumb or stroking her face.

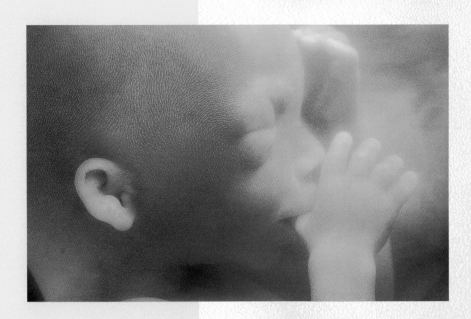

WEEK 22

...of your pregnancy.
Your baby is 20 weeks old.

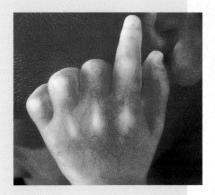

Your baby measures about 7½ inches (19 cm) from crown to rump and weighs about 12¼ oz (350 g).

Your baby now has sweat glands and his skin is less transparent, although blood vessels can still been seen. His fingernails are fully formed and continuing to grow. If your baby is a boy, his testes have begun their descent from the pelvis to the scrotum. Primitive sperm have already formed in the testes.

Your baby's brain has begun to grow very quickly now, especially in the germinal matrix, a structure in the center of the brain that manufactures brain cells. This structure vanishes before birth but your baby's brain will keep on expanding until the age of 5.

WEEK 23

...of your pregnancy.
Your baby is 21 weeks old.

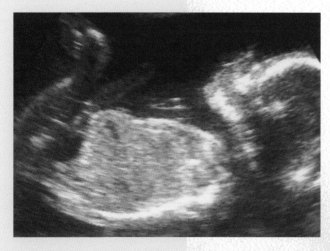

Your baby measures about 8¾ inches (22 cm) from crown to rump and weighs almost 1 lb (455 g).

Your baby's body is becoming better proportioned each day and looking like a full-term baby, but her bones and organs are still visible beneath her transparent skin.

Her hearing is much more acute now, as the bones of her inner ear have hardened. She can distinguish different noises from outside the uterus and from inside your body. You'd be surprised just how noisy your body is, with the gurgling of your stomach, the thump of your heartbeat, and the rushing of your blood around your body.

At birth, your baby will recognize your voice by its pitch and cadences, so talk to her as much as possible now. Fathers should talk to their unborn babies as well. Research shows that deeper "male" voices are easier for your baby to hear than high-pitched "female" voices. Playing games such as patting your belly and talking, may elicit a kick in response and help neurological stimulation.

WEEK 24

...of your pregnancy.
Your baby is 22 weeks old.

Your baby measures 8½ inches (21 cm) from crown to rump and weighs about 1¼ lbs (540 g).

If your baby was born now, he'd have a one in four or five chance of survival. But he's still quite thin and covered in fine body hair. His body is starting to produce white blood cells to fight infection.

His lungs have developed just enough to give him a chance of surviving in a neonatal intensive care unit. But he continues to practice breathing by inhaling amniotic fluid into his developing lungs. Airway passages form tubes in order to take in and expel air. Blood vessels and air sacs start to develop in the lungs—these will eventually exchange oxygen and circulate it to all parts of his body. The cells in your baby's lungs begin to produce surfactant, a substance that keeps the sacs from sticking together.

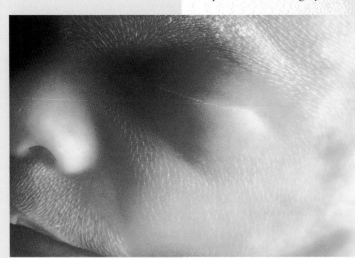

WEEK 25

...of your pregnancy.
Your baby is 23 weeks old.

Your baby measures about 8¾ inches (22 cm) from crown to rump and weighs 1½ lbs (700 g).

Your baby can now hold her feet and curl her hand into a fist. The components that form her spine—33 rings, 150 joints, and 1000 ligaments—begin to form. Blood vessels continue to develop in her lungs, and her nostrils begin to open. High inside the gums, your baby's permanent teeth are developing in buds. These adult teeth won't descend until the baby teeth—also called primary teeth—start to fall out around age 6. Meanwhile, nerves around the mouth and lip area are showing more sensitivity now, preparing your baby for the essential task of finding her mother's nipple once she is born.

That crucial lifeline, the umbilical cord, is thick and resilient now. A single vein and two arteries run through it, encased in a firm jellylike substance that prevents kinking and knotting, protecting the blood flow between placenta and baby.

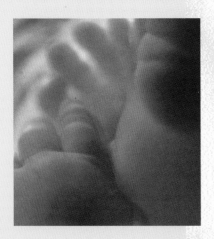

WEEK 26

...of your pregnancy.
Your baby is 24 weeks old.

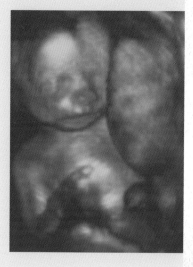

Your baby measures about 9¼ inches (23 cm) from crown to rump and weighs almost 2 lbs (910 g).

Your baby's lungs are still maturing and he still has some growing to do. His spine is getting stronger and more supple to support his growing body, and a friend can hear his heartbeat just by putting an ear to your abdomen. Your baby can inhale and exhale. His eyes have completely formed. His pulse quickens as he reacts to sounds; he'll even move in rhythm to music. Studies of unborn babies' brain activity shows that your baby can now respond to touch.

WEEK 27

...of your pregnancy.
Your baby is 25 weeks old.

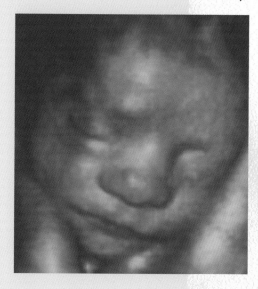

Your baby measures about 9½ inches (24 cm) from crown to rump and weighs a little over 2 lbs (1 kg).

Your baby is becoming plumper and rounder as the amount of fat under her skin increases. Thumb-sucking may now be one of your baby's favorite activities, strengthening her cheek and jaw muscles and possibly soothing her. Her lungs continue to grow. She now has fully functioning taste buds on her tongue and inside her cheeks, and her higher brain functions are becoming more sophisticated.

About this time, your baby's eyelids begin to open, and the retinas begin to form. Babies now seem to be able to detect changes in light, and studies have shown that when a flashlight is shone against a mother's abdomen, the baby may move toward—or sometimes away from—its beam. Your baby's first visual impressions outside the uterus will be sorted into light and dark, too—that's why many toys designed for newborns are black and white. Her eyelashes are fully grown now, and will protect her delicate eyeballs from harmful matter once she's born.

WEEK 28

...of your pregnancy.
Your baby is 26 weeks old.

Your baby measures about 10 inches (25 cm) from crown to rump and weighs about 2½ lbs (1.1 kg).

At week 28, your baby's getting fatter and rounder and his muscle tone is getting better.

Your busy baby is growing and developing at top speed. His lungs are capable of breathing air, but if he's born now, he would find it hard to breathe properly. He will enjoy hearing your voice now so carry on talking to him. Next week you officially enter the third trimester, when your baby's main job will be to put on weight.

In baby boys, the testes are beginning their descent into the scrotum by this point. In baby girls, the labia are still small and don't yet cover the clitoris. The labia will grow closer together in the last few weeks of pregnancy.

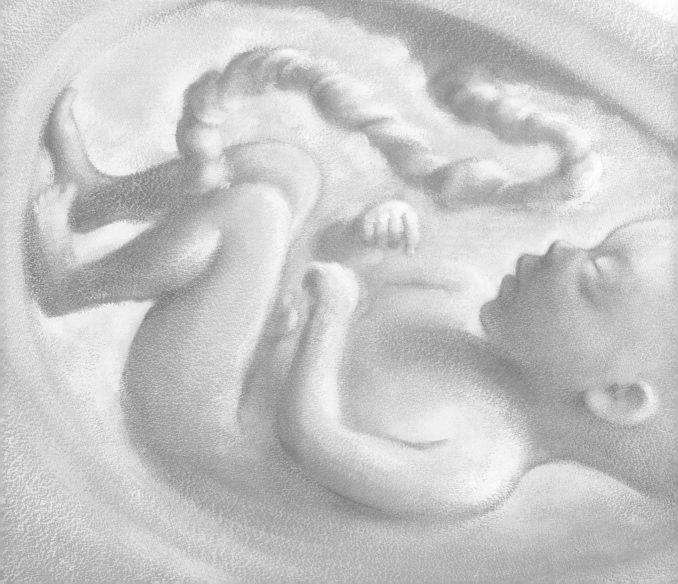

WEEK 29

...of your pregnancy.
Your baby is 27 weeks old.

Your baby measures about 10½ inches (26 cm) from crown to rump and weighs about 2¾ lbs (1.25 kg).

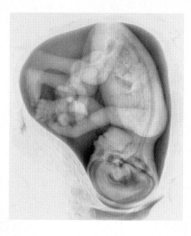

Your baby continues to fatten up as her brain and organs carry on growing. These soft tissues show up clearly on a magnetic resonance image (MRI) scan, which uses magnetic fields and radio waves. She doesn't have as much room now so she can't show off her acrobatic skills, but she's still managing to stretch and kick you from inside.

Your baby's brain is growing so quickly that the soft skull bones are being pressed outward, and her head is now in proportion to the rest of her body. Her brain is looking more wrinkled as it gets faster and more powerful, building up connections between nerve cells. Her brain can control her breathing and body temperature. Her eyes can move in their sockets, and she's becoming more sensitive to light, sound, taste, and smell. Through the wall of the uterus she can tell the difference between sunlight and artificial light.

WEEK 30

...of your pregnancy.
Your baby is 28 weeks old.

Your baby measures about 10¾ inches (27 cm) from crown to rump and weighs about 3 lbs (1.36 kg).

Your baby's lanugo (early body hair) is disappearing. The few fuzzy patches left at birth will rub off over the following weeks. The hair on his head is thicker, and his eyelids open and close, and his toenails are growing. The bone marrow has taken over the task of red blood cell production from the liver. His skeleton hardens even more and the brain, muscles, and lungs continue to mature.

Many babies adopt the head-down position in the uterus now, the most common and most straightforward position for birth. Prepare to feel strong kicks under your rib cage and pressure on your pelvic floor when your baby presses down on it.

WEEK 31

...of your pregnancy.
Your baby is 29 weeks old.

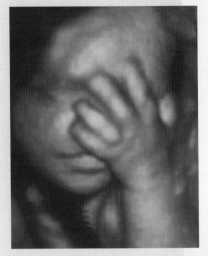

Your baby measures about 11¼ inches (28 cm) from crown to rump and weighs about 3½ lbs (1.59 kg).

While your baby's overall growth starts to slow, she will continue to put on weight. Her brain is continuing its growth spurt. Her lungs will be the last major organ to become fully mature.

Her eye color begins to appear around now, but the real color won't show for six to nine months after birth, as eye pigmentation needs light exposure to complete its formation. Dark-skinned babies usually have dark gray or brown eyes at birth, developing into a true brown or black after the first six months or year. Most Caucasian babies are born with dark blue eyes and their true eye color may not be apparent for weeks or months. In the meantime, her eyes are being prepared for life after birth. Her pupils start to dilate in reaction to the reddish light that filters into the uterus. Her eyelids are frequently open during active times and closed during sleep.

WEEK 32

...of your pregnancy.
Your baby is 30 weeks old.

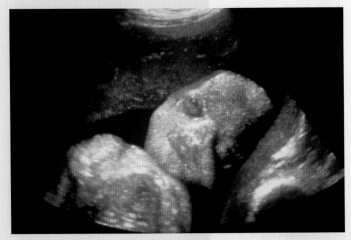

Your baby measures about 11½ inches (29 cm) from crown to rump and weighs 4 lbs (1.8 kg).

All of your baby's five senses are working and he can show off a new skill—turning his head from side to side. His organs are continuing to mature, his toenails are complete, and hair on his head is still growing. He continues to practice opening and closing his eyes, but he sleeps 90 to 95 percent of the day.

Your baby's "breathing lessons" continue to help his lungs strengthen and mature. Recent studies have shown that this vital practice also encourages the lungs to produce more surfactant, the protein that's essential for the lungs' healthy development.

WEEK 33

...of your pregnancy.
Your baby is 31 weeks old.

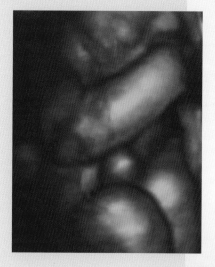

Your baby measures about 12 inches (30 cm) from crown to rump and weighs almost 4½ lbs (2 kg).

The amniotic fluid is at its highest level and will remain at this level until the birth. Rapid brain growth has increased the size of your baby's head by approximately ⅜ inch (9.5 mm) this week. Fat continues to accumulate, and this turns her skin from red to pink.

Your baby doesn't have much elbow room these days, as you can see from this 3D ultrasound scan, so her movements will feel more like rolls than kicks, and you'll be spared all those digs in the ribs. You may also notice that your actions affect her movements—how much and when you eat, what position you are in, and sounds from the world outside can all influence your baby's activity level.

Take some time each day to relax and check her movements. Your healthcare provider will be able to give you guidelines on how much movement you should feel—for example, you may be told to expect about six movements in one hour, but not every hour of the day.

WEEK 34

...of your pregnancy.
Your baby is 32 weeks old.

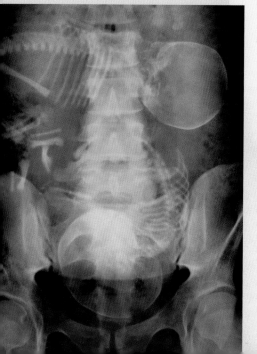

Your baby measures about 12¾ inches (32 cm) from crown to rump and weighs almost 5 lbs (2.275 kg).

Your baby's developing his immune system to fight mild infection. The ends of his fingers are tiny, but he has sharp fingernails.

He's too big to float about in the amniotic fluid now and his movements are bigger and slower. He may have settled into the head-down position, although 3 to 4 percent of all babies will be lying with their bottoms or legs toward the cervix in the "breech presentation." A healthcare provider may sometimes encourage a baby to turn into the correct position with a procedure called "external cephalic version." This involves manipulating the lower abdomen manually, and is best carried out in a hospital so that mother and baby can be closely monitored.

With twins, as can be seen on the colored X-ray, left, only one baby may be able to fit into the head-down position, while his twin fits around him as best he can.

WEEK 35

...of your pregnancy.
Your baby is 33 weeks old.

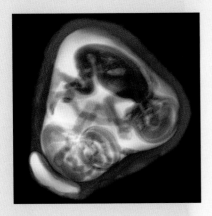

Your baby measures about 13¼ inches (33 cm) from crown to rump and weighs over 5½ lbs (2.55 kg).

Ninety-nine percent of babies born now survive without any major problems. The central nervous system is maturing, the digestive system is almost complete, the lungs are usually fully mature, and respiratory problems, which "preemies" (babies born before 37 weeks) never used to survive, are much more easily vanquished now.

Your baby's arms and legs are plumping up nicely—in fact she's big enough to take up most of the uterus, and there's less room to move around. With twins, the conditions are even more cramped, as can be seen on this MRI scan—the pink area is the shared placenta.

WEEK 36

...of your pregnancy.
Your baby is 34 weeks old.

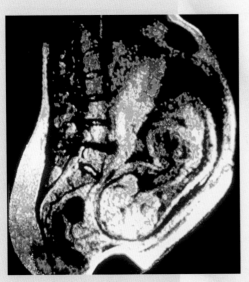

Your baby measures over 13½ inches (34 cm) from crown to rump and weighs about 6 lbs (2.75 kg).

No doubt you've noticed a change in your baby's movements by now, as your uterus is getting very tight for space. He may wriggle about less because of this constriction, but his movements will generally be stronger and more defined. You may be able to see the outline of certain body parts such as an elbow or a heel appearing under your skin.

By this stage, most babies will have assumed the head-down position ready for birth. This magnetic resonance image (MRI) scan shows the baby resting with its head in the lower part of the uterus.

WEEK 37

...of your pregnancy.
Your baby is 35 weeks old.

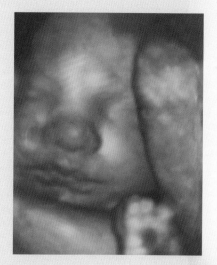

Your baby measures about 14 inches (35 cm) from crown to rump and weighs almost 6½ lbs (2.95 kg).

Your baby is now considered full term, meaning that she can be born any day. As shown by a 3D ultrasound scan, she looks like a newborn. If labor starts now, no effort will be made to delay it. Research suggests that it's actually your baby who triggers labor, producing hormones as a reaction to her cramped surroundings. These hormones start biochemical reactions which initiate labor.

Through most of the pregnancy, your baby has relied on you for protection against infections, but gradually her own immune system has begun to develop. It will carry on developing after birth, and breastfeeding will boost your baby's immunity. At first, your breasts produce colostrum, a substance rich in nutrients and antibodies. The breast milk that follows is nutritionally balanced and will help protect your baby against infections and build her immunity.

WEEK 38

...of your pregnancy.
Your baby is 36 weeks old.

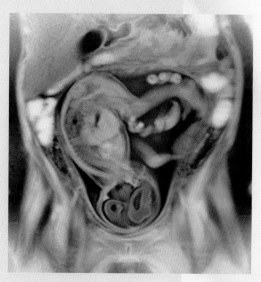

Your baby measures about 14 inches (35 cm) from crown to rump and weighs about 6¾ lbs (3.1 kg).

Your baby is clinically mature, and he's ready to be born any time now. All his body systems have developed, it may be possible to see them on an MRI scan. His intestines have been accumulating waste material, a greenish-black sticky substance called meconium, which he may pass before or after birth. His head and abdomen have about the same circumference.

Your healthcare provider will probably be able to give you an idea of your baby's size at this point, but be aware that this will just be an estimate—no one knows just how big a baby will be until birth.

The placenta starts aging now, as its role of sustaining your baby comes to an end. It becomes less efficient at transferring nutrients, and blood clots and calcified patches begin to show.

WEEK 39

...of your pregnancy.
Your baby is 37 weeks old.

Your baby measures about 14½ inches (36 cm) from crown to rump and weighs just over 7 lbs (3.25 kg).

Most of your baby's lanugo is gone now as she prepares for birth. Your baby will swallow her lanugo, along with other secretions, and store them in her bowels. These will add to your infant's first bowel movement, a blackish waste called meconium. Her lungs are maturing and surfactant production is increasing. You may not feel all her movements at this stage. At 20 inches (51 cm) long, the umbilical cord is about as long as your baby from head to toe.

Pregnancy hormones produced by your body may cause the breasts in both newborn boys and girls to be swollen at birth and even produce tiny quantities of milk. The genitalia—the labia in girls and the scrotum in boys—may appear enlarged as well. All these side effects should disappear shortly after birth, when your baby's detached from your blood supply. At the time of birth, your baby has no fewer than 300 bones—more than adults, who possess 206. Some of these bones will fuse together as your baby grows.

At week 40, your baby is fully formed and ready to be born any day now.

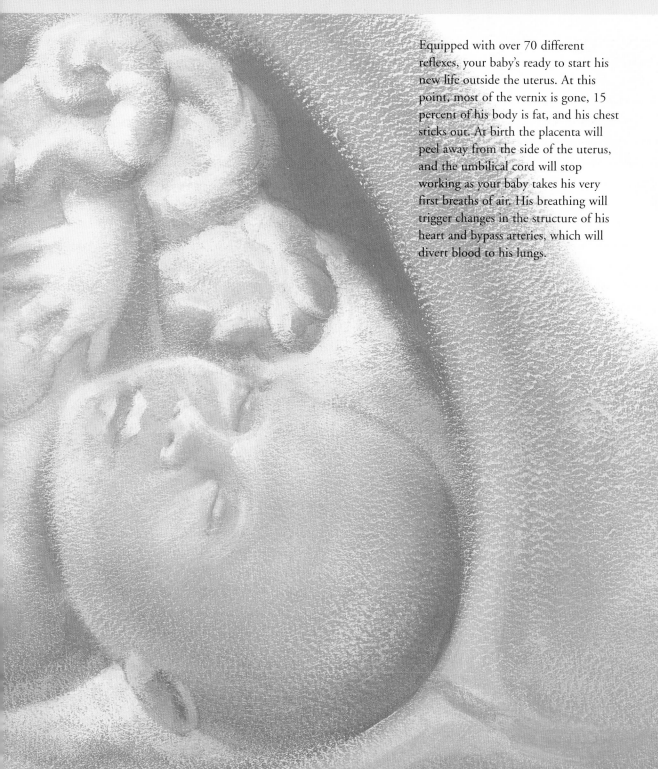

WEEK 40

...of your pregnancy.
Your baby is 38 weeks old.

Your baby measures about 14¾ to 15¼ inches (37 to 38 cm) from crown to rump, with a total length of about 21½ inches (48 cm).

Equipped with over 70 different reflexes, your baby's ready to start his new life outside the uterus. At this point, most of the vernix is gone, 15 percent of his body is fat, and his chest sticks out. At birth the placenta will peel away from the side of the uterus, and the umbilical cord will stop working as your baby takes his very first breaths of air. His breathing will trigger changes in the structure of his heart and bypass arteries, which will divert blood to his lungs.

YOUR PREGNANT BODY

Weeks

Mentally and physically this is an exciting but demanding time, as you enter the last three months of your pregnancy. Some women feel great during this last trimester, others feel exhausted. Anxiety about the impending birth is very common, too. Expect to put on between 10 and 12 lbs (4.5 kg and 5.4 kg) during this last trimester, 7 to 8 lbs (3 to 3.6 kg) of which is due to your baby.

You will be offered a prenatal check at least every two weeks, until week 36.

Your uterus has grown around 1½ inches (4 cm) in the past month and will now be pushing up against the bottom of your rib cage, making the lower ribs spread out, which may cause discomfort.

Between now and week 32, you may be offered a glucose screen and blood test for anemia.

Sometimes pressure on the veins that take blood from the legs to the heart can cause varicose veins.

If you want to have a birth plan, now is the time to start writing it, including issues such as the kind of birth you want and your views on pain relief.

Your prenatal check is a good time to discuss any concerns you have about the birth.

The weight of your growing baby and changes to your center of gravity can put increasing strain on your back.

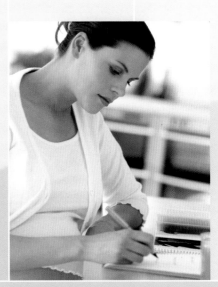

You may find that you are becoming unusually forgetful. Your baby takes up more and more of your concentration as you approach the birth.

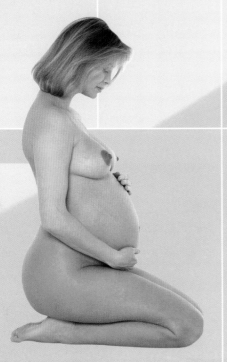

28-31

- Your belly button may be stretched and elongated, and may start to protrude, but it will return to normal after the birth.
- Your legs can feel heavy and tired in late pregnancy, and you will need to rest more often.
- Breathlessness is common, due to the increased effort needed to move around. Your lungs also have to absorb about 20 percent more oxygen and expel more carbon dioxide with each breath as you breathe for your baby.

32 | 33 | 34 | 35 | 36

As your pregnancy progresses you continue to put on weight and may be doing so faster than at any other time in your pregnancy. Your uterus is approaching the highest position it will reach, with the top sitting about 5 inches (12 cm) above your navel.

If this is your first baby, he may have moved into the head-down position as he gets ready to be born.

Once this happens, your breathing will become easier and any indigestion should start to improve.

Tests on blood pressure and urine will be carried out at each prenatal check.

You may notice that the rings on your hand feel tight, or that your feet and hands are swollen. This is due to fluid retention, but it can be made worse if tight clothing restricts your blood flow.

The pregnancy hormone relaxin, coupled with the weight of your baby, causes your pelvic joints to expand in readiness for the birth. You may experience a few aches and pains in this area.

Prenatal checks are recommended every week now until you give birth. This prenatal check may include a test for Group B strep (see page 363).

You may find that you dream a lot and that your dreams are extremely vivid.

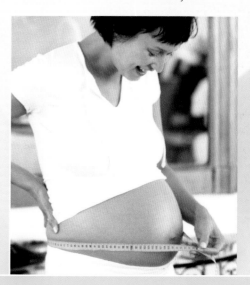

You will be putting on weight faster than at any other time in your pregnancy and you may be surprised at how big your belly is growing.

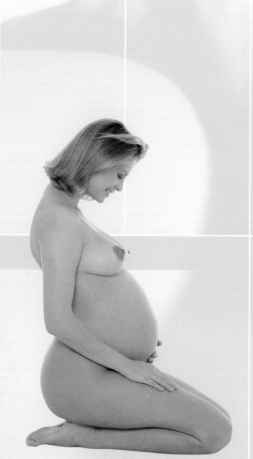

32–36

- ◆ The placenta reaches maturity at around 34 weeks, and from then on it starts to age.
- ◆ The amount of blood in your body has increased by 50 percent during the first two trimesters. After 34 weeks it remains constant until you give birth.
- ◆ A common symptom at this stage is a tingling sensation or pressure in the pelvic area, due to your baby moving down the uterus.
- ◆ Your nipples enlarge and your breasts become heavier.

traveling down the birth canal

At full dilation, the cervix, uterus, and the vagina run together seamlessly to form the birth canal. *Your baby has completed a 90-degree rotation and is now facing your back.* During the second, "pushing" stage, the wavelike sensations of contractions are replaced by an intense urge to push. *Your baby is actively helping himself to be born by pushing himself away from the wall of your uterus with his feet and by wriggling his head through your cervix and vagina.*

As your baby passes down the vagina he goes under the pubic bone and through the opening in the pelvic-floor muscles. Although the journey is, literally, a tight squeeze, he is helped by the fact that his skull bones are soft and can overlap—the skull can be made up to 1 cm smaller. *Your baby positions his head sideways, chin down, so it's at its narrowest when passing through the pelvic outlet.* Once the top of his head has "crowned" (can be seen at the entrance to the vagina), the next few contractions push your baby's head out of your body.

HOW YOUR BABY IS BORN

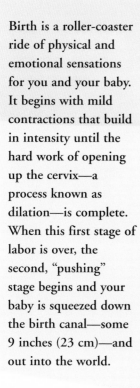

Birth is a roller-coaster ride of physical and emotional sensations for you and your baby. It begins with mild contractions that build in intensity until the hard work of opening up the cervix—a process known as dilation—is complete. When this first stage of labor is over, the second, "pushing" stage begins and your baby is squeezed down the birth canal—some 9 inches (23 cm)—and out into the world.

the journey begins

The birth process begins with the onset of contractions. These are the rhythmical tightening and flexing actions of the uterus, the largest muscle in the female body. With each contraction, the uterus pulls upward and squeezes your baby down onto the cervix. The pressure of your baby's head gradually effaces (thins) and dilates (opens up) your cervix. *At first, your baby is facing your side, with the widest part of his head in the widest part of your pelvis.*

By the end of the first stage of labor the cervix has transformed from a thick, sealed exit to a soft, thin opening. Once the cervix is fully dilated to 10 cm, it feels something like the rim of a teacup, with your baby's head—if it's properly engaged—usually filling the center. *Your baby now has his chin on his chest, as his head and upper body begin to twist to face your back.*

37

Your baby's size and position will be checked at each prenatal check.

You are likely to experience "practice contractions" known as Braxton Hicks contractions from now on. This is when your uterus hardens for around 30 seconds, then relaxes. These contractions should not be painful.

38

Your prenatal check will include all the routine tests that you have at each check-up.

Some women experience depression in late pregnancy, the result of a mixture of emotions—anxiety about the forthcoming birth, fatigue due to lack of sleep, and a desire for the pregnancy to end. If you feel this way, talk through your feelings with your healthcare provider and try to take time out for yourself.

39

Your uterus is taking up all the space in your pelvis and a great deal of room in your belly so you may be feeling very uncomfortable.

Discuss any concerns you may have at your prenatal check.

40

This is the week you are due to give birth but only around 5 percent of babies are born exactly on the estimated date of delivery (EDD). You could give birth two weeks either side of it.

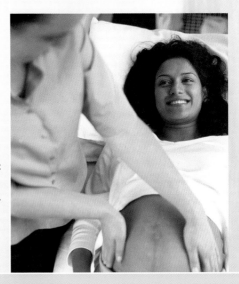

The baby usually gets into the birth position at around 33 to 36 weeks. Your healthcare provider will examine you at each visit to check how your baby is lying.

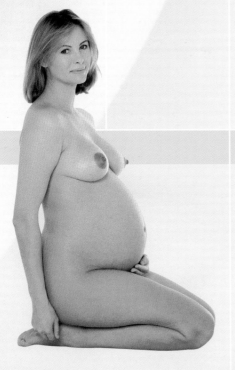

37-40

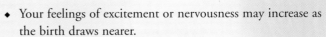

- Your feelings of excitement or nervousness may increase as the birth draws nearer.
- Your weight is likely to plateau, and a few women actually lose weight in the last week or so before the birth.
- As the uterus presses against the rib cage you may experience some discomfort.
- You may look a little flushed as your circulation works harder than ever before.

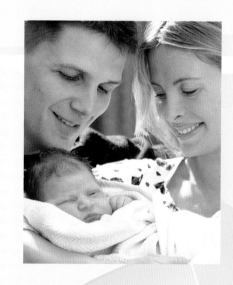

the moment of birth

Once his head is born *your baby turns to straighten his neck so that he is facing your* *side once again.* With the next contraction his shoulders are born, one before the other, with his arms held close to his body. Once his shoulders are through, the rest of the body slips out quickly—your baby has arrived at last.

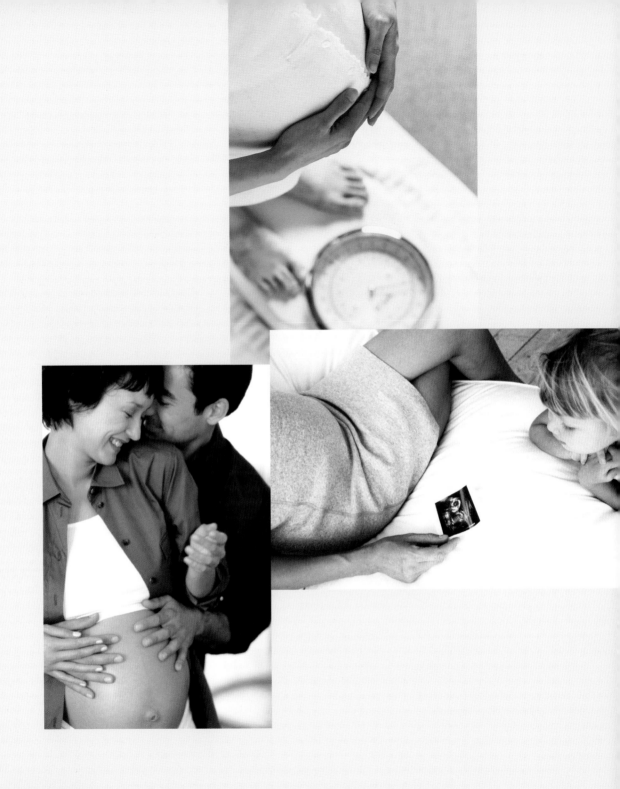

PART II   ENJOYING YOUR PREGNANCY

2

CHAPTER

YOUR PREGNANT BODY

Your body will be going through incredible changes

over the nine months of pregnancy, but your busy

lifestyle may continue at much the same pace. With

a little guidance and some minor adjustments, you

can carry on with most of your everyday activities,

safe in the knowledge that you're protecting your

baby's well-being.

INNER CHANGES

From the moment you conceive, your body begins to make adjustments to nourish and nurture your growing baby. While some of these changes can be discerned, others are subtler and may not be noticeable right away.

Around the time of your first missed period, early pregnancy symptoms usually start to occur. You may notice tenderness in your breasts, fatigue, and feelings of nausea. These, and other changes that you may experience during pregnancy (see page 67), can be an irritation and may even cause discomfort, but in many cases they can be relieved. However, any unusual discomfort or pain should never be ignored, so speak to your healthcare provider.

HORMONAL CHANGES
Pregnancy is a time of great hormonal activity. Production of existing hormones is raised dramatically and new hormones are made specifically for pregnancy.

Human chorionic gonadotropin (HCG)
This hormone, released by the developing placenta as it begins to implant within the uterus, is widely known as the "pregnancy hormone," because it's the one that is tested for in pregnancy tests. HCG is very important because it triggers other hormonal activity needed to maintain your pregnancy and prevent menstruation from occurring. However, HCG does have some noticeable effects; in particular, it's thought to be partly responsible for the nausea and vomiting—morning sickness—that occurs in the first trimester.

Progesterone
This hormone is present in non-pregnant women, but at much lower levels. Produced first by the ovaries, and then by the placenta at around 8 to 9 weeks, progesterone plays an important role in sustaining your pregnancy including preventing the uterus from contracting strongly and endangering your unborn baby. Some pregnant women who have

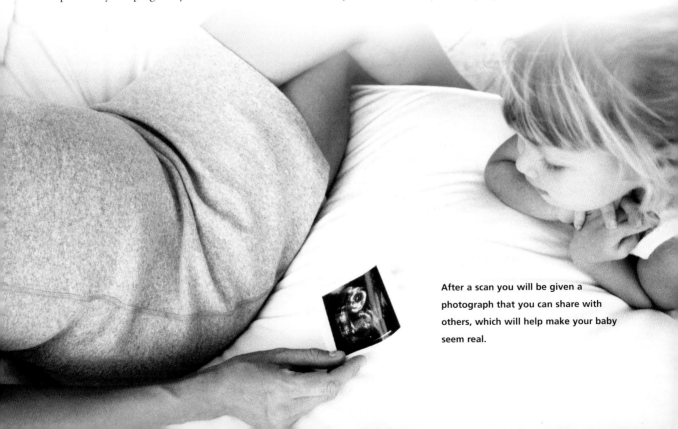

After a scan you will be given a photograph that you can share with others, which will help make your baby seem real.

had problems maintaining a pregnancy in the past are put on progesterone supplements, in the form of pills, suppositories, vaginal gel, or injections.

Progesterone maintains the functions of the placenta, strengthens the pelvic walls in preparation for labor and relaxes certain ligaments and muscles in your body. This relaxant effect can cause some unwelcome side effects.

Progesterone makes your bowel muscles sluggish, leading sometimes to constipation as well as a feeling of "fullness" after eating. Progesterone also relaxes the sphincter (ring of muscle) between the esophagus and the stomach, at times causing heartburn. It also causes veins to dilate, which can lead to varicose veins.

Another key role of progesterone is that of preparing your breasts for milk production. The hormone helps stimulate and develop the duct system in your breasts, so that by the second trimester there is milk available. Early on you may feel its effects as breast tenderness.

Estrogen

This is another hormone present in high levels during pregnancy. Very early on, estrogen helps prepare the lining of the uterus for the pregnancy, increasing the number of blood vessels and glands present within the uterus. Estrogen also is responsible for some increase in blood volume, which can lead occasionally to bleeding gums or nosebleeds. Its most noticeable effect is an increased flushing, or redness of the skin, resulting in the familiar "glow" of pregnancy.

Other significant hormones

Besides HCG, progesterone, and estrogen, a number of other hormones have specific roles to play throughout pregnancy:

- *Human chorionic somatomammotropin (HCS)* Also called human placental lactogen (HPL), this hormone is regulated by estrogen and is produced

HEALTH FIRST

Pre-eclampsia Increased levels of progesterone can lead to blurred vision and headaches in pregnancy. However, if you develop persistent symptoms of blurring vision and headaches in late pregnancy tell your healthcare provider immediately—these are two of the symptoms of pre-eclampsia, which can lead to eclampsia, a life-threatening condition unique to pregnancy (see page 254).

within the placenta in very large amounts. It plays a part in the development of your baby and helps your breasts develop the glands needed for breastfeeding. It also mobilizes fat for energy and may promote the growth of your baby.

- *Calcitonin* This conserves calcium and increases vitamin D synthesis, which enables your calcium and bone strength to remain stable despite an increased need for calcium for your baby.
- *Thyroxine (T4 and T3)* This hormone is needed for the development of your baby's central nervous system. It also increases your oxygen consumption, and helps your baby process proteins and carbohydrates. Moreover, it interacts with growth hormones to regulate and stimulate your baby's growth.
- *Relaxin* This encourages your cervix, pelvic muscles, and ligaments and joints to relax, in preparation for birth.
- *Insulin* This helps your baby store food in his body and regulates glucose levels. If you are diabetic and your condition is not well controlled, your baby can grow too much and have problems balancing his own glucose levels.
- *Oxytocin* This hormone works in a kind of positive feedback loop. Released in response to the stretching of your cervix during labor it, in turn, causes your uterus to contract further.

Similarly, oxytocin is released in response to stimulation of your nipples during breastfeeding and causes your milk to flow in the letdown reflex (see page 297).

- *Erythropoietin* Produced in the kidneys, this hormone increases the total red blood cell mass and plasma volume by retaining salt and water.
- *Cortisol* This helps your baby use various foods properly within his body.
- *Prolactin* This hormone helps prepare your breasts ready for breastfeeding and promotes the growth of your baby.

CIRCULATION CHANGES

Shortly after conception, profound changes begin to occur in your body's circulatory system. One of the most significant of these is that your blood volume increases during pregnancy so that by week 30 you'll have 50 percent more blood circulating within your bloodstream. This massive increase is necessary for your body to provide an adequate blood supply to your developing baby, your enlarging uterus, and the growing placenta.

Despite this increase in blood volume, some women's blood counts decrease during pregnancy. This is because a blood count is a reading of the proportion of blood cells in relation to the amount of plasma—the fluid in which the blood cells are suspended—and the plasma tends to increase in volume more than the number of blood cells. Such a condition is called "dilutional anemia." Anemia can also be caused by iron deficiency, in which case your healthcare provider may recommend that you take an iron supplement.

You also may notice that your heartbeat is a little faster. This is perfectly normal and an indication that your body is adapting to pregnancy. No one knows for certain why a woman's heart rate increases during pregnancy. One theory is that it's nature's way of making sure that the extra blood volume gets circulated throughout the body.

Changes in blood pressure

Another change to your circulation, and one that you might notice, is a difference in your blood pressure. Some pregnant women's blood pressure begins to fall in the first trimester, reaching its lowest levels midway through pregnancy. A sudden drop in blood pressure—for example, when you stand up quickly—can give you a feeling of dizziness, or you might even faint. This is nothing to worry about, but you should mention it to your healthcare provider.

Although it is usually symptomless, some women experience an increase in blood pressure. Your healthcare provider might pick this up at a routine check-up, and it is a condition that he or she will want to watch closely (see page 253).

RESPIRATORY CHANGES

You may find that you become short of breath toward the end of pregnancy. This is because your growing baby prevents your lungs from fully expanding. If you get short of breath, sit down and breathe steadily, consciously pushing your lungs up and down. If, however, you suddenly develop shortness of breath or get a sudden chest pain, you should let your healthcare provider know right away.

CHANGES IN METABOLISM

If you feel hungry all the time, or especially late at night, you'll be glad to know that there really is a physiological reason for this. During pregnancy your growing baby extracts glucose and other nutritional substances from your bloodstream throughout the day and night. So, in between your own meals, or at bedtime, your own blood sugar levels may well drop, leaving you feeling hungry. If you find yourself constantly foraging for food, try eating frequent, small healthy snacks, instead of fewer, large meals.

OUTER CHANGES

Of course, most women expect a burgeoning belly and enlarging breasts when they're pregnant, but you may not be aware that the texture of your skin may alter, and that your teeth, hands, and feet might undergo changes.

Many of the physical changes you experience during pregnancy will be flattering: Softer curves, a rosy complexion, and thick, shiny hair can make you feel sexier than ever before. However, be prepared, too, for a few changes that aren't so attractive: Swollen ankles, varicose veins, and flaky skin are also common in pregnancy.

FULLER BREASTS

One of the earliest and most amazing changes in your body happens to your breasts. As soon as you find out that you're pregnant, you may begin to notice that your breasts are fuller and more tender. From about week 16, the nipples and areola (the darkened area surrounding the nipples) will be noticeably darker. Your nipples will become more prominent and the little glands on the areolas—known as Montgomery's tubercles—enlarge, resembling goose bumps.

These changes are caused by the large amounts of estrogen and progesterone your body produces during pregnancy. These hormones cause the duct system inside your breasts to grow and branch out, in preparation for milk production and breastfeeding after your baby is born.

As your pregnancy advances, the veins on your breasts will become more prominent, stepping up the blood supply to these areas. Your nipples may secrete a clear or golden-colored liquid from time to time. This is known as colostrum, and is the liquid that your baby will ingest initially before your real milk is produced. Taking good care of your breasts throughout pregnancy will help prepare them for breastfeeding, and will also help ease any discomfort you may experience.

HAIR AND NAIL GROWTH

While you're pregnant, your fingernails and toenails are likely to become stronger than they've ever been before and will grow at an unprecedented rate. This is due to the increase in metabolism and circulation caused by pregnancy hormones. For information about caring for your nails, see page 134.

Pregnancy also speeds up hair growth, usually causing the hair on your head to grow faster and look thicker. However, sometimes hair might grow in places where it hasn't done before, such as on your abdomen or face. The best way to remove it is by plucking or waxing. It is probably best to avoid using depilatory creams or bleach as your skin may not react well to the chemicals they contain. Electrolysis and laser hair removal are not recommended during pregnancy even though there are no documented risks.

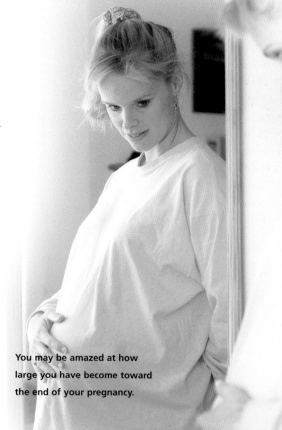

You may be amazed at how large you have become toward the end of your pregnancy.

A healthy weight gain

Starting pregnancy at a healthy weight and gaining weight at a moderate pace can help ensure that your baby grows and develops normally and that you stay healthy. Exactly how much weight you should gain depends on several factors including your pre-pregnancy weight and how many babies you're carrying.

Before you can figure out your ideal weight gain during pregnancy (see chart, opposite), you need to know your body mass index.

Your body mass index Locate your pre-pregnancy weight on the vertical line of the chart and your height on the horizontal line. The place where the points intersect is your body mass index (BMI).

The cream-colored area indicates the ideal BMI range at which a woman should start pregnancy.

- If your BMI is 19 or below, you're underweight.
- If your BMI is between 19 and 26, you're a healthy weight.
- If your BMI is between 27 and 30, you're overweight.
- If your BMI is over 30, you're clinically obese.

BODY MASS INDEX

LBS	KG																	
203	92	39	38	37	36	36	35	34	33	32	31	31	30	29	29	28	27	27
		39	38	37	36	35	34	33	33	32	31	30	30	29	28	28	27	27
		39	38	37	36	35	34	33	32	32	31	30	29	29	28	27	27	26
196	89	38	37	36	35	34	34	33	32	31	30	30	29	28	28	27	27	26
		38	37	36	35	34	33	32	32	31	30	29	29	28	27	27	26	26
		37	36	35	34	34	33	32	31	30	30	29	28	28	27	27	26	25
189	86	37	36	35	34	33	32	32	31	30	29	29	28	27	27	26	26	25
		36	35	35	34	33	32	31	30	30	29	28	28	27	27	26	25	25
		36	35	34	33	32	32	31	30	29	29	28	27	27	26	26	25	25
182	83	35	35	34	33	32	31	30	30	29	28	28	27	26	26	25	25	24
		35	34	33	32	32	31	30	29	29	28	27	27	26	26	25	24	24
		35	34	33	32	31	30	30	29	28	28	27	26	26	25	25	24	24
175	79	35	33	32	32	31	30	29	29	28	27	27	26	26	25	24	24	23
		34	33	32	31	30	30	29	28	28	27	26	26	25	25	24	24	23
		34	32	32	31	30	29	29	28	27	27	26	25	25	24	24	23	23
168	76	33	32	31	30	30	29	28	28	27	26	26	25	25	24	23	23	22
		33	32	31	30	29	29	28	27	27	26	25	25	24	24	23	23	22
		32	31	30	30	29	28	28	27	26	26	25	24	24	23	23	22	22
161	73	32	31	30	29	29	28	27	26	26	25	25	24	24	23	23	22	22
		32	30	30	29	28	27	27	26	26	25	24	24	23	23	22	22	21
		31	30	29	28	28	27	26	26	25	25	24	23	23	22	22	21	21
154	70	31	30	29	28	27	27	26	25	25	24	24	23	23	22	22	21	21
		30	29	28	28	27	26	26	25	24	24	23	23	22	22	21	21	20
		30	29	28	27	27	26	26	25	24	23	23	22	22	21	21	21	20
147	67	29	28	28	27	26	26	25	24	24	23	23	22	22	21	21	20	20
		29	28	27	26	26	25	25	24	23	23	22	22	21	21	20	20	19
		29	27	27	26	25	25	24	24	23	22	22	21	21	21	20	20	19
140	64	28	27	26	26	25	24	24	23	23	22	22	21	21	20	20	19	19
		28	27	26	25	25	24	23	23	22	22	21	21	20	20	19	19	19
		27	26	25	25	24	24	23	22	22	21	21	20	20	20	19	19	18
133	60	27	26	25	24	24	23	23	22	22	21	21	20	20	19	19	18	18
		26	25	25	24	23	23	22	22	21	21	20	20	19	19	19	18	18
		26	25	24	24	23	22	22	21	21	20	20	19	19	19	18	18	17
126	57	26	24	24	23	23	22	22	21	21	20	20	19	19	18	18	18	17
		25	24	23	23	22	22	21	21	20	20	19	19	18	18	18	17	17
		25	24	23	22	22	21	21	20	20	19	19	18	18	18	17	17	17
119	54	24	23	23	22	21	21	20	20	19	19	19	18	18	17	17	16	16
		24	23	22	22	21	21	20	20	19	19	18	18	17	17	17	16	16
		23	22	22	21	21	20	20	19	19	18	18	18	17	17	16	16	16
112	51	23	22	21	21	20	20	19	19	18	18	18	17	17	16	16	16	15
		23	22	21	20	20	19	19	19	18	18	17	17	16	16	16	15	15
		22	21	21	20	20	19	19	18	18	17	17	16	16	15	15	15	15
105	48	22	21	20	20	19	19	18	18	17	17	17	16	16	15	15	15	14
		21	20	20	19	19	18	18	17	17	17	16	16	15	15	15	14	14
		20	20	19	19	18	18	17	17	17	16	16	16	15	15	15	14	14
98	45	20	19	19	18	18	18	17	17	16	16	16	15	15	15	14	14	14
		19	19	18	18	18	17	17	16	16	16	15	15	15	14	14	14	13
		19	19	18	18	17	17	16	16	16	15	15	15	14	14	14	13	13
91	41	19	18	18	17	17	16	16	16	15	15	15	14	14	14	13	13	13
		18	18	17	17	16	16	16	15	15	15	14	14	14	13	13	13	12
		18	17	17	16	16	16	15	15	15	14	14	14	13	13	13	12	12
		17	17	16	16	16	15	15	15	14	14	14	13	13	13	12	12	12

FEET	5'0	5'1	5'2	5'3	5'4	5'5	5'6	5'7	5'8	5'9	5'10	5'11	6'0
METERS	1.52	1.56	1.6	1.64	1.68	1.72	1.76	1.80	1.84				

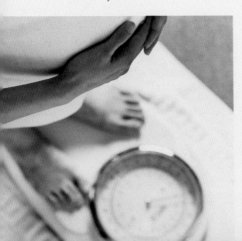

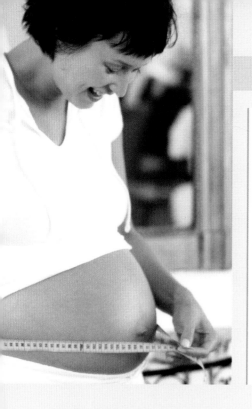

BODY MASS INDEX	RECOMMENDED TOTAL WEIGHT GAIN
Less than 19 (underweight)	28 to 40 lbs (12.5 to 18 kg)
19 to 26 (normal weight)	25 to 35 lbs (11.5 to 16 kg)
27 to 30 (overweight)	15 to 25 lbs (7 to 11.5 kg)
30 or more (obese)	15 lbs (7 kg) or less

These numbers refer to total weight gain during the entire pregnancy, so you won't know whether you hit the target until delivery day. These recommendations are for women expecting one baby. If you're expecting twins or triplets you'll need to gain more. Many healthcare providers recommend an average total gain of 34 to 45 lbs (15.5 to 20.5 kg) for twins and 45 to 50 lbs (20.5 to 23 kg) for triplets.

Your weight gain The chart above gives the recommended weight gain for your body mass index. Keep in mind, however, that the figures refer to a singleton pregnancy. The rate at which you gain weight may vary from week to week. And, unfortunately, little is known about the best time to put on weight in pregnancy. Some research suggests that gaining very little weight early on—when you may be suffering from morning sickness—has less effect on fetal growth than poor weight gain late in the second or third trimester. Some women gain weight very inconsistently, piling on the pounds early and then much less later on. Nothing is necessarily unhealthy about this pattern.

It's important not to become fanatical about how much you weigh. Even if the amount you gain is somewhat off course, if your healthcare provider says your baby is growing normally, you have nothing to worry about. Women who gain more than average can still have healthy babies, and so can women who gain very little.

If your weight gain is way too high or low, your healthcare provider can check your baby's growth by measuring the fundal height (see page 91) or, if there's cause for concern, by scheduling you for a series of ultrasounds (see page 92). If necessary, you may be advised to see a nutritionist or dietitian for specific advice on what and how much you should eat. See Chapter 4 to find out more about healthy eating in pregnancy.

HOW WEIGHT GAIN IS MADE UP IN PREGNANCY

- BABY 39%
- BLOOD 22%
- AMNIOTIC FLUID 11%
- UTERUS 11%
- PLACENTA 9%
- BREASTS 8%

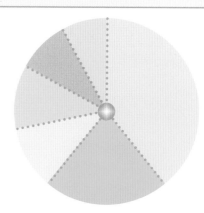

SKIN CHANGES

Overall, you may find that your skin becomes softer, due to its increased ability to retain moisture, and that you have the characteristic "glow" of pregnancy, which is partly due to an increase in hormone levels. However, you may notice other changes to your skin. Most of these go away in the first six months after the birth, but some may remain permanently.

Linea nigra

You may notice a dark line running from your pubic bone up to your navel. Called the linea nigra, this is usually more prominent in darker-skinned women.

Chloasma

The skin around your cheeks, nose, and eyes may also darken. This is called chloasma or "the mask of pregnancy" and appears dark in fair-skinned women and light in dark-skinned women. Chloasma is due to hormonal influences on skin pigment cells. Exposure to the sun can make these changes darker.

Spider angiomas

Tiny red spots, called spider angiomas or spider veins, may suddenly appear anywhere on your body. These spots, which turn white when you press on them, are concentrations of blood vessels caused by the high level of estrogen in your body.

Acne

Some women who suffer from acne find that their skin improves during pregnancy. Others find that the condition becomes worse, and women who do not normally have acne may develop it or be subject to pimples. You may be able to control pimples by cutting down on fats in your diet and exercising regularly. Always consult your healthcare provider before taking any acne medication, as it may contain chemicals that could affect your baby. Acne and pimples usually clear up around mid-pregnancy.

Itchy hands and feet

Your palms and sometimes the soles of your feet may become red and itchy. Known as palmar erythema, this is caused by increased levels of estrogen. If your skin is itching unbearably, make sure you see your healthcare provider as this could be a symptom of cholestasis (see page 273).

Skin flaps

Minuscule tags of skin are also a common occurrence in high-friction areas, although it isn't totally clear why they occur. It's not a good idea to rush to the dermatologist to have them removed.

MORE **ABOUT** | stretch marks

Stretch marks occur when fibers of the skin protein collagen are broken due to the rapid stretching of the skin or to hormonal changes that disrupt the fibers. They affect three in five pregnant women. They're most likely to appear on your stomach, the sides of your breasts, and your thighs—those areas where it's most common to put on weight. Stretch marks initially appear as pinkish-red streaks, which fade to silvery gray or white several months after birth. You are more likely to get stretch marks if you've had more than one baby, gain an excessive amount of weight during pregnancy, or have a genetic disposition to getting them.

There's no surefire way of preventing stretch marks. Your best bet is to avoid excessive weight gain and to exercise regularly to maintain muscle tone, which eases the pressure of the uterus on the overlying skin.

COMPLAINT	WHAT YOU CAN DO ABOUT IT

Morning sickness

Feelings of nausea and vomiting can occur at any time throughout the day, so the term "morning sickness" is somewhat of a misnomer. Something like 75 percent of women suffer from it from as early as week 5 or 6. Morning sickness usually goes away—or becomes much less severe—by the end of the first trimester. No one knows exactly what causes it, but most experts believe that it's related to the hormone HCG (see page 60).

Even when nausea doesn't actually cause you to vomit, it can be extremely unpleasant and truly debilitating. If your queasiness gets out of control—if you experience weight loss, if you can't keep down food or liquids, or if you feel dizzy or faint—speak to your healthcare provider, who will want to rule out hyperemesis gravidarum (see page 256).

Above all, don't compound the problem by worrying about it—the nausea is harmless to you and your baby. Your optimal weight gain for the first three months is only 4 lbs (1.8 kg). Even losing weight probably isn't a big problem in early pregnancy.

- ◆ Eat small, frequent meals so that you never have an empty stomach.
- ◆ Don't worry too much about adhering to a balanced diet for this short period; just eat whatever you can.
- ◆ If nausea gets worse when you brush your teeth, switching toothpaste brands may help.
- ◆ If your nausea is made worse by the accumulation of saliva in your mouth, suck lemon candies.
- ◆ Ginger—in the form of tea, tablets, or cookies—helps some women.
- ◆ Try eating dry toast, potatoes, and other bland, easy-to-digest carbohydrates.

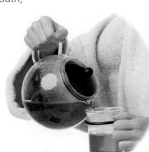

- ◆ Keep crackers by your bedside—eating them before getting out of bed can ease nausea.
- ◆ Try acupressure wrist bands, sold in drug stores and health food stores.

Fatigue

Many women are astonished at how exhausted they feel in the first trimester; this is completely normal. Fatigue may be a side effect of all the physical changes taking place, including the dramatic rise in hormone levels. You'll probably find that your exhaustion goes away somewhere around weeks 12 to 14. As fatigue lessens, you'll begin to feel more energetic and almost normal, until about 30 to 34 weeks when you may feel tired again. At this point, part of the fatigue is due to carrying around extra weight. Try to rest when you can, and recognize that it's natural to reduce your physical activity and get more sleep at this time. Women often find their second or third pregnancies more tiring than their first because they have to care for other children.

- ◆ Try to be realistic about what you can do, and don't feel guilty about what you can't get done. No one expects you to be Superwoman.
- ◆ Get as much rest as you can by sitting with your feet up during the evenings and going to bed earlier.
- ◆ Whenever possible, let other people help with household chores and other responsibilities. This is especially important if you already have children and can't just put your feet up when you feel like it.
- ◆ Make sure you are eating a healthy pregnancy diet (see Chapter 4) and avoid caffeine and candy, which will give you a quick energy lift and then leave your body feeling more fatigued as the blood-sugar level drops.
- ◆ Take some gentle exercise each day.

COMPLAINT	WHAT YOU CAN DO ABOUT IT

Stress incontinence

During the last months of pregnancy, some women begin to leak a little urine when they cough, sneeze, laugh, or move suddenly. Referred to as stress incontinence, this is perfectly normal and is caused by the growing uterus putting pressure on the bladder.

- Practice your Kegel exercises (see page 122) regularly to help strengthen pelvic-floor muscles and support the urinary sphincter.
- Urine loss can be a sign of a urinary tract infection (see page 259), so discuss it with your healthcare provider.
- Continuous loss of fluid may also be a sign of ruptured membranes (see page 212). Your healthcare provider can determine if this is the case.

Dizziness and fainting

Feeling lightheaded is common in pregnancy. In the early stages, it may occur as your blood flow strives to catch up with your increased circulation; later on, dizziness can be a result of the uterus pressing on large blood vessels. Low blood-sugar levels, low blood pressure, getting up too quickly, or becoming overheated can all contribute to dizzy spells.

Fainting during pregnancy is rare, but if you do faint it's because the flow of blood to your brain is reduced temporarily. This will not harm your baby. Report fainting to your healthcare provider right away as this may be a sign of severe anemia (see page 252).

- Always get up slowly from sitting or lying down so that the blood has time to flow to your brain.
- When you're lying down, rest on one side or the other whenever possible; don't lie flat on your back.
- Drink plenty of liquids—dizziness can be a sign of dehydration—and don't avoid salt.
- Eat protein at every meal or try eating smaller, more frequent meals to maintain your blood-sugar levels.
- Carry raisins, a piece of fruit, or some whole wheat crackers in your bag for a quick blood-sugar lift while you are out.
- If you feel too warm, get some fresh air and loosen your clothes, especially around the neck and waist.
- If you feel faint, try to increase the circulation to your brain by sitting with your head between your knees or lying down with your feet higher than your head.

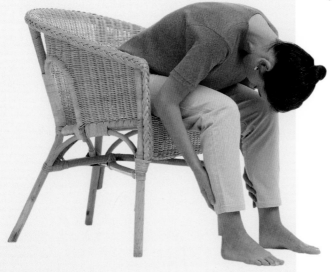

COMPLAINT	WHAT YOU CAN DO ABOUT IT

Hemorrhoids (piles)

Essentially varicose veins of the rectum, hemorrhoids are caused by the uterus pressing on major blood vessels, making the veins enlarge and swell. Progesterone relaxes the veins, allowing the swelling to increase. Even if you avoid getting hemorrhoids during pregnancy, it is possible to develop them during delivery.

Hemorrhoids sometimes bleed. While this bleeding isn't harmful, if it becomes frequent, talk to your healthcare provider, who may refer you to a colorectal specialist. If your hemorrhoids become very painful, you may want to discuss further treatment.

- ◆ Avoid becoming constipated (see page 72). Straining during bowel movements puts added pressure on the blood vessels.
- ◆ Exercise every day to help stay regular.
- ◆ Sit in a warm bath two or three times a day to help relieve the muscle spasms that often cause the pain.
- ◆ Soothe the area with witch hazel or special pads.
- ◆ Speak to your healthcare provider about medications.
- ◆ Take pressure off the area by sleeping on your side, and avoid standing for long hours.
- ◆ Do pelvic-floor exercises (see page 122) regularly, as these will help improve circulation to the area.

Round ligament pain

Between 18 and 24 weeks, you may feel a sharp pain or a dull ache on one or both sides of your lower abdomen or near your groin. It's often stronger when you move quickly or stand, and it may fade if you lie down. This is called round ligament pain. The round ligaments are bands of fibrous tissue on each side of the uterus that attach the top of the uterus to the labia. As the uterus enlarges in the second trimester, the stretching of these ligaments may cause discomfort. While it can be quite uncomfortable, it's perfectly normal. The good news is that it usually goes away or at least decreases considerably after 24 weeks.

- ◆ Take breaks from standing or walking, and put your feet up when sitting.
- ◆ Always mention any abdominal pain to your healthcare provider so that you can be reassured that there is nothing wrong.

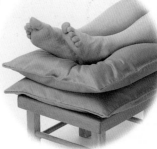

Excessive salivation

Over-production of saliva, which is sometimes called ptyalism, can be a problem but only in the first half of pregnancy. The symptoms include: producing double the amount of bitter-tasting saliva; a thickened tongue; and swollen cheeks, caused by enlarged salivary glands. Ptyalism appears to be more common in women who have morning sickness, and it can make the nausea worse temporarily.

- ◆ Cut down on starchy foods or dairy products, but still follow a healthy, balanced diet (see Chapter 4).
- ◆ Eat fruit, as this can ease symptoms.
- ◆ Mints, chewing gum, frequent small meals, and cracker snacks can help reduce the amount of saliva produced.
- ◆ Try brushing or rinsing your teeth with minty products to freshen your mouth.
- ◆ Suck on a piece of lemon or a lemon candy.

COMPLAINT	WHAT YOU CAN DO ABOUT IT

Nasal stuffiness and nosebleeds

High levels of progesterone and estrogen result in increased blood flow throughout your body, causing the lining of your nasal passages to become swollen. This can lead to congestion and over-production of mucus. This increased blood flow also puts pressure on your nose's delicate veins, making you more prone to nose-bleeds. Nasal stuffiness is likely to get worse before it gets better, after the birth.

- ◆ Increase your intake of fluids.
- ◆ Humidify your home, especially your bedroom, at night.
- ◆ Prop your head up when you sleep.
- ◆ With severe congestion, consider breathing steam from a simmering water pan, or use a saline nasal spray. Don't use medication or medicated nasal sprays unless they are prescribed by your healthcare provider.
- ◆ Blow your nose gently to avoid inducing bleeding.
- ◆ Eat vitamin C-rich foods, as these will help strengthen your capillaries and help prevent nosebleeds.

Gas and bloating

Burping and passing gas at inopportune times can be highly embarrassing but are inescapable complaints in pregnancy. Even before the end of the first trimester, you may find that your belly looks bloated and distended—an unwelcome side effect of the hormone progesterone, which causes you to retain water. This hormone slows down the bowels also, causing them to enlarge. Estrogen, the other key pregnancy hormone, causes your uterus to enlarge, which also makes your belly feel bigger.

- ◆ There's very little you can do to prevent burping or passing gas, but try to avoid becoming constipated (see page 72), because that may make things worse.
- ◆ Avoid eating large meals that may leave you feeling bloated and uncomfortable, or foods you know make the problem even worse. These vary from person to person, but some common offenders include onions, cabbage, fried foods, rich sauces, and beans.
- ◆ Don't rush your meals. This can cause you to swallow air, which can form painful pockets of gas in your gut.

Heartburn

A burning sensation, which occurs in the upper part of your abdomen, near the sternum (breastbone), is very common in the latter part of pregnancy. It's the result of acids produced in the stomach being pushed up into the lower esophagus (the tube connecting your mouth to your stomach).

Heartburn is more pronounced during pregnancy for two reasons. The high level of progesterone that your body is producing can slow digestion and relax the sphincter muscle between the esophagus and the stomach, which normally prevents the upward movement of stomach acids.

- ◆ Eat small, frequent meals.
- ◆ Take an antacid after meals—always check that this is suitable for use in pregnancy.
- ◆ Munch on dry crackers when you feel heartburn. They may neutralize the gas.
- ◆ Avoid spicy, fatty, and greasy foods.
- ◆ Avoid eating just before bedtime—heartburn occurs most readily when you lie down.
- ◆ Try sleeping with your head elevated on several pillows.
- ◆ If your heartburn becomes intolerable, talk to your healthcare provider about suitable medications that have been shown to be safe during pregnancy.

COMPLAINT	WHAT YOU CAN DO ABOUT IT

Shortness of breath

Two-thirds of all pregnant women occasionally experience breathlessness. This is caused by increased production of progesterone, which speeds up your breathing rate, and, in the last trimester, by your enlarged uterus, which presses against your diaphragm and lungs. Your breathing should improve as your baby descends into your pelvis in the final weeks.

- Relax and try to avoid stress. Try not to panic if you get breathless—it can make it worse.
- Don't slump. Stand tall and allow plenty of room for your chest to expand.
- Call your healthcare provider if you experience wheezing, tingling lips or fingers, blueness of lips or fingers, or chest pain, as these could be signs of a problem such as anemia, which may require treatment.

Insomnia

Many women complain of difficulty sleeping during the last few months of pregnancy. This may be due in part to normal anxiety about having a baby, but also may be due to the physical discomforts that can occur later in pregnancy. As your uterus grows, finding a comfortable sleeping position can sometimes be quite a challenge.

- Invest in a number of pillows to tuck under your belly, and under and between your legs, making it easier to find a comfortable position.
- Take a warm, relaxing bath before going to bed.
- Drink warm milk. Warming the milk releases tryptophan, a naturally occurring amino acid that makes you feel sleepy.
- Don't eat a heavy meal before bedtime; eat earlier in the evening and then have a light snack before bed.
- Get plenty of fresh air. Open a window so that you are not sleeping in a stuffy environment.
- Try to exercise on a regular basis.

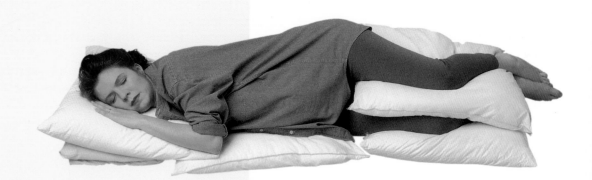

COMPLAINT	WHAT YOU CAN DO ABOUT IT

Back pain

Half to three-quarters of pregnant women experience back pain at some stage. Fortunately, only one third of these will be significantly affected by it. There are two main reasons for back discomfort in pregnancy. In preparation for the birth, your joints are more relaxed than usual, and this, along with your growing belly, puts your body off balance.

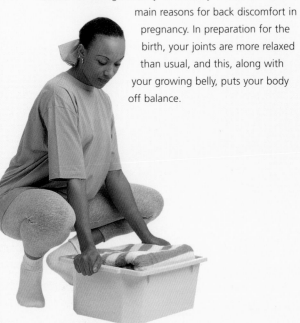

- ◆ Adjust your posture when standing to compensate for the shift in your center of gravity (see page 116).
- ◆ Sit on chairs with good back support. Also, make sure your knees are elevated above your hips.
- ◆ Sleep on your side on a firm mattress. Keep a pillow between your legs and under your abdomen to support your back.
- ◆ Lift properly so that you don't strain your back: Place your feet shoulder-width apart. Don't bend at the waist but at the knees. As you lift, push up with your thighs and keep your back straight.
- ◆ When carrying bags, make sure the weight is evenly distributed: If you're carrying groceries in your hands, divide the load into two bags and carry one in each hand; and if you're carrying a small backpack with straps, carry it on both shoulders.
- ◆ Wear low-heeled shoes.
- ◆ Apply a heated pad to painful areas. Massage can also be very effective.

Constipation

Hard and difficult-to-pass stools may be the result of high levels of progesterone, which relaxes the bowel, meaning that waste matter passes through your system more sluggishly. At the same time, your expanding uterus squashes your intestine. The extra iron in your prenatal vitamin can make matters worse.

- ◆ Eat plenty of high-fiber foods such as bran cereals, fruit, and vegetables. Some women find it helpful to eat popcorn, but go for the natural kind, without added butter, oil, or salt. Too much high-fiber food can cause discomfort, bloating, or gas so you may have to experiment to see which foods you tolerate best.
- ◆ Drink plenty of fluids—watered-down fruit juice, milk, and water are fine.
- ◆ Eat prunes or drink a glass of prune juice every day.
- ◆ If necessary, take a stool softener. Stool softeners containing docusate sodium may be used in pregnancy, and you can take them two to three times a day. It's best to avoid laxatives, as they can cause abdominal cramping and, occasionally, uterine contractions.
- ◆ Exercise regularly. It encourages the bowels to become more active and promotes daily bowel movements.

COMPLAINT	WHAT YOU CAN DO ABOUT IT

Fluid retention and swelling

Your body swells due to the accumulation of fluid in the tissues. The swelling is connected to the normal increase in body fluids in pregnancy, and three out of four pregnant women will develop edema (swelling) at some time. Usually the swelling appears in feet and ankles, hands, and fingers. It's most noticeable at the end of the day or after prolonged standing or sitting and in warm weather. Swelling could be a sign of pre-eclampsia, so you should mention it at your check-ups.

- ◆ Don't stand for long periods. Take regular breaks and sit with your legs elevated.
- ◆ If your hands are swollen, keep them elevated above your heart rather than down by your sides.
- ◆ Avoid wearing tight clothing or shoes.
- ◆ Wear support stockings or talk to your healthcare provider about special prescription elastic stockings.
- ◆ Drink plenty of fluids to help expel excess fluid.
- ◆ Don't restrict your salt intake unless your blood pressure is high (see page 265).

Varicose veins

Swollen veins often appear just under the surface of the skin of your legs and sometimes in the vulva and as hemorrhoids around the anus. They occur when the uterus puts pressure on the pelvic veins, increasing pressure on the veins in the legs and causing backflow. Blood pools in the veins in the legs causing them to distend. You may be more likely to get varicose veins if they run in the family, if you're overweight or stand or sit for long periods of time. They're usually painless, but occasionally they may be associated with discomfort, achiness, or pain. Varicose veins usually regress after delivery, but sometimes not completely.

- ◆ Avoid standing still for long periods of time.
- ◆ Try to take several rest periods throughout the day so that you can get off your feet.
- ◆ Sit with your legs elevated as much as you can.
- ◆ If you have to sit still for long periods, move your legs around from time to time to stimulate circulation. Flex your feet up and down to keep the blood from pooling.
- ◆ Wear support stockings or talk to your healthcare provider about special prescription elastic stockings.
- ◆ Avoid wearing stockings or socks with tight elastic tops that grip around one part of your leg.

Leg cramps

Often worse when you've gone to bed, leg cramps occur more frequently and painfully as pregnancy progresses. No one's sure exactly what causes cramps— one theory links them to low levels of magnesium or calcium. Fatigue and a buildup of fluid in the legs at the end of the day are also thought to be contributory factors. Some healthcare providers believe that leg cramps may be related to a decrease in circulation, which gets worse when you're sitting down.

- ◆ Walking about in bare feet can help ease the pain of leg cramps.
- ◆ Stretching and extending your legs and feet should help diminish the cramping (see page 118).
- ◆ Leg massage may help minimize the cramps.

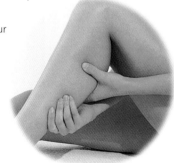

Complementary therapies

Many women use complementary medicine to promote relaxation and help cope with pregnancy complaints. Although generally safe, you should always consult a fully qualified practitioner before embarking on any treatment.

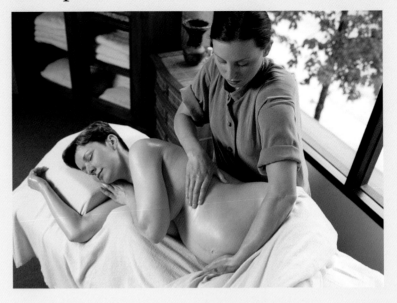

Herbal remedies

Pure fruit or mint teas are good alternatives to caffeine during pregnancy, and a slice of ginger in boiling water can ease morning sickness. However, teas and remedies containing herbs should be treated with caution, as herbs can be extremely potent, and in some cases, toxic. You should always consult your healthcare provider before taking any herbal remedy and ask an expert to recommend a particular brand, as the quality of herbs can vary.

Reflexology

This therapy operates under the premise that points on the feet and hands correspond to other parts of the body. It may help relieve a number of pregnancy complaints including backache and circulatory problems, and reflexology has been used during labor to ease the pain of contractions. However, deep pressure should be avoided near the ankles, which correspond to the uterus and ovaries, as this may bring on premature labor. Some reflexologists also recommend it should be avoided during the first trimester if the woman has a history of miscarriage.

Aromatherapy

Essential oils derived from plants are often applied with massage in the practice of aromatherapy. It can be very effective in combating stress and promoting relaxation. However, a number of essential oils can be harmful to the extent that some experts advise against the use of all oils during pregnancy. The safest course is to consult a qualified aromatherapy practitioner.

Acupuncture

This ancient Eastern practice is usually perfectly safe during pregnancy provided the treatment is carried out by a properly qualified acupuncturist. It may be especially useful for alleviating morning sickness, or reducing low back pain during pregnancy. However, special precautions should be taken because certain acupuncture points may stimulate uterine contractions.

Homeopathy

This therapy can be effective in combating minor pregnancy complaints such as heartburn, nausea, and vomiting, and some women find it can help during labor. Homeopathic remedies are unlikely to cause side effects to either mother or baby, as only a very minute amount of the active ingredient is used in a specially prepared form. However, you should always consult a professional homeopath in pregnancy, as pinpointing the right remedy can be quite difficult.

WILL IT HARM MY BABY?

Now that you're pregnant you'll probably want to take greater care of yourself in order to protect and nurture the little one inside you. With only a few minor adjustments, you can probably carry on as you have been.

When pregnant, many women become more aware of how their lifestyles affect their bodies. The things you see in the media or hear from friends and family may make it seem that health hazards lurk everywhere. However, there are really only a few areas in which you need to make changes. One vital area you need to pay attention to is what you take into your body; apart from food and drink (see page 110), this means considering the amount that you smoke, and the other drugs and medications that you might use. And, as certain illnesses can affect your baby, you need to be aware of their effects.

RECREATIONAL DRUGS

Drugs used for pleasure—whether legal or illegal—all have the potential to affect and possibly harm your baby. Alcohol consumption is a major concern of many pregnant women, and many experts agree that the best advice is to avoid alcohol during pregnancy. If you do drink, limit your intake to one or two alcoholic drinks a week at most (see page 111). With caffeine, despite what you may have heard, there is no evidence that it causes birth defects, and drinking one or two cups of coffee or tea each day won't cause your baby any harm. However, large amounts of caffeine may affect your baby (see page 112). Other drugs—smoking in particular—are more risky.

Smoking

When you smoke, you run the risk of developing lung cancer, emphysema, and heart disease, among other illnesses. Smoking when you're pregnant, however, means that you're subjecting your baby to very serious health risks as well.

If you smoke during pregnancy, the nicotine contained in cigarette smoke will decrease blood flow to your baby, while carbon monoxide decreases the amount of oxygen this blood contains. As a result, women who smoke during pregnancy stand an increased chance of delivering babies with low birth weights. Babies weighing less than 5½ lbs (2.5 kg) at birth are 20 times more at risk of dying in their first year than babies of normal birth weight. They're also more likely to experience developmental problems. Babies born to smokers are expected to weigh ½ lb (0.25 kg) less, on average, than those born to nonsmokers. The exact difference in birth weight depends on how much the mother smokes.

Smoking during pregnancy is also associated with a greater risk of pregnancy complications like miscarriage, preterm delivery, placenta previa, placental abruption, and preterm rupture of the membranes. Research has suggested that smoking during pregnancy may even be linked to sudden infant death syndrome (SIDS) once the baby's born.

Quitting smoking can be extremely difficult, but it's the very best thing you can do for your baby. If you stop smoking in the first trimester, the risk of low birth weight drops to a similar level as that for a nonsmoker. If you find that you can't quit completely, even cutting back on the number of cigarettes you smoke is a benefit to your baby. Nicotine substitutes and anti-smoking medications are not suitable for use during pregnancy.

Illegal drugs

You should avoid taking all illegal drugs during pregnancy. Many studies have shown that they put you at a higher risk of delivering a premature or low-birth-weight baby. Also, some drugs can cause developmental and behavioral problems in the baby.

◆ *Marijuana* The data on marijuana isn't clear-cut, but it does suggest that pregnant women who use it stand a higher-than-average risk of delivering their babies prematurely or at low birth weights.

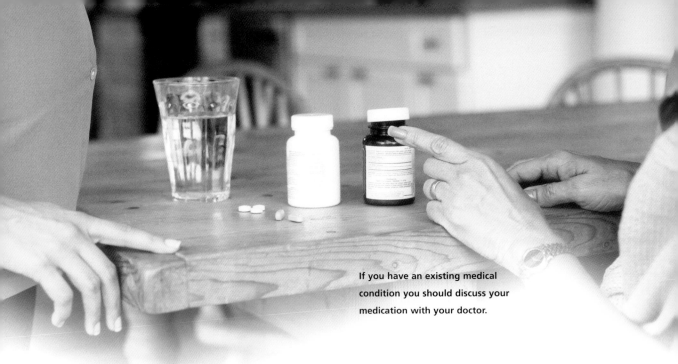

If you have an existing medical condition you should discuss your medication with your doctor.

◆ *Cocaine and crack cocaine* These are highly addictive drugs. Using them during pregnancy puts you at higher risk of premature delivery and placental abruption. Cocaine also has been found to increase the chance of birth defects, neurological problems, seizures, developmental problems, and SIDS. In addition to these adverse effects on the baby, a pregnant woman who uses cocaine is at greater risk of having a stroke, heart attack, or very high blood pressure.

◆ *Narcotics and opiates* This group of drugs includes heroin, methadone, codeine, Demerol, and morphine. Taking narcotics to treat medical conditions and under medical supervision—for example, to provide pain relief after surgery—won't harm your baby; taking narcotics continually and in substantial amounts will. Narcotic addiction puts you and your baby at a very serious risk. It's associated with fetal growth problems, preterm delivery, fetal death, and small head size. Perhaps even more importantly, narcotic addiction places the baby at a high risk of complications after the birth—even death—due to withdrawal from the drug. If you're addicted to narcotics or opiates, beginning a treatment program during your pregnancy can minimize the effects of the drugs on your baby.

◆ *Amphetamines and "uppers"* This group includes crystal methamphetamine and blue ice. Because these substances historically haven't been used as widely as narcotics and cocaine, there's less information available about their side effects during pregnancy. However, they do decrease the appetite, which in turn, could lead to poor fetal growth. Also, evidence shows that the drugs themselves can increase the risk of fetal growth problems, including small head size, placental abruption, and fetal stroke or death.

It is worth keeping in mind that there are additional risks associated with drug-taking. Women who abuse drugs are more likely to be malnourished than other women, and generally suffer a higher incidence of sexually transmitted diseases. All of these factors, independent of drug use, can cause problems for pregnancy and for the baby.

PRESCRIBED MEDICATIONS

Some women are reluctant to take any sort of medication in pregnancy, for fear that it might harm their babies. Many medications are safe during pregnancy, but it's always a good idea to discuss with your healthcare provider, perhaps at your first prenatal visit, the type of drugs you are likely to take over the next nine months—both over-the-counter medications and prescriptions you might need. If you visit a different healthcare provider, be sure to tell him or her that you're pregnant.

If you have an existing medical condition such as high blood pressure or a thyroid condition (see page 271), you will most likely need to continue taking your medication during pregnancy. Stopping medication for a chronic condition will probably pose a greater risk to a growing baby than any possible side effects of the medication itself. Make sure you discuss your dose with your healthcare provider as soon as you find out that you're pregnant, as it may need to be adjusted. Don't stop taking a prescription medication or change the dosage without talking to him or her first.

Many medications are labeled "Do not take during pregnancy" because they haven't been adequately studied in pregnant women. However, this doesn't necessarily mean that adverse affects have been reported, or that you can't use them. Whenever you have a question about a particular medication, ask the advice of your healthcare provider. Don't be surprised if opinions vary among practitioners, because there is not always only one right answer. If you require further information you can try contacting your regional office of The Food and Drug Administration, or writing to the US Public Health Service. In Canada, get in touch with Health Canada.

ILLNESSES

You are still susceptible to illness when you are pregnant. Serious illnesses that can affect your baby are covered in the Prenatal Reference section, but even common problems may have repercussions. It is important to tell your healthcare provider if you have come in contact with any infectious diseases.

Colds

As miserable as it can make you feel, a cold won't harm your baby. However, you need to check with your healthcare provider before taking any cold treatments, as some aren't recommended in pregnancy. Meanwhile, rest as much as you can and take in plenty of fluids in the form of juices, soups,

and water. If you have a respiratory infection that does not improve after a week, let your healthcare provider know.

Fever

While fever is your body's defense against illness, it can pose a threat to your baby, especially in the very early weeks when all the crucial development is going on. If you have a fever you need to bring it down, by bathing in tepid water, wearing fewer clothes, and taking cold drinks. If you're running a temperature of 102°F (38.9°C) or over, call your healthcare provider for advice on treatment.

Stomach upsets

Gastroenteritis is unlikely to affect your baby. Fortunately, it's normally short-lived, lasting only a day or two, but it's always best to consult your healthcare provider and report any other symptoms you may have, such as fever, abdominal pain, or blood in your stools. It's important to rule out other illnesses such as food poisoning or an infection picked up when traveling; if either of these are diagnosed you may need medical treatment. Rest and plenty of fluids are the best treatments for stomach bugs. You can carry on eating, but it is best to stick to bland, easily digestible foods.

HEALTH FIRST

Flu The US Centers for Disease Control and Prevention and Health Canada both recommend that pregnant women who will be in their second or third trimester during the flu season—which usually peaks in late December and early March—should have an annual flu shot. Speak to your healthcare provider to arrange it.

EVERYDAY HAZARDS

You and your baby can both be affected by pollution and chemicals found in everyday products, so you should try to maintain a healthy environment, both at work and at home.

Maintaining a healthy environment for you and your growing baby also involves considering the activities you do every day and the effects they may have on your body.

HOUSEHOLD PRODUCTS

Everyday household cleaners won't harm your baby, but try and avoid using highly toxic products, such as oven cleaners. If you can't, avoid using products with strong fumes. Make sure the room is well aired and take frequent breaks to get some fresh air.

If you're seized with an irresistible urge to decorate your baby's room, try to resist it in the last weeks of pregnancy, or get someone else to do the painting. Pregnant women should avoid exposure to paint that may contain lead, and some latex paints, which may contain mercury. Most water-based paints can be used, but always check the label for contents that could be harmful. Painting should always be done in a well-ventilated room.

INSECTICIDES

Occasional contact with an insecticide shouldn't harm you or your baby. What is harmful is repeated exposure to a chemical over a period of time. High levels of exposure have been linked with birth defects. There are plenty of environmentally friendly products on the market that won't pose a risk to your unborn baby. If you have unwanted insects in the house, try and avoid spraying, if possible, and use non-chemical alternatives.

HOUSEHOLD PETS

Many pregnant women wonder if their household pets pose any risk for their pregnancy, but the reality is that having a pet usually doesn't cause any problem. Even if your large golden retriever jumps up to your belly occasionally, it's unlikely to hurt you or your baby. The one pet that may carry some risk is a cat, since some outdoor cats carry a rare infection known as toxoplasmosis (see page 257)—indoor cats are not affected. As this organism is present in a cat's feces, you should avoid changing your cat's litter box. If this is impossible, you should wear gloves and wash your hands immediately after cleaning the box.

HOT TUBS, SAUNAS, AND STEAM ROOMS

Studies suggest that pregnant women whose core body temperatures rise above 102°F (38.8°C) for more than 10 minutes during the first seven weeks of pregnancy stand an increased risk of miscarriage or having babies with neural tube defects such as spina bifida. For this reason, it's vital to avoid overheating when you're pregnant. However, after your first trimester, occasional use of hot tubs, saunas, and steam rooms for less than 10 minutes is reasonable and safe.

POLLUTION

Air quality becomes a big issue for some pregnant women, especially those who live in a city, and you may suddenly become acutely conscious of how dirty and polluted the air is. There's no evidence that city life is harmful to a developing baby, but what you can do for your baby is minimize the time you spend in highly polluted areas. Keep in mind, too, that air quality can be up to two to five times worse in the home than outdoors. For this reason, keep your use of toxic household products to a minimum (see above), check for any signs of mold or damp, and have heating appliances checked to ensure that they're not emitting carbon monoxide.

WORKING SAFELY

With the exception of a few physically demanding or high-risk jobs, it's perfectly safe for most women who have no complications to continue working throughout pregnancy. And there are ways to make your day even more comfortable.

Many women find that work is a good distraction from some of their uncomfortable pregnancy symptoms. And, if you plan to return to your job after the birth, balancing the demands of work and the physical challenges of pregnancy now will be great practice for managing your future career when you have your kids.

ADAPTING YOUR ROUTINE

Speak to your employer as soon as you know that you're pregnant so you can discuss ways to make your day more comfortable. It may be possible to arrange more flexible working hours to help you cope with times when you're suffering from fatigue or morning sickness. You also should be given time off to attend prenatal tests.

If your job is physically very demanding, your healthcare provider may advise you to make more drastic changes to your routine. If your job involves long hours, long periods on your feet, or working with any hazardous materials, you are within your rights to ask your employers to get you some additional help or give you alternative duties.

Minimize stress

Rushing to get to work on time, meeting deadlines, or working late can exaggerate pregnancy symptoms, making you feel tired or down. Although there may be little you can do to reduce stress that's inherent in your work—for example, you can't change deadlines or stop dealing with customer complaints—you can change your own attitude to work. Always keep in mind that your baby comes first, and for the sake of your baby's well-being, as well as your own, try to find ways to eliminate any extra stress. For example, delegate when possible and learn to say "no" to overtime, excessive traveling, or entertaining. Take plenty of breaks throughout the day, walking around

5 ways to make your work place more comfortable

1   Most companies have a nonsmoking policy, but if there are smoking areas in your company try to avoid them.

2   Keep your desk drawer topped up with healthy snacks such as dried fruit, vegetable strips, and granola bars.

3   If you work in a place where there are extremes of heat, such as a kitchen, ask to work elsewhere—overheating may damage your baby.

4   If you work in front of a computer screen all day, take frequent breaks to get up and move around.

5   Make sure that your workstation is properly set up. Sit in a height-adjustable chair with a backrest, and use a wrist support and footstool, if necessary.

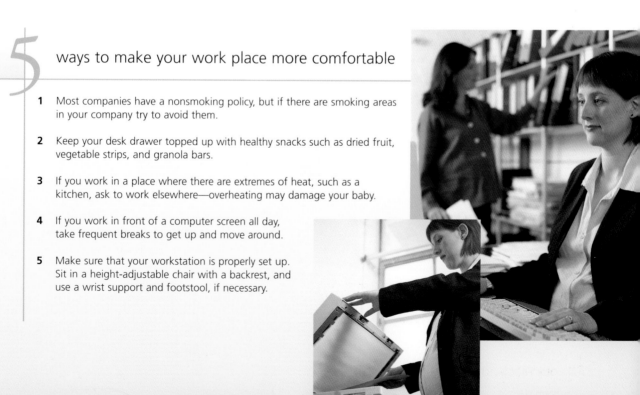

and stretching if you've been sitting at a desk, or sitting down and putting your feet up if you've been standing up all day.

Deciding when to stop

If your pregnancy proceeds without complications, there's no medical reason why you can't continue to work right up until your delivery date. Although most women find they are too exhausted to carry on working past eight months, this is very personal. Some women are happy to carry on with their daily routine; others feel the need to stop earlier in the last trimester. If you want to stop work earlier than you'd planned, discuss it with your employer; you may be able to work part-time your last few weeks.

Occasionally, complications arise during pregnancy that make it advisable to reduce your workload or stop altogether. For example, if you develop high blood pressure or if there are problems with the baby's growth, your healthcare provider may advise you to stop working.

AVOIDING HAZARDS

As jobs are so diverse and individual pregnancies are so different, you'll need to do a bit of research to find out if there are specific hazards in your workplace. Contact the US Occupational Safety and Health Administration or The Canadian Centre for Occupational Health and Safety for information. At your first prenatal visit, talk to your healthcare provider about the type of work you do.

Your daily tasks

Think about what you do each day. Do any of your tasks put you at risk of strain or injury? For example, if you work at a computer, incorrect seating can contribute to pregnancy backache, while prolonged typing or using a mouse may increase your risks of carpal tunnel syndrome (see page 260). Both of these can be minimized with correct seating and positioning of equipment, and by the use of wrist supports. Speak to your employer to have your workstation assessed. If your job involves lifting or carrying, check that you know how to lift correctly (see picture, page 72), and avoid carrying heavy objects. If your job involves standing for long periods, take frequent breaks to reduce the chances of swelling and varicose veins (see page 73).

The equipment you use

In the office, there is little chance that any equipment you use will cause you any harm. Some women worry that computer monitors may emit harmful radiation. However, research has shown that the levels of radiation involved are well below international safety limits. The jury's still out on whether or not cell phones cause brain damage, but to be safe, use your cell phone sparingly and limit conversations to less than 20 minutes.

In other industries, risks are dependent on the type of work you do. Consider in particular any chemicals or biological agents you work with, such as drugs, laboratory specimens, or pesticides. These are potentially harmful to pregnant women, so take all necessary steps to avoid contamination. If any machinery you use puts you at risk, ask about doing another job during pregnancy.

Your work environment

Most companies today have a nonsmoking policy in the workplace, so this is unlikely to be a problem. But if there are smoking areas at your place of work, try to avoid them. If you work in a place where there are extremes of heat, perhaps in a factory or kitchen, you may need to ask for work in a different area, as this can be damaging for your baby.

TRAVELING SAFELY

Being pregnant doesn't mean you have to cocoon yourself and never venture farther than two blocks away. As long as your pregnancy is progressing normally and you follow a few precautions, you can still explore the world, if you want.

Keep in mind that going away puts distance between you and your healthcare provider, so discuss your plans with your healthcare provider as far in advance of your trip as possible. You should talk about medications for common problems such as traveler's diarrhea; and immunizations you might need. It's also advisable to avoid traveling to areas at high altitudes—adjusting to the reduction in oxygen could be too taxing for you and your baby, especially during the last trimester.

WHEN TO GO

One of the key questions is when is it safe to go away? In general, you're best off traveling during the mid-second trimester, between about 18 and 24 weeks, when the risk of miscarriage or premature labor is low. Obviously, you need to take into account your own particular circumstances—if you're expecting triplets, for instance, it wouldn't be advisable to travel at this time as you will require frequent medical check-ups.

EATING SAFELY

Be careful of what you eat and drink in underdeveloped countries. Make sure that you stick to the healthy eating guidelines in Chapter 4, avoiding any potential hazards (see page 110). Choose restaurants that look hygienic, and make sure that you know what you're eating—if you're unsure of what a dish contains, don't eat it. Be wary of food bought from stalls and markets, where dishes, and meats in particular, may be only semi-cooked. Peel fruit before eating. Before you travel, find out what the water supply is like. You'll need to keep up your water intake, so if you're at all unsure about the safety of the drinking water, drink still, bottled water. You should even use bottled water to brush your teeth. Avoid drinks containing ice.

Travelers' diarrhea

It's very common to get diarrhea when you're traveling. While not serious in itself, the dehydration it causes can lead to weakness, fainting, preterm labor, and reduced blood flow to your baby. If you do develop serious diarrhea while traveling, drink plenty of liquid, and seek medical advice.

LOOKING AFTER YOUR HEALTH

It may be hard to find a drug store where you're traveling, so take along any medications that you feel you may need, provided that you have checked their safety with your healthcare provider. If you usually take prescription medications, for asthma or hypertension for example, make sure you carry enough to last you for your entire trip—and a little extra isn't a bad idea either. Again, discuss this with your healthcare provider.

If you're planning to be away for any length of time, you need to be in touch with a prenatal care provider in the area you're visiting, and make sure that whatever tests you would need to have done—

HEALTH FIRST

Malaria It's not recommended for pregnant women to travel to countries where malaria is common. Malaria is a serious disease, which can pose a serious threat for a pregnant woman and her developing baby. While medications are available for the prevention of malaria, they aren't 100 percent effective. If you cannot avoid the trip, ask your healthcare provider for advice.

for example, glucose screen for gestational diabetes, or ultrasound for anatomy—can be performed at the appropriate time. If you're traveling in the third trimester, you should find out whether there are adequate labor and delivery facilities nearby. Can the facility handle such complications as emergency cesareans or pre-eclampsia? Will anesthesia be readily accessible if it is required?

Traveling to tropical countries

If you plan to visit tropical countries, where some diseases are particularly prevalent, you may need to be vaccinated before you travel. Your healthcare provider will be your best source of information about vaccines you may need for the area you're visiting and whether they're safe during pregnancy.

It's not recommended for pregnant women to travel to areas in which malaria is prevalent (see page 81). However, other diseases can also be transmitted by insects. You can help avoid bites and stings by wearing long sleeves and pants, shoes, and socks. Use an insect repellent containing a substance called DEET, but use it sparingly.

TRAVELING BY CAR

This poses no special risk in pregnancy, except for the fact that you can be sitting in one place for a long time. On long trips, stop every couple of hours to get out and walk around a bit. Wear your seat belt and shoulder strap; they keep you safe, and they won't hurt the baby, even if you're involved in an accident. The amniotic fluid surrounding the baby serves as a cushion against any constriction from the lap belt. Not wearing restraints clearly poses a greater risk; studies show that the leading cause of fetal death in auto accidents is death of the mother.

FLYING

Airline travel is permitted by most airlines up until 36 weeks of pregnancy, although you may need a letter from your healthcare provider to state that you are safe to travel. Check with the airline well in advance of your trip.

- *Stretch your legs* Get up from your seat occasionally during longer flights and walk around the plane. Prolonged periods of sitting can cause blood to pool in your legs. Walking around keeps your circulation going and helps prevent deep vein thrombosis (DVT).
- *Sip water frequently* Carry a water bottle with you and drink from it frequently. Air travel can make you incredibly dehydrated—the relative humidity in airplanes is typically lower than it is in the Sahara Desert.
- *Sit near the aisle* Try and book an aisle seat, so you don't have to worry about disturbing your neighbor when you need to use the bathroom for the umpteenth time.

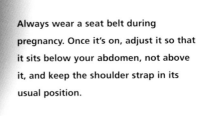

Always wear a seat belt during pregnancy. Once it's on, adjust it so that it sits below your abdomen, not above it, and keep the shoulder strap in its usual position.

YOUR PRENATAL CARE

Throughout your pregnancy, you and your baby will

be closely monitored to make sure everything is

progressing as it should. This prenatal care is a vital

part of your pregnancy and can provide you with a

lot of information and reassurance.

THE BASICS OF GOOD CARE

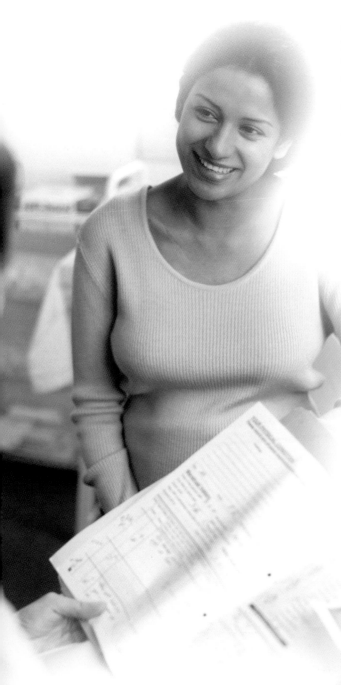

After that first rush of excitement on finding out you're pregnant, you need to start taking proper care of yourself and your baby, and that means organizing your prenatal care.

The ultimate goal of any prenatal care program is a healthy pregnancy, for both mother and baby, and the successful birth of a new life. It's never been safer to have a baby than today—if you're currently healthy, your chance of giving birth to a healthy baby is over 95 percent. But this isn't a reason to skip your regular check-ups; in fact, the opposite is true—studies have shown a strong link between early involvement in prenatal care and healthy babies of a good birth weight.

THE PURPOSE OF PRENATAL CARE

The tests and check-ups that make up prenatal care are designed to provide as much information as possible about your pregnancy. They will:

- *Assess your general health* Examinations and tests will uncover any existing medical problems, such as kidney failure (see page 270) or high blood pressure (see page 265). If a problem surfaces, it will be monitored at subsequent visits and you'll be advised on how the condition may affect your baby and how your condition may change as a result of your pregnancy.
- *Check on your well-being* Professionals on your prenatal team can monitor your physical and emotional well-being when they see you.
- *Check on your baby's well-being* Your schedule of tests, which may include an ultrasound scan between weeks 18 and 20, is designed to monitor the normal development and growth of your baby. If anything unusual is found, you'll be offered other tests to confirm the problem and determine the exact cause. Your healthcare provider can then explain your options and help you take whatever steps are necessary to safeguard your baby's health.

- *Detect complications* Common pregnancy complaints such as heartburn or hemorrhoids are minor, but a nuisance all the same. Your healthcare provider can give you advice on how to treat these and, if possible, prevent them from recurring. Prenatal checks are designed to detect "invisible" conditions, such as gestational diabetes (see page 253) or pre-eclampsia (see page 254), so that they can be treated successfully and therefore have minimal effects on your developing baby.
- *Educate and prepare you for parenthood* There's so much to learn about becoming a parent—in fact, you never stop learning—and your healthcare provider will give you advice on joining a parenting class.
- *Prepare you for the birth* It may seem a long way off now, but you'll be surprised how quickly your due date arrives. Your team is there not only to help you and your partner make informed choices about the sort of birth you want but also to support you both throughout the miraculous birth experience.

CHOOSING A PRACTICE

Your family doctor may be able to offer you the care that you need throughout your pregnancy, but if your doctor doesn't attend births or if you prefer to go to a specialist, such as an obstetrician or midwife, he or she may be able to recommend a good practice. Also, talk to friends who have recently had babies, or contact a pregnancy and child birth organization and ask them for a list of practitioners in your area.

Depending on where you live, you may have several types of practice from which to choose. You might opt for a solo practice, in which the doctor or obstetrician works alone. This has the advantage that you always see the same person at each visit. In a partnership or group practice, there may be one or more doctors, obstetricians, or midwives responsible for your care. A combination practice is similar to a group practice in that a number of healthcare professionals work together.

MORE **ABOUT** | your schedule of visits

Your first visit to your healthcare provider—for many women at around week 6 to 8—will probably be to confirm the news that you're pregnant. Then, either at this visit or at one scheduled in the next few weeks, you'll have a full physical. This will probably include an internal exam, routine blood tests, and a blood pressure test, and your medical history will be taken. An ultrasound may be given to confirm the due date.

After that, your schedule of visits will vary depending on your healthcare provider and medical needs. With a normal, low-risk pregnancy, you'll probably have monthly visits until weeks 28 to 32, when you'll start to go for more frequent visits, every one or two weeks. At each visit, it's likely that your blood pressure will be taken, your urine will be tested for protein and perhaps glucose, and the baby's size and position will be checked. The baby's heart rate may be monitored from week 16 onward.

Special tests will be given at particular stages. For example, an ultrasound will usually be given around week 16 to 20 to check the baby's anatomy. Your rhesus status (see page 90) will be tested at the first visit and in the third trimester. At week 36 to 37 you may have a swab for Group B strep culture (see page 363). And if you go past your due date— from week 41 onward—you may be booked in for an induction.

Who's who in your prenatal team

Everyone involved in your prenatal care wants what's best for you and your baby, and they'll do whatever they can to ensure you feel informed, comfortable, and safe. For information on who'll attend the birth, see page 177.

Family practitioner Some doctors provide obstetric care.

Obstetrician-gynecologist This practitioner specializes in pregnancy and childbirth as well as in women's general healthcare, such as giving Pap smears and breast exams.

Perinatologist or maternal-fetal medicine specialist This is an obstetrician who specializes in high-risk pregnancies, for example, if a woman has heart disease or diabetes, or a history of recurrent

miscarriages. Many perinatologists are trained in prenatal diagnosis—for example, performing obstetrical ultrasounds and invasive procedures such as chorionic villus sampling (see page 242).

Midwife Most US midwives are Certified Nurse-Midwives (CNMs). A nurse-midwife is a registered nurse who is specially trained and certified in the care of pregnant women, and licensed to perform deliveries. A nurse midwife often works in conjunction with an obstetrician so that he or she has appropriate back-up should complications arise.

Direct-entry midwives are trained without first becoming nurses, although they may have degrees in other healthcare areas. They attend hospital and home births, calling on medical help if complications arise.

In Canada, midwives belong to the Canadian Association of Midwives (CAM) and have hospital privileges.

Residents It's accepted practice at big teaching hospitals for residents (physicians undergoing special training in obstetrics and/or gynecology) to be present during prenatal visits. You can refuse to have residents in the room, but their presence is usually taken for granted, and you can request that certain procedures be performed only by the attending doctor.

Anesthesiologist This specialist doctor is responsible for providing pain relief. An anesthesiologist can play a crucial role if complications arise in the birth process. For example, if a woman is bleeding heavily, an anesthesiologist will monitor her vital signs, or if a woman has severe pre-eclampsia, he or she may be involved in helping control her hypertension.

Other health practitioners Ultrasound technicians and radiologists may carry out and review ultrasound examinations. Physical therapists can give you advice and support about pregnancy-related aches and pains and also recommend exercises to speed your recovery after delivery (see page 334). Phlebotomists are specialists in taking blood samples.

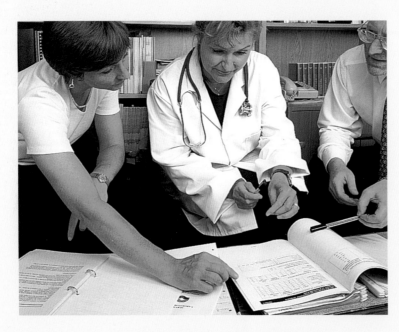

YOUR FIRST VISIT

As soon as your pregnancy is confirmed, you'll need to set up a visit with your healthcare provider. This should take place between weeks 5 and 9 and is one date you shouldn't miss.

At the initial visit you'll be asked what can sometimes seem like a barrage of questions, but if you're prepared for this, you'll feel less overwhelmed and more receptive to the information you're given.

Your healthcare provider will probably start with a review of your and your partner's past and current health, and this is usually followed by a sequence of checks, such as your weight and blood pressure. Be forewarned: you will be asked to give a urine sample and some blood will have to be taken from a vein in your arm for various laboratory tests. For more on routine blood tests, see page 89. At the end of this visit, you'll agree on a schedule of further visits depending on your medical needs (see page 85).

Medical history

Gathering information about your health and that of your partner is one of the goals for your healthcare provider at your first visit. This questioning process is called taking your medical history. Your healthcare provider will ask you various questions about all aspects of your life; so have the answers to the questions in the box on page 88.

It's important to be honest and accurate: all the details you give help build a complete picture of your history so that any risk can be more easily spotted and support provided, as necessary. Don't be embarrassed about answering personal questions and becoming upset when revealing certain sorts of information, such as if you had a previous miscarriage; your healthcare provider is there to offer support and understanding. If you can't remember all the details of a previous episode, give as much information as you can, and your healthcare provider can try to expand on this information from records elsewhere.

Physical examination

Most women don't need a top-to-toe check-up, but there are certain aspects of your health that your healthcare provider will want to assess. First, he or she will want to listen to your heart and lungs, to make sure they're strong and healthy, and may take this opportunity to check your breasts. Do discuss your feelings about breastfeeding, if you wish, particularly if you have any concerns, such as if you think your breasts are too small, your nipples are an unusual shape, or you have had breast surgery.

Your healthcare provider may wish to perform a pelvic examination at your first visit to assess pelvic and uterine size. An ultrasound scan may be offered to determine the length of your pregnancy or the presence of twins. A Pap smear test will then be performed if you haven't had one recently along with a check to make sure that you have no cervical abnormalities.

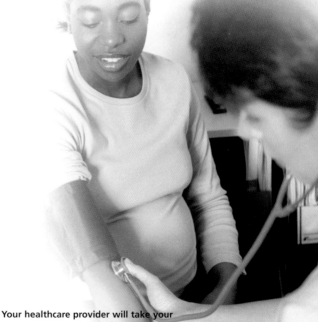

Your healthcare provider will take your blood pressure at each check-up—high blood pressure is a common complication in late pregnancy.

Measuring your weight

You may be weighed at every prenatal visit. But some healthcare providers weigh you only if you were over- or underweight when you started your pregnancy or if you don't seem to be gaining weight at a reasonable rate. Gaining too much weight can make it difficult for your healthcare provider to discern how your baby is growing, and if you're overweight you're more likely to experience complications such as gestational diabetes (see page 253). Being underweight isn't healthy either—your healthcare provider will want to monitor your baby's growth more closely if you're below average weight, because your baby may not be growing as well as expected (see page 261).

Blood pressure

Your healthcare provider will check your blood pressure at every visit; it's an essential part of prenatal care because high blood pressure is an important—and common—complication, especially in late pregnancy. The reading taken at your first visit will form the baseline against which any fluctuations can be measured. You may become familiar with the numbers your healthcare provider writes down for your blood pressure reading—a typical measurement is 120/70. Blood pressure is measured in millimeters of mercury—written as mmHg; the first number represents the systolic pressure (when the heart contracts), while the second number represents the diastolic pressure

 subjects to discuss at your first appointment

Your first visit will be a successful and productive one if you prepare in advance. As well as considering the questions below, it's a good idea to talk to your mother to find out about her pregnancies—were they straightforward or were there complications, and if so, what sort? Ask your partner to obtain similar information from his mother, too.

1   What is your medical history? Do you or your partner have any conditions that seem to run in the family? Have you had any operations—and therefore anesthetic—or stayed in hospital for any length of time? Are you allergic to any medications?

2   Do you have any pre-existing medical conditions? Are you taking medication—and were you when you discovered your pregnancy—for a chronic condition, such as asthma or high blood pressure?

3   If this isn't your first pregnancy, how long ago was your last one? Was it a healthy, normal pregnancy or were there any complications? You should let your healthcare provider know about any previous terminations or miscarriages as well.

4   Do you exercise regularly? How healthy is your diet? Do you smoke? How much and how often do you drink alcohol? Do you use any recreational drugs?

5   What is your ethnic origin? Because certain medical conditions are more prevalent in particular ethnic groups, your healthcare provider may want to know from where your family and that of your partner originate (see page 240).

6   What sort of job do you have? Could your job pose any risks or hazards to your unborn baby? Do you work with chemicals or X-rays? Do you work in a hot or cold environment? Do you travel extensively? Do you have a hectic work schedule?

7   Do you have a secure, permanent place to live? Is it clean and safe?

8   What date was the first day of your last period? Your due date is calculated from this date (see page 22). Typically, how regular were your periods and how far apart were they?

9   Were you using any form of contraception before you discovered that you were pregnant? If you have an intrauterine contraceptive device (IUCD) alert your healthcare provider to this fact, as there's a potential for it to cause complications. If you were on the Pill when you got pregnant, it shouldn't be harmful for your pregnancy or your baby, but your dates may not be accurate.

(when the heart relaxes). Your blood pressure will probably decrease during the first 24 weeks of pregnancy, with the systolic measurement dropping by about 5 to 10 mmHg and the diastolic by 10 to 15 mmHg. As you progress toward your third trimester, however, your blood pressure should return to your pre-pregnancy levels. If it starts to increase further, your healthcare provider will assess you for pre-eclampsia. Occasionally, blood pressure medication may be administered.

Urine tests

Changes within your body may mean that you're more prone to kidney and urinary tract infections during pregnancy—about 4 percent of women are found to have bacteria in their urine samples. Recognizing and then treating infection while you're expecting is important, because these types of infection can cause preterm labor (see page 250).

To discount a bacterial infection, you'll be asked at your first visit to give a sample of urine, which will be sent off to a laboratory for testing. At your first and all subsequent visits, your urine is tested for the presence of protein, which could mean you have an infection or, more seriously, pre-eclampsia (see page 254) or kidney failure (see page 270). Normally, urine tests are done quickly on site using a specially impregnated dipstick; your healthcare provider may give you a supply of these dipsticks so that you can monitor your urine at home on the day of your prenatal check and then report the result. It's imperative that you report any positive results of protein in your urine.

Your urine will also be tested for the presence of glucose. Pregnant women have sugar in their urine from time to time, but if it's found at consecutive visits or if your baby is very large for her dates, you'll

DID YOU KNOW…

About white-coat hypertension
Some women's blood pressure goes up only when they're having it taken at a hospital or doctor's office. If your healthcare provider suspects that a high reading may be brought on by your clinical surroundings, you may be given a machine that can measure your blood pressure at home; it uses an automated cuff that takes a reading every 15 minutes for 24 hours. If you have high blood pressure or are at risk of pre-eclampsia, you may need to check your blood pressure once a day.

be checked for gestational diabetes—a type of diabetes seen only in pregnant women, which disappears after their babies are born (see page 253).

Routine urine cultures aren't usually sent off, unless the dipstick indicates a possible infection, or the presence of white blood cells, blood, or protein. Routine cultures may be done for women with a history of recurrent urinary tract infections, kidney infections, diabetes, or sickle-cell disease.

ROUTINE BLOOD TESTS

You may have already received information from your healthcare provider explaining what blood tests are done and why, but if you're unsure about a specific test ask for clarification. At your first visit you'll be asked to give a blood sample from a vein in your arm; you might need to give further samples during your pregnancy but this depends on your health and if any complications occur. Fortunately, a whole host of tests can be performed on just one sample of blood.

Rubella (German measles)

It's likely that you have either had rubella or been vaccinated against it as a child—in which case you can't be reinfected and your baby is safe. If you develop rubella infection in early pregnancy, which is quite rare, your baby can suffer from serious abnormalities, such as mental retardation. If, on testing, you're found not to be immune, you can be vaccinated after your baby is born to protect any future pregnancies. Most women are instructed not to get pregnant for three months after receiving the vaccine. If you do become pregnant less than three months after vaccination, don't feel concerned, as there have been no reports of adverse outcome in children born under these circumstances.

Complete blood count

As the name implies, this blood test checks the level of each type of blood cell: red blood cells (which carry oxygen), white blood cells (which fight infection), and platelets (which are involved in blood clotting). If you're anemic (see page 252), for example, the level of red blood cells—and therefore hemoglobin, of which iron is an essential component—is low and your healthcare provider will prescribe an iron supplement to remedy the problem. You may also be advised to include more iron-rich foods in your diet such as dark green, leafy vegetables; red meat, including small amounts of liver; cooked shellfish, particularly clams; dried fruit, fortified cereals, enriched pastas and breads, and eggs. Because iron-deficiency anemia develops most often after 20 weeks—and especially in the third trimester—this check for low iron levels is normally repeated as your pregnancy progresses.

Blood group and rhesus status

This blood test, carried out at the beginning of pregnancy and again in the third trimester, identifies your blood group—A, B, AB, or O—and tests for blood antibodies, in particular rhesus antibodies. Your genes determine your blood group; 85 percent of the US population is rhesus positive. Your rhesus status is vitally important during pregnancy because if your baby is rhesus positive and you're rhesus negative, you can form antibodies to your baby's red blood cells, which will destroy the blood cells of your next rhesus-positive baby. This puts the baby at risk of developing a serious form of anemia, called Rhesus disease (see page 244).

However, thanks to modern treatment this disease is now quite rare. Rhesus-negative mothers are regularly given an injection of Rh immuno-globulin (anti-D) at 28 and 34 weeks as well as after delivery. It can also be given if the woman experiences vaginal bleeding during the pregnancy. It's also given after chorionic villus sampling (CVS), amniocentesis, or attempts to turn the baby. This completely safe injection prevents the mother from making antibodies that can cross the placenta and attack her baby's red blood cells. A woman who is Rh negative should receive the injection, unless she knows for certain that the father is Rh negative too. If the fetus' father is also Rh negative, the baby will be Rh negative.

MORE **ABOUT** | testing for HIV

Although you cannot be tested for HIV without your consent, some women choose to go for a voluntary HIV test, as it's possible to be infected and not know that you have it. It's important to find out this information, as immediate treatment can reduce the risk of transmission of the virus to the baby, as well as keep the mother healthy. If you think you could have been exposed to any risk factors in the past—unprotected sex or sharing needles—ask your healthcare provider to arrange a test for you.

If you do have HIV, your healthcare provider can drastically reduce the chance of your baby being infected—from around 1 in 4 to around 1 in 50—with the antiretroviral treatments currently available and by arranging an elective cesarean. You'll also be advised not to breastfeed your baby because the virus can transfer to your baby in breast milk. It's worth knowing, too, that in some US states, doctors have the right to perform HIV testing on a newborn without parental consent.

SUBSEQUENT VISITS

In sharp contrast to the detailed and lengthy first prenatal visit, later appointments are shorter and involve fewer checks.

If, for any reason, you can't make an appointment, make sure you reschedule; don't be tempted to skip it because you feel alright—regular checks are in place because they're the best way to keep an eye on you and your developing baby.

At each visit your healthcare provider will ask you how you're coping and give you the opportunity to discuss any pregnancy-related complaints (see page 67) or concerns you may have. As with the first visit, a series of checks are performed—some every time and others at key stages—to keep a close eye on your baby's health and development.

Screening tests

Healthcare providers can now detect a disease or problem before obvious signs or symptoms indicate that there's something wrong. A whole range of screening tests exist, including ultrasound scanning, nuchal translucency screening, amniocentesis, chorionic villus sampling, alphafetoprotein testing, and cord blood sampling. These tests are covered in detail in the Prenatal Reference section.

Blood pressure and urine protein

At every visit your blood pressure will be measured and your urine tested for protein—or you will be asked for your home result—to detect signs of pre-eclampsia (see page 254). Pre-eclampsia is almost unheard of before 20 weeks, and usually doesn't develop until the third trimester. If your blood pressure rises or your urine test is positive for the presence of protein, your healthcare provider will refer you for further tests, and you may need to be admitted to hospital. You may have certain blood tests to check for blood abnormalities that can occur with pre-eclampsia, such as low platelets and abnormal liver function tests.

Growth and fetal position

To follow the growth of your baby, your healthcare provider will palpate your abdomen at each visit and will measure your fundal height. This measurement is the distance from the top of your uterus to your pelvic bone. The distance lengthens as your baby grows and so gives an estimate of her size for her age. If your healthcare provider thinks your baby is either too big or too small, you'll probably be referred for an ultrasound scan for a more accurate measurement. If your baby isn't growing well or is growing too fast—for example if you've developed gestational diabetes—you may need to deliver her early. With twins or triplets, your babies' growth will be assessed with ultrasound about every four weeks.

At each of your visits after 35 weeks your abdomen may be checked to ascertain the position of your baby. Usually, your baby will take up a

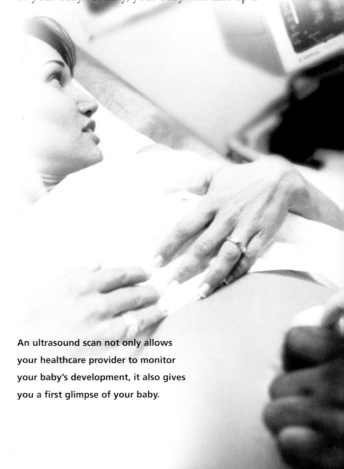

An ultrasound scan not only allows your healthcare provider to monitor your baby's development, it also gives you a first glimpse of your baby.

head-down position in the last few weeks. During your pregnancy, however, she's been somersaulting around and may adopt many different positions before finally settling into her "finishing position." Because of natural constraints—such as the shape of a woman's pelvis and the shape of a baby's head—over 95 percent of babies are born head first. It's common for babies not to be in the head-down position before 36 weeks; however, after this time, it's more unusual and your healthcare provider may advise you to take steps to try to turn your baby around into the correct position (see page 204) so that you can have a normal delivery.

Fetal movements

You'll be asked about your baby's movements, how often you feel them, and how strong they are. In some practices your healthcare provider will listen to your baby's heart rate at each visit. However, if everything seems fine, this may not be necessary—although if you want to hear your baby for reassurance, just ask. You may also be given a kick-count sheet (see page 207) on which to record your baby's movements.

Your first scan

That first momentous ultrasound can be carried out in a hospital or in a special center or office, and is often done by a perinatologist or a radiologist. Watching your baby moving around inside and seeing her tiny heart beating is truly mesmerizing and breathtaking. It may be the first time your pregnancy feels "real," especially if you've been lucky enough not to have morning sickness and don't have any other obvious signs.

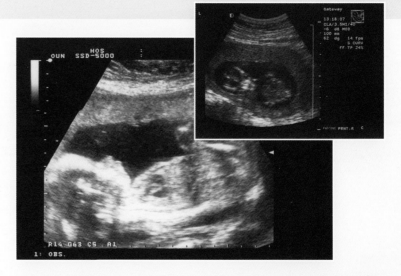

As wonderful as it may be to see your baby, the purpose of the scan is to make sure that your baby is developing properly and that there aren't any problems. Several measurements will be taken to check that she's growing well and to check for neural tube defects (see page 375) or other abnormalities. You can be given an idea of the sex of your baby at around 16 weeks—but it is only an idea and shouldn't be relied on for decorating your baby's room.

By the end of the appointment, your healthcare provider should be able to confirm your due date or give a more accurate estimation based on your baby's size. As with all your prenatal visits, taking your partner, or a close friend or relative, is enormously important, both for support and for sharing the joyous experience. You'll almost always be offered a printout.

SPECIAL PREGNANCIES

Every pregnancy is special, of course, but there may be circumstances in which you need to be more closely monitored to ensure your and your baby's continued well-being.

The questions you're asked as part of your medical history (see page 88) will identify whether or not you're more likely to need closer monitoring and extra care during your pregnancy. If, for instance, you're over 35, have an existing medical condition such as asthma or diabetes, or have had a previously complicated pregnancy, your healthcare provider may offer you more screening tests and want you to attend extra visits. Also, if you're carrying twins or more, your prenatal team will want to keep an especially close eye on you all.

BEING AN OLDER MOTHER

If you're over 35, your prospects of a smooth and trouble-free pregnancy and birth have never been better. These days you're more likely to be in good health and improvements in medical technology have increased the chances of having a healthy baby.

If you hear your healthcare providers referring to you as an "elderly" or "mature primip," don't be insulted; this is simply a medical term that describes the fact that you're over 35 and having your first baby. "Primip" is the shorthand form of primiparous, which means this is your first baby; if you're having your second or third baby you will be referred to as "multip," standing for multiparous.

Research shows that if you've waited to have children, you're more likely to make more of a conscious effort to promote your baby's well-being by eating healthily, exercising regularly, and avoiding hazards. If you are fit and healthy, you're likely to have a good pregnancy.

Age	Risk of Down syndrome
25	1:1500
30	1:900
35	1:350
40	1:100
44	1:30

Health risks

The main risk for older mothers is the increased chance of chromosomal abnormalities. Chorionic villus sampling (CVS) or amniocentesis are the diagnostic tests used to identify such abnormalities. The good news is that many studies looking at neonatal outcome indicate that as long as the chromosomes are normal, the outcome for the babies is the same as it is for women under 35.

Older women also have a slightly increased risk of developing gestational diabetes (see page 253), pregnancy-induced hypertension (see page 253), and pre-eclampsia (see page 254). Because of this, you may be offered more prenatal visits and more ultrasound scans to monitor your baby's development closely and to detect any problem as early as possible.

Down syndrome

Any woman can have a baby affected by a chromosomal disorder, such as Down syndrome, although this is more common as you get older. If you're 35, the chance of having a child with Down syndrome is about 1 in 300. From a positive point of view, though, that means you have a 99.7 percent chance of having a normal, healthy baby.

If you so wish, your healthcare provider can arrange for tests to detect the likelihood of your baby being affected. Before you undergo any extra prenatal test, however, your healthcare provider will offer you counseling to discuss the full implications should results come back positive. You may be offered any of the following tests:

◆ *Chorionic villus sampling* Ultrasound is used to insert either a catheter or a thin needle into the placenta to take a sample of chorionic tissue—the chorion is part of the placenta—for analysis.

- *Alpha-fetoprotein (AFP) test* Also known as a maternal serum alpha-fetoprotein (MSAFP) test, this blood test measures the level of a protein made by your baby and can indicate whether he is at risk of Down syndrome or spina bifida.
- *Triple screen* This blood test usually combines the results of your AFP test with measurements of other key chemicals found in your blood.
- *Amniocentesis* First, an ultrasound scan identifies the position of your baby and then a needle is inserted into the amniotic sac to remove a small sample of amniotic fluid for analysis.
- *Nuchal translucency test* This specialized ultrasound scan specifically examines and measures the thickness of the fluid-filled region

on the back of your baby's neck. This measurement can indicate whether you baby is affected by Down syndrome.

For more information about prenatal tests, see page 236. Your prenatal team is there to support you throughout your pregnancy, so don't hesitate to contact them between visits if you need more information, reassurance and/or advice.

EXPECTING TWINS OR MORE

Discovering you're going to have more than one baby can come as a shock and be overwhelming. Some women, especially if they're a twin themselves or if they've already had one baby, have an inkling that "something's up" but can't quite believe it until

 ways to take double care of yourself

Whether you're expecting twins—and triplets or more—you need to be extra careful. The tips below are designed to avoid or alleviate common complaints that are part and parcel of a multiple pregnancy, and so make your pregnancy as safe and as comfortable as possible.

1 Eat little and often. Don't be surprised if you start feeling full even after a glass of fruit juice and an oatmeal bar—your stomach will have less space as your babies fill out and jostle for room. Nibble food on a little-and-often basis to keep up energy levels and obtain your essential nutrients.

2 Take a nap. Physically you'll need more rest as you may find daily life more tiring, so it's vital to build in some rest periods every day—especially in later months—in which you can sleep or practice some relaxation techniques. If you don't do this, you'll be exhausted before you know it and may even have to be admitted to hospital for the last month or so.

3 Beat backache. Be superconscious of your posture—remember to stand and sit tall—as carrying the extra weight of your babies can exaggerate the curve of your spine and exacerbate backache, especially in your lower back. Ask your partner or a friend to try his or her hands at doing a back massage.

4 Swim for support. Being in water reduces the effect of gravity on your babies and offers some much-needed support. Swimming, especially crawl and

backstroke—which don't cause you to arch your back as breaststroke does—is great exercise and can soothe pressure on your pubic bone and help alleviate any backache.

5 Make your pillow a friend. To relieve and prevent the extreme backache common in multiple pregnancies, buy or borrow a specially designed pillow to support your lower back. Carry it with you wherever you go.

6 Enlist your partner, friends, and family in helping out around the house and in doing strenuous chores. In addition, try not to lift anything heavy, including bags of groceries and small children.

7 Take things slowly. You may feel dizzy or faint as your blood vessels are more dilated (open) than usual and blood rushes to your feet when you stand up—so don't leap up, get up slowly and learn how to get up from a lying-down position by rolling over onto your side first.

8 Sleep easy. When sleeping or resting, you may want to keep yourself propped up with pillows or a beanbag to avoid putting pressure on the major blood vessels, which could restrict the blood supply to the placenta. You'll probably have to try out a few positions until you find the one that is right for you.

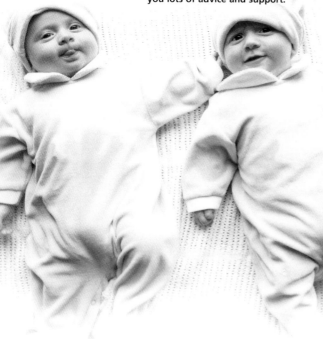

You may be a little apprehensive about giving birth to twins, but your healthcare provider will be able to give you lots of advice and support.

they see conclusive proof on the ultrasound scan. Occasionally, if you're expecting twins, you'll experience exaggerated pregnancy symptoms—compared with carrying a singleton—so severe morning sickness and extreme tiredness in the early days could be clues that something is different.

Today 90 percent of multiple pregnancies are diagnosed by an early ultrasound scan; this early "warning" enables you and your prenatal team to plan a specially tailored schedule of tests and check-ups. An ultrasound scan at 12 to 14 weeks can identify how many babies are present. Sometimes it is possible to determine if the twins are identical, but not always (see page 16).

How you feel

The unexpected news of a multiple pregnancy may make you feel extremely "special": one of the few parents of twins, triplets, or more. But after this exciting start, fears and ambivalence about the idea

of having more than one baby may emerge. If you and your partner are first-time parents, your natural apprehension about approaching parenthood may be intensified further when you consider the reality of how you're going to cope with two babies at once. There's no denying it will be hard work initially but you'll soon find your feet and establish routines to nurture and love the new budding personalities in your life. For parents who had planned to have more than one child, finding out that twins are on the way is fantastic news—everything they wanted in one pregnancy and delivery.

Finding out that you're carrying twins early on in pregnancy allows time for you and your partner to adjust emotionally, so that you can get on with the practicalities that preparation for two babies requires. Of course, you'll need extra equipment—cribs, clothes, car seats, diapers, and so on—so double the number when making a list of everything you need (see page 199). This preparation also helps reduce extra anxiety about the approaching births, because you feel more in control and ready to respond as necessary.

Your healthcare provider may be able to recommend support organizations for specific advice and information. You'll discover all sorts of handy hints and tips from chatting to other parents of twins and listening to their stories.

What can you expect?

Carrying twins can be much more complicated than carrying a singleton, so your medical team will want to keep a close eye on how everything is progressing. You can expect:

♦ *More frequent check-ups* Your blood pressure and urine protein will be checked more regularly for signs of pre-eclampsia (see page 254), a common complication of a multiple pregnancy. If your initial blood test showed that your hemoglobin has dropped—not only because twins need more nutrients but also because your blood becomes more diluted—your healthcare provider may recommend a daily iron supplement—60 to 100 mg—and folic acid—4 mg—to normalize your levels and prevent further anemia.

- *More ultrasound scans* Because it's difficult to monitor the growth and development of twins with a simple examination, your healthcare provider will want accurate and regular updates on how your babies are getting on in their uterine world. If your twins are nonidentical you'll probably have a scan every four weeks, or every two weeks if they're identical twins as complications are more common.
- *Preterm labor and early delivery* Babies are born early—by week 37—in 50 percent of twin pregnancies. Contact your healthcare provider immediately if you have any signs of pain, bleeding or watery vaginal discharge.
- *A hospital delivery* If you were planning to have your baby at home before you discovered that you're carrying two, you may initially be disappointed that you'll require a hospital delivery, but keep focused on the fact that your healthcare providers are thinking of your best interests. Although you can have twins normally, if the first baby is head first, keep in mind that it's not unusual for women carrying twins to require delivery by cesarean (see page 188), so be flexible in your approach to birth. For more on twin positions and vaginal delivery see page 226.
- *Extra maternity leave* If you work, both your tiredness and your increased need for rest may mean you have to stop working earlier on in your pregnancy and take more time off.

COMPLICATED PREGNANCIES

If you suffered complications in any previous pregnancies, there's a risk that the same problem could recur, and you should alert your healthcare provider to your history at your first prenatal visit. Of particular importance is severe pre-eclampsia (see page 254) and preterm delivery. Having one previous miscarriage doesn't affect your chances for a normal and healthy pregnancy this time around; even after three miscarriages, you still stand a good chance of getting pregnant again and carrying your baby the full nine months. Talk through any concerns with your healthcare provider, who may arrange more intensive prenatal care.

Pre-eclampsia recurs in up to 30 percent of pregnancies, although it's likely to be less severe and to occur later on in the pregnancy. If there is concern about you, you'll be offered more frequent prenatal clinic visits to check that your blood pressure is normal and to look for signs of edema, such as swollen ankles and hands. Your healthcare provider may prescribe a small dose of aspirin—75 mg daily—to be taken all through pregnancy. Some studies suggest that this may help reduce the risk of developing pre-eclampsia, or at least delay its onset.

If your last baby was born more than three weeks early, the same could happen again, although it depends on the cause of the previous premature delivery. Your healthcare provider may want to see you more often, especially in your last trimester, and may also recommend that you take plenty of rest to lessen the chance of going into labor too far ahead of your due date. Ask what signs or symptoms could indicate a preterm labor so that you can alert your healthcare provider as soon as possible, if the problem recurs.

CHRONIC CONDITIONS

Even though you may manage a long-term condition such as diabetes or high blood pressure excellently, you may be worried initially about how it will affect your baby. What's also important is how your pregnancy will affect your condition. It's imperative to discuss your condition with your healthcare provider, as you may need to visit another specialist for more frequent check-ups.

Depending on your condition, you may be offered more frequent visits for regular checks of your blood pressure, urine protein, and your baby's growth. With diabetes, it's worth discussing your plans with your healthcare provider before getting pregnant next time around, so your body can be in the best possible shape healthwise for conception. For information on how your condition could affect your pregnancy, see the Prenatal Reference section.

CHAPTER

NINE MONTHS OF HEALTHY EATING

Eating a varied and balanced diet will give you the

energy and nutrients you need for a healthy

pregnancy. It also will be one of the biggest gifts you

can ever give your baby, providing him with a firm

foundation for his future health and well-being.

MAKING HEALTHY ADJUSTMENTS

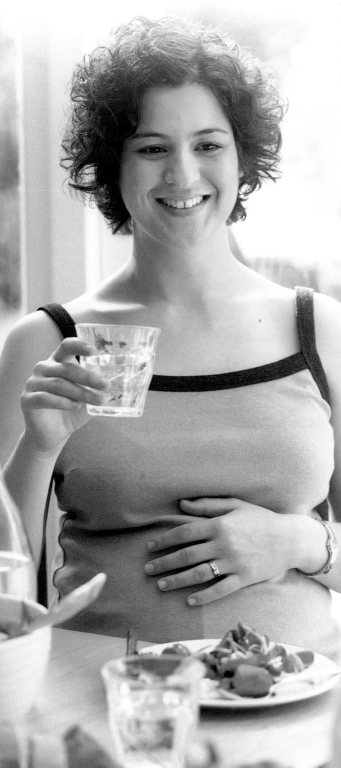

There's probably no other time at which you'll feel better motivated to adopt healthy eating habits than in pregnancy—and with good reason. Eating a varied and nutritious diet provides the best start for your baby and benefits you at the same time.

There's no great mystery to eating well in pregnancy; you simply need to eat a diet that's balanced in terms of the different food groups and that contains sufficient nutrients. Analyze what you eat each day using the food groups chart on page 102, and you'll probably discover that you're already following a fairly healthy diet. You may have to make some minor adjustments to this—for example, if you're not eating enough iron-containing foods, or eating too many sugary foods—and there are a few foods that you should avoid (see page 112), but there's no need to set yourself impossible targets.

SMALL CHANGES FOR GREAT REWARDS

Food is for enjoying, and this doesn't change even though you're pregnant. However, you will want to consider whether there are any improvements you could make to your eating habits. Maybe, for example, you usually skip breakfast, don't eat much fruit, or are often too busy to cook a meal when you finish work. While it's perfectly okay to have the occasional take-out or pre-prepared meal, these should be the exception rather than the rule, since they may not contain as many nutrients as fresh foods. When you find out how eating a good breakfast and sufficient fruit will benefit you and your baby, you'll want to make sure you get your fill.

Providing a nurturing diet for you and your baby doesn't mean you have to spend the whole day in the kitchen: Cook meals in batches to store in the freezer; experiment with quick and healthy cooking methods, such as stir-frying, broiling, and steaming; and if you're tired or nauseous, it'll be particularly helpful if your partner or a friend takes over some of the cooking or brings over the occasional meal.

Avoid drastic changes

Bear in mind that pregnancy isn't a time for radical change, so don't switch from being a meat-eater to a vegetarian or vice versa; it can take your body months to adjust to such a drastic difference in diet. It's much better to adapt your current eating habits so your baby receives the best nourishment possible. If you're concerned that you're not eating enough from a particular food group, speak to your doctor or a nutritionist who will be able to advise you on your individual requirements.

YOUR NEW EATING PATTERNS

During pregnancy, your taste buds, appetite, and digestive system can be a little erratic, so prepare yourself for some weird and wonderful eating patterns. Initially, and particularly if you're suffering from morning sickness, you may not feel like eating at all. Also, you might find yourself craving the strangest foodstuffs while shunning your favorite foods. Later on, in your second and third trimesters, you may feel like you're eating constantly, as you move onto a little-and-often regime. Eventually, as your baby grows to take up most of your abdominal space, you may feel full even after a glass of milk and a banana.

Food cravings and aversions

Don't be surprised if you suddenly develop a passion or violent dislike for foods you felt differently about before you got pregnant. This is very common, particularly in early pregnancy. If you find you suddenly can't live without spicy or pickled items, candy and chocolate, milk, fruit and fruit juices, and very cold foods like ice cream, you're in

good company, as these are the most common cravings. On the other hand, you may develop a sudden aversion to some things, such as tea, coffee, even some meats, too.

Some people believe that food cravings are a sign that your body is lacking in a particular nutrient, but this theory has yet to be proved. The exact reasons for pregnancy food fads aren't known, but changes in hormone levels, such as estrogen, are often thought to be responsible.

In general, as long as your cravings or aversions don't prevent you from following a sensible diet most of the time, indulge yourself and don't worry. Sometimes these feelings can work in your favor, for example, if you develop an aversion to coffee or alcohol, which aren't very good for your baby

MORE **ABOUT** | strange cravings

Some pregnant women develop a very rare condition called pica, which is a compulsion to eat substances such as ice, clay, chalk, coal, toothpaste, or burnt matches. Many theories have been put forward to explain this strange habit, but none has been widely accepted. One theory is that some pregnant women eat non-food substances because they are subconsciously trying to correct a deficiency in certain nutrients—some studies have linked pica to iron deficiency, even though the craved items don't contain significant amounts of iron. What is known, however, is that pica can interfere with the absorption of essential minerals, and if you fill up on pica substances, your intake of nutritious foods is reduced. If you're having any extreme cravings, discuss them with your healthcare provider.

anyway (see page 111). However, if you find that you're missing out on a food that's a valuable source of nutrients, try to make up for any lack by substituting it for a food of similar nutritional value from the same food group (see page 102).

Eating for two?

You'd assume that with a baby on the way, you'd need to eat twice as much food. In fact, you need only about 300 calories a day over your pre-pregnancy needs—a total of 2300 to 2500 calories a day. In general, you'll need fewer calories during your first trimester and more later in your pregnancy, when your baby grows quickly. These extra calories could be met easily with:

◆ A bowl of cereal and low-fat milk.
◆ Two slices of toast and butter or margarine.
◆ A glass of milk and a banana.
◆ A glass of fruit juice and a boiled egg.

However, requirements do vary with individual circumstances, and if you're concerned about your weight, speak to your healthcare provider. If you were underweight when you started your pregnancy, are expecting twins or triplets, or are a teenager, you'll need more calories. If you're overweight, you'll probably be advised to keep your weight gain to a minimum until the last trimester.

Pregnancy isn't a time to diet, and you should never restrict your calorie intake to lose weight—sufficient calories are essential both to give you energy and to help your baby grow. If you find that you're putting on too much weight, it will help to exercise regularly, limit your fat intake, and base your diet on fruit and vegetables and unrefined carbohydrates (see page 101). If you have an eating disorder, talk to your doctor or a dietitian who'll be able to help you plan a good pregnancy diet.

200-CALORIE SNACKS: A COMPARISON

	5 semi-sweet cookies	Branflakes with low-fat milk
energy (kcal)	200	200
protein (g)	2.9	8.4
fiber (g)	0.7	6.5
vitamin B_1 (mg)	0.06	0.5
vitamin B_2 (mg)	0.04	0.8
vitamin B_3 (mg)	0.7	7.6
vitamin B_6 (mg)	0	1.3
folic acid/folate (mcg)	5.7	130
calcium (mg)	53	145
iron (mg)	0.9	10.1
zinc (mg)	0.3	2.1

Healthy choices

As well as making sure you get enough calories, you need also to make sure they're from a healthy source. Eating nutritionally "empty" foods, such as high-sugar or high-fat snacks, may satisfy your energy requirements but it won't meet your nutritional needs. There's no need to obsess about every mouthful, but wherever possible, aim to eat a variety of fresh food. When choosing foods, study the nutritional information to find out what—apart from calories—you're gaining. The chart above shows how the values of two 200-calorie snacks can vary.

Managing meal times

If you have a busy schedule you may have got into the habit of skipping lunch or breakfast. But, just as pregnancy isn't a time to diet, it isn't a time to miss meals either, so make a conscious effort to eat properly at least three times a day.

At times, you may find that you can't manage to eat much at meals, so snack to make up your daily calories. Rather than eating nutritionally empty snacks like cookies and candy, go for fresh or dried fruit, raw vegetables, granola bars, yogurts, and fruit smoothies. If you're working, keep a supply of healthy snacks in your desk drawer or your bag so you've always got something to nibble on.

HOW TO EAT A BALANCED DIET

Eating for optimal health doesn't depend on some magic formula or a definitive list of dos and don'ts—it's about balancing your intake from the different food groups and choosing the foods you want from within that framework.

An easy way to choose foods and plan your meals is to make use of the chart on page 102. This shows you the contribution that each of the five food groups should make to your daily diet.

WHAT ARE THE ESSENTIAL FOODS?

Most nutritionists divide food into five groups: carbohydrates; fruit and vegetables; dairy foods; meat, fish and protein foods; and oils, fats and sugars. Carbohydrates and fruit and vegetables are the two most important food groups, and they should constitute the bulk of all your meals and snacks, together with smaller amounts of dairy and protein foods. Oils, fats, and sugars do contain some valuable nutrients, but should be eaten only in moderation. Within each food group, eat a wide variety of foods in order to take in all the nutrients you and your baby need.

Carbohydrates

Breads, breakfast cereals, pasta, rice, and potatoes should form roughly a third of your diet. Choose unrefined cereals, such as brown rice and wholewheat breads and pastas, as they're extremely nutritious. They contain both the bran, which is the outer protective coat of grain, and the germ, the small area at the base of each grain. When cereals are refined—to make white flour or polished rice, for example—most of the B vitamins, vitamin E, and essential fatty acids are removed. In addition, about 20 percent of the protein content and a high proportion of fiber is lost. Adequate fiber intake is important for your digestion and can help prevent common pregnancy complaints such as constipation (see page 72).

Contrary to popular opinion, carbohydrates in themselves aren't particularly high in calories, but they are often served with or accompanied by high-fat, high-calorie toppings such as butter and creamy or oily sauces. If your healthcare providers are concerned that you are gaining too much weight during your pregnancy, cut down on the toppings and sauces but not on the carbohydrates, which help you feel full and energized for longer, as they take longer for the body to break down.

Fruit and vegetables

A variety of fresh fruit and vegetables should form a major part of your diet, too. As well as providing water and fiber, fruit and vegetables contain many important vitamins and minerals (see page 106). Frozen and dried produce is a great standby—it often has more nutritional value than fresh produce that has been been displayed in the supermarket for a day or two, because it will have been picked at its

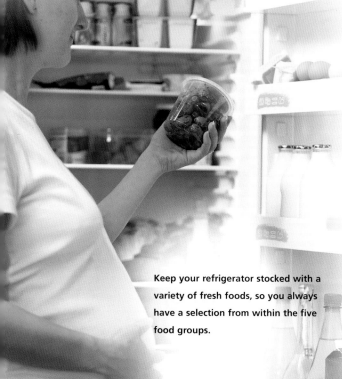

Keep your refrigerator stocked with a variety of fresh foods, so you always have a selection from within the five food groups.

A HEALTHY BALANCE OF FOOD

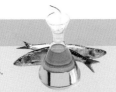

Oils, fats, and sugars Limit your intake to less than 30% of your daily calories.

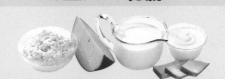

Proteins Eat 2 to 3 portions a day. A portion = 3 oz (85 g) meat, 4 oz (115 g) fish, or 5 oz (140 g) cooked lentils.

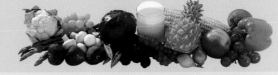

Dairy products Have 3 portions a day. A portion = ⅓ pint (200 ml) of milk, 5 oz (140 g) yogurt, or 1½ oz (40 g) cheese.

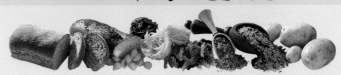

Fruit and vegetables Aim to eat 5 to 6 portions every day. A portion = 1 glass of orange juice, 1 large piece of fruit, or 3 tablespoons of cooked vegetables.

Carbohydrates These should form the largest part of your diet. Eat 6 to 7 portions daily. A portion = 2 slices of bread, 5 oz (140 g) potatoes, 4 tablespoons cooked rice, or 6 tablespoons cooked pasta.

---

prime and preserved within hours. To maximize your nutrient intake, eat a wide variety of fruits and vegetables, including, for example:

- Citrus fruit, strawberries, kiwi fruit, and guavas, are rich in vitamin C, which boosts your body's absorption of iron.
- Yellow fruit, such as mangoes, peaches and apricots, which are good sources of beta-carotene, the plant-based form of vitamin A.
- Oranges, tangerines, blackberries, raspberries, and bananas, which contain moderate amounts of folic acid. This is important throughout your pregnancy but particularly in your first trimester.
- Dried fruit, which can be a good source of iron and other trace elements.
- Green leafy vegetables, especially dark green varieties such as spring greens, purple sprouting broccoli, brussels sprouts, and spinach, which contain significant quantities of folic acid, vitamin C, and beta-carotene, as well as iron and other important trace elements.

- Root vegetables, such as carrots, turnips, and beets, which are good sources of vitamin B_1.
- Dried peas and beans, including lentils, which contain protein, fiber, B vitamins, and minerals.
- Fruit and vegetable juices, such as apple, cranberry, orange, tomato, and carrot, which contain lots of water, as well as being packed with vitamins and minerals.

Dairy products

Milk, cheeses, and yogurt, are rich in calcium, which is one of the most important pregnancy minerals. Calcium helps your baby grow strong bones and teeth, and protects your bones, too. Reduced-fat dairy products retain all the minerals and water-soluble vitamins (see page 106) of full-fat versions, so choose these when you can. Unless you buy enriched milk, all that is removed, besides fat, are the fat-soluble vitamins A and D, but milk isn't a major source of these vitamins, so don't worry that you're missing out. An 8-oz (225-ml) glass of cow's milk contains one-third of your daily recommended calcium requirements—drink three glasses and you've reached 100 percent. Dairy foods are rich also in B vitamins and protein. However, some cheeses should be avoided during pregnancy (see page 111).

Protein foods

Meat, poultry, fish, eggs, cheese, cereals, pulses (peas, beans, and lentils), and nuts contain protein, an essential constituent of all living organisms. Protein is needed to build your baby's cells, tissues, and organs. Protein foods are rich also in vitamins and minerals, such as B vitamins, iron, and zinc.

The amino acids that make up protein can't be made by the body and are provided only by food. But not all protein foods are equal in the amount and quality of amino acids they contain. Animal proteins—found in meat, fish, milk, and cheese—contain a good range of essential amino acids. Plant proteins—in dried peas and beans, nuts, seeds, and bread and other cereal products—tend to be low in one or more amino acids, so if you're vegetarian or vegan you'll need to eat a combination of plant-based proteins to get your full complement of essential amino acids (see page 104).

Oils, fats, and sugars

This group includes foods that are high in calories and low in nutrients—so-called "empty calories"—and, consequently, should make up the smallest proportion of your daily intake. Eating too many fatty or sugary foods on a regular basis may mean you eat less from the four other nutrient-rich food groups. You don't have to exclude fried foods, potato chips, sodas, sugar, candy, and cookies completely—you can have them as an occasional treat—but don't let them become a regular feature in your diet. Over-indulging in these foods can lead to other health problems, such as obesity and heart disease.

However, small amounts of sugars and fats are essential to your health and that of your baby. They provide energy, help maintain healthy skin and hair, and transport the fat-soluble vitamins (see page 106). More importantly, the fats in vegetables, seeds, and nuts and their oils, lean meat, and fish and fish oils supply you with essential fatty acids, which are compounds that the body can't make and must get from foods (see box, below).

Where possible, choose fats that are high in mono- or polyunsaturated fatty acids and low in saturated fatty acids. Unsaturated fatty acids come mostly from plant and fish sources and are generally liquid at room temperature. They are a healthy source of fats in your diet. Highly saturated fatty acids generally come from animal sources and are solid at room temperature. Eating too much saturated fat can contribute to heart disease.

Don't forget your fluids

An adequate fluid intake is essential during pregnancy, to help your blood volume increase and to supply your baby with nutrients. Also, pregnancy boosts your body temperature so it's easy to become dehydrated. Aim to drink at least eight 8-oz (225-ml) glasses of fluids every day. As much as possible of this should come from water, but milk, herbal teas, and fruit and vegetable juices are also good choices. Limit your intake of caffeinated drinks and alcohol, as they can dehydrate you and have an effect on your baby (see page 111).

DID YOU KNOW...

Some fat is good for you Oily fish, such as herring, sardines, salmon, and mackerel, are rich in omega-3 essential fatty acids, which are known to be important in the development of your unborn baby's brain and visual system. Sixty percent of your baby's brain is, in fact, made up of essential fatty acids, so it's particularly important to eat such foods during the last three months of your pregnancy, when your baby's brain increases in weight by four or five times. A diet rich in essential fatty acids is good for you, too, as it has been linked with a reduced risk of high blood pressure during pregnancy.

BALANCING A VEGETARIAN DIET

While you're probably eating a healthy diet already, during pregnancy you may have to top up your nutritional reserves and you should make doubly sure that you're getting enough protein, iron, calcium, vitamin D, and vitamin B_{12}. If you're concerned that you're missing out on any nutrients, ask your doctor or dietitian for advice.

Boost your protein

If you eat cheese and eggs, they will be valuable sources of protein, but make sure they're not your only sources. To obtain the full range of essential amino acids, make sure you eat protein-rich foods from a variety of sources. For example, try combining legumes (peas, beans, and lentils) with wholegrain cereals. Also, any foodstuffs made from soybeans, such as tofu, tempeh, or miso, are great protein providers.

Pump up your iron

Iron is essential for nourishing you and your baby (see page 108), particularly for producing new blood cells, and you need about 30 mg of iron a day during pregnancy. As it's more readily absorbed from dairy products and eggs than from plant sources, consume more of the former during your pregnancy, if possible. Also increase your intake of rice, legumes, spinach, and soy products, and snack on dried fruit for an iron boost. Remember, too, that vitamin C enhances iron absorption, so drink orange juice with an iron-rich meal.

Go calcium-rich

If you don't eat dairy products, you'll need to boost your calcium intake by eating plenty of green vegetables (such as broccoli), soy products, dried figs, and sesame seeds. Topping up on vitamin D will help you absorb calcium more efficiently, so eat

Pregnancy meal planner

If you're tired, it can be easy to opt for a take-out or TV dinner, which may not give you the best balance of nutrients. Planning your meals in advance may save you some time and effort. Here are some suggestions for a week's worth of all-around healthy menus.

If you work and there aren't many healthy lunch options available locally, take a packed lunch. Dinner will probably be your main meal, so try to cook your favorite wholesome recipes then, including lots of fresh produce.

Try also to balance out your meals. For example, follow a rich main course with a light dessert, or eat a vegetable-based main dish followed by a protein-based dessert, such as yogurt or cheese.

Breakfasts
- Fortified breakfast cereal topped with low-fat milk and fruit.
- Slices of hard-boiled egg with a bagel and low-fat spread.
- Banana and strawberries, sprinkled with wheatgerm.
- Strips of lean bacon broiled with tomatoes and mushrooms.

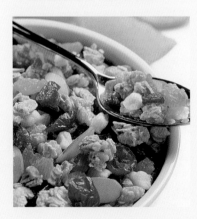

- Oatmeal with bran, served with low-fat yogurt and sprinkled with raisins or other dried fruit.
- Scrambled eggs on two slices of wholewheat toast with polyunsaturated margarine.
- Dried apricots in low-fat yogurt.

Lunches
- A large jacket potato topped with tuna, cucumber, and green beans.
- Chickpea or broccoli soup accompanied by a bagel.
- A roast chicken and salad sandwich on wholewheat bread
- Salmon steak with a salad of lettuce, tomato, bell peppers, and sesame seeds.
- Mushroom and broccoli omelet with lettuce and tomato.

eggs and dairy products, too. If you're a vegan, you can obtain vitamin D from fortified cereals, or speak to your doctor about taking a supplement.

Safeguard your vitamin B_{12}

This vitamin is primarily found in animal products such as eggs and dairy foods. However, fermented foods such as tempeh also contain vitamin B_{12}. Some yeast extracts, soy milk, and vegetarian cheeses and spreads are fortified with vitamin B_{12} so stock up on these, too. If you're a vegan, you may find it difficult to fulfill your vitamin B_{12} daily requirement, so speak to your healthcare provider about taking a supplement throughout pregnancy.

OTHER TYPES OF DIET

If you are following a restrictive diet for medical or other reasons, seek specialized support and advice from a dietitian or your doctor during pregnancy.

He or she will be able to tell you how you can maximize your nutrient intake so that your baby has access to all the essentials he needs. The following dietary tips are worth bearing in mind:

- If you're unable to tolerate lactose, you can boost your calcium levels by eating sesame seeds, broccoli, canned fish with bones, peanuts and dried fruit, and by drinking fortified soy milk.
- If you have a gluten intolerance you need to stock up on carbohydrates in the form of potatoes, gluten-free bread, rice, and corn.
- If you're diabetic or develop gestational diabetes (see page 253), your healthcare provider will monitor you closely. As a rule, about half of your daily intake should come from carbohydrates, such as pasta, brown rice, and whole grains.

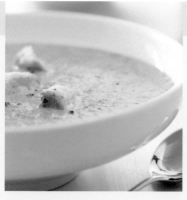

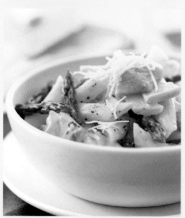

- An open grilled-cheese sandwich on wholewheat bread with a tomato and raw spinach salad.
- Rice and wild rice salad with walnuts, raisins, and green onions, dressed with olive oil.

Dinners

- Steamed salmon and asparagus, tossed with penne pasta and pasteurized hollandaise sauce.
- Mediterranean vegetables (eggplant, tomato, zucchini, and yellow bell peppers) roasted in olive oil and tossed with pasta.
- Baked or roasted sweet potato with cottage cheese, lima beans, and steamed vegetables, such as carrots or broccoli.
- Roasted cod, with green beans, mashed potato, and salsa verde.

- Cauliflower with a cheese and sundried tomato sauce and a fresh green salad.
- Thai-style green chicken curry with bamboo shoots and zucchini, served on steamed rice.
- Stir-fry with lean pork or tofu, ginger, and mushrooms on rice.

Desserts

- Baked apple, stuffed with dried fruit.
- Passion fruit with natural yogurt poured over meringue pieces.
- Crackers and a selection of cheeses (see page 111).
- Lemon tart, with low-fat crème fraîche.

THE ESSENTIAL NUTRIENTS

Nourishing your baby means more than eating the all-important body-building proteins and energy-providing carbohydrates; it means also giving him a range of vitamins and minerals.

Although your body can manufacture one or two vitamins, it relies mainly on the food you eat to provide it with nutrients. Refer to the chart on page 108 to find out the recommended daily intakes of vitamins and minerals during pregnancy, and familiarize yourself with the good sources of each. Some foods are great providers of a range of nutrients, such as green vegetables (vitamins A, B_2, and C, folate, and calcium) and whole grains (B vitamins, iron, and zinc).

ESSENTIAL PREGNANCY VITAMINS

There are 13 known vitamins, each with its own role to play in your and your baby's health. You can store some vitamins in your body and these are the fat-soluble vitamins A, D, and E. However, your body cannot store the water-soluble variety—the B vitamins and vitamin C—so these have to be supplied on a regular basis.

If you were consuming ideal levels of all your vitamins before you were pregnant, then, theoretically, you could continue to eat the same diet throughout your pregnancy and still provide your baby with enough of each vitamin. This is because after 8 weeks, the placenta actively starts to concentrate the nutrients in your bloodstream. In reality, however, this can leave the mother with a deficiency—albeit a slight one. While it's important to take sufficient amounts of all vitamins during pregnancy, a few vitamins are especially important to the health of both you and your developing baby.

Vitamin A

This vitamin occurs naturally in two forms: retinol, which is a mature version found in animal products, and beta-carotene, which can be converted to vitamin A in the body and is found in plant foods. Vitamin A is involved in the development of your baby's cells, heart, circulatory system, and nervous system. Consequently, when your baby's weight gain is at its greatest—in the last three months—the need for an adequate supply of vitamin A increases. Luckily, most women easily achieve their recommended daily intake of this vitamin.

Very large doses of retinol have, in fact, been associated with an increased risk of birth defects, but it is very unlikely that you will be consuming too much. Liver is the only food that provides high amounts of retinol, so pregnant women are advised to minimize their intake of liver and liver products such as pâté. Check that any supplements you take do not contain retinol.

B vitamins

This family of vitamins includes thiamin (B_1), riboflavin (B_2), niacin (B_3), pyridoxine (B_6), and cobalamin (B_{12}), as well as folates (see below). B vitamins, which help convert food into energy, have a major part to play in new cell formation. They are particularly important in the early part of pregnancy when the rate of cell division is highest. At this stage, a good intake of B vitamins—notably thiamin and niacin—may be a strong predictor of a good birth weight. You need also to step up your intake of vitamin B_6, which is involved in the development of your baby's nervous system, and vitamin B_{12}, which is vital for the manufacture of red blood cells. Foods rich in B vitamins include vegetables, whole grains, meat, fish, eggs, and milk.

Folates and folic acid

Belonging to the B vitamin family, folates and folic acid are particularly important during your first trimester. Studies have shown that women can reduce drastically the risk of giving birth to a baby with a neural tube defect such as spina bifida (see page 375), by taking a folic acid supplement before conception and during the first trimester. By 12 weeks, the baby's neural tube has formed completely and so the vulnerable period has passed.

Although folates are found naturally in foods such as green leafy vegetables, oranges, and bananas, these alone can't provide adequate amounts. So it's advisable to take a folic acid supplement and to eat foods fortified with folic acid, such as bread and breakfast cereals. In contrast to other vitamins, folic acid (the synthetic version of the vitamin) is more readily absorbed than the natural version.

Vitamin C
Your need for this vitamin increases during pregnancy, as it helps you manufacture new tissues. Your baby needs vitamin C for proper growth and development. Vitamin C also helps your body absorb iron from food, so drink fruit juice with an iron-rich meal. Cranberries, citrus fruits, and potatoes are all great vitamin-C providers.

Vitamin D
Synthesized in the skin when exposed to the sun's ultraviolet light, vitamin D is vital for the absorption of calcium and for your baby's bone and tooth development. People whose skins are exposed to sunlight are usually able to synthesize enough vitamin D during the spring and summer months to build up a reserve for the winter. However, if you don't expose your skin to much sun, your healthcare provider may recommend you take a supplement to guarantee an adequate intake.

Vitamin E
This is an antioxidant, which helps counteract cell damage. Low levels of vitamin E have been linked to pre-eclampsia (see page 254), so make sure you eat plenty of avocados, seeds, nuts, and vegetable oils.

ESSENTIAL PREGNANCY MINERALS
Your body can't manufacture minerals; they have to be consumed within foods. Certain minerals—iron, calcium, and zinc—are particularly important during pregnancy, and these are discussed below. However, you should also make sure that you get an adequate intake of iodine, magnesium, and selenium, which are involved in a range of functions, from the regulation of your metabolism to the development of genetic material.

Calcium
This is the most abundant mineral in the body with around 99 percent of calcium being found in your bones and teeth. It is essential for blood clotting, muscle contraction, and nerve signaling. It may also help prevent high blood pressure, a major cause of pre-eclampsia (see page 254).

5 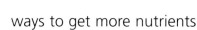 ways to get more nutrients

1 Much of the fruit we buy today is under-ripe, so wait until fruit softens and the color changes before you eat it—it will be at its tastiest and the vitamin content will be at its peak.

2 Fresh vegetables lose their nutrients quickly, so shop frequently and eat vegetables on the same day or soon after you bought them.

3 A high proportion of the nutrients in vegetables are stored just under the skin, so eat them with the skin on, if possible. Scrub root vegetables, such as carrots, rather than peeling them.

4 Fruit and vegetables lose vitamins wherever they're cut, so eat them whole or in large pieces.

5 Nutrients leach out into cooking liquid, so eat vegetables raw or cook them in a steamer. Cook meat and poultry using dry-heat methods, such as broiling and roasting, or use the liquid from braised or stewed dishes in sauces or gravies.

During pregnancy, your body adapts to absorb more calcium from your food, and your own calcium stores are used to supply your baby. However, because many women have a lower intake than is recommended, it's vital to boost your levels throughout pregnancy, especially during the last trimester when the finishing touches are being put to your baby's bones and teeth. If you're under the age of 25, it's even more important that you get enough calcium, as peak bone health isn't reached until around this age.

Iron

This mineral is vital for new cell and hormone formation, and constitutes a large part of hemoglobin, the oxygen-carrying protein in red blood cells. During pregnancy your blood volume may double, so iron is in great demand.

The recommended intake of iron is 30 mg a day for both menstruating and pregnant women. After conception, menstruation ceases and your body becomes more efficient at extracting iron from food, so in theory you shouldn't need extra iron during pregnancy. But because many women—particularly teenagers, those with heavy periods, or women who don't eat enough iron-rich foods—are already slightly deficient in iron, boosting iron levels can reduce your chances of developing iron-deficiency anemia (see page 252).

Iron is present in both animal- and plant-based foods. Animal sources, such as red meat, poultry, and fish, contain a form called heme iron, which is more readily absorbed than the non-heme iron from plant-based sources such as vegetables, pastas, fruit, grains, nuts, eggs, and fortified breakfast cereals.

Vitamin C enhances iron absorption, so have citrus fruit juice or another source of vitamin C with meals containing iron. As tea and coffee are believed to inhibit iron absorption, wait for an hour or so after meals before drinking them.

Zinc

Essential for growth, wound healing, and immune function, zinc is involved in cell replication. Low intakes during pregnancy have been associated also

HOW TO MEET YOUR DAILY VITAMIN NEEDS

Vitamin	Daily requirement
A (retinol/beta carotene)	770 mcg
B_1 (thiamin)	1.4 mg
B_2 (riboflavin)	1.4 mg
B_3 (niacin)	18 mg
B_6 (pyridoxine)	1.9 mg
B_{12} (cobalamin)	2.6 mcg
folic acid/folate	600 mcg (first trimester) 400 mcg (last two trimesters)
C (ascorbic acid)	80 mg
D (calciferol)	5 mcg
E (tocopherol)	15 mg

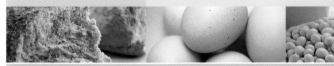

HOW TO MEET YOUR DAILY MINERAL NEEDS

Mineral	Daily requirement
Calcium	at least 1000 mg
Iodine	220 mcg
Iron	27 mg
Magnesium	350 mg
Selenium	60 mcg
Zinc	11 mg

mg = milligrams
mcg = micrograms, sometimes written as µg

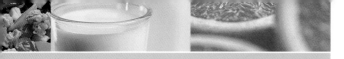

Good food sources

fish oils, kidney, dairy produce, egg yolk, yellow and red fruit, and yellow, red, and dark green vegetables

fortified breakfast cereals, wholegrain breads, dried peas and beans, pork, bacon, milk, yeast extract, and eggs

milk, wholemeal bread and cereals, egg yolk, cheese, and green leafy vegetables

wholewheat bread and cereals, fortified breakfast cereals, dried peas and beans, lean meats, fish, and nuts

meat (especially pork), chicken, fish, eggs, and wholewheat bread and cereals

lean meat, oily fish, milk, cheese, and eggs

fortified breakfast cereals and breads, green leafy vegetables, bananas, orange juice, berries, wholegrains, and dried peas and beans

citrus fruit and juices, rosehips, kiwi fruit, cranberries, strawberries, papaya, cauliflower, green vegetables, potatoes, and bell peppers

oily fish, eggs, polyunsaturated margarine, and butter

wheatgerm, egg yolk, seeds and seed oils and margarines, nuts, and green vegetables

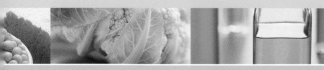

Good food sources

milk, cheese, yogurt, canned fish with bones in (such as salmon and sardines), tofu, and green leafy vegetables

saltwater fish, iodized salt, dairy products, and eggs

lean red meat, fish, egg yolks, wholegrain cereals, spinach, fortified breakfast cereals, and legumes

legumes, nuts, wholegrains, spinach, and peanut butter

oily fish, meats, wholewheat flour, and brazil nuts

lean red meat, eggs, canned sardines, wholegrain cereals, and dried peas and beans

with low birth weights. As with iron and calcium, your body becomes more efficient at processing this mineral, so if you were getting enough before, you probably won't need to increase your intake during pregnancy. However, if you're taking an iron supplement, this can interfere with zinc absorption. Generally speaking, zinc is associated with protein-rich foods such as meat and fish. Zinc from plant sources is less well absorbed.

SUPPLEMENTS: DO YOU NEED THEM?

In theory, of course, if you eat a healthy, well-balanced diet, taking vitamin and mineral supplements shouldn't be necessary. But as it's quite possible to be deficient in some nutrients, how do you decide if you should take one or not?

Your best source of advice about supplements will be your healthcare provider, who will probably recommend a daily prenatal supplement containing a balance of vitamins and minerals. If your healthcare provider suspects that you're not getting enough calcium from your diet he or she may advise you to take an additional supplement.

Although you may be tempted to take other supplements to make up for what you think you lack in your diet, never do so without first checking them with your healthcare provider. Not only is this potentially dangerous, but relying on supplements can create a false sense of security that you're meeting all your nutritional needs. An adequate intake of vitamins and minerals is only a part of what a healthy diet has to provide. You also need to have energy-rich carbohydrates, protein, essential fatty acids, and fiber. Some experts also question the effectiveness of nutritional supplements. The nutrients in foods are absorbed alongside other constituents, some of which may speed their journey to the bloodstream. If you do decide to take a vitamin or mineral supplement, remember that it is no substitute for a healthy diet, and you should continue to follow your regime of healthy eating.

AVOIDING FOOD HAZARDS

During pregnancy, and particularly in your first trimester, you're susceptible to infections in food that can be transmitted to your baby. But by following some simple rules you can cook and eat meals that are nutritious and completely risk-free for you and your baby.

Bacterial toxins, contained in certain foodstuffs or caused by poor preparation techniques, can pass from your blood to your baby's via the placenta. Also, during pregnancy your natural immunity is slightly lower, because of metabolic and circulatory changes in your body. This is why it's paramount to minimize the risk of food-borne infections.

BUYING WISELY
Food safety starts in the supermarket. Always choose dairy products, meat, poultry, and fish with the longest 'best before' date and try to select these products at the end of your shop, so they'll be out of a refrigerated environment for less time. Never eat

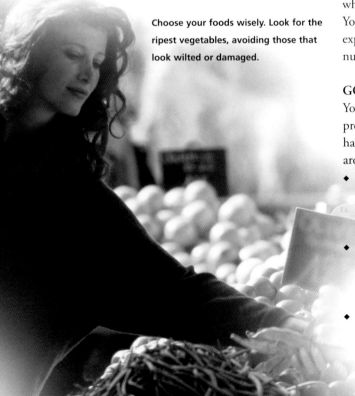

Choose your foods wisely. Look for the ripest vegetables, avoiding those that look wilted or damaged.

foods past their "best before" date. When selecting other items during your shop, reject or discard any products with damaged packaging, such as a dented can or torn plastic bag, so that the preservation of the food is guaranteed.

Should I choose organic?
Increasingly, you may have the choice between organic and regular foods. Organic foods are popular because many people believe they are healthier since they are grown without the use of chemical pesticides and herbicides. They believe that not only do such pollutants undermine the environment but that the cumulative effect of these chemicals and other pollutants—from the environment, smoking, and drinking—can be damaging for your body.

However, this doesn't mean that conventionally produced food is unsafe: Farmers' use of chemicals is strictly controlled, and you can minimize your intake by thoroughly washing any fruit and vegetables you eat. Ultimately, the question of whether to 'go organic' is one of personal choice. You might consider, too, that organic food is more expensive and may not contain any more protein, nutrients, or fiber than regular food.

GOOD FOOD HYGIENE
You may already be aware of the safest ways to prepare food, but now that you're pregnant, you have a good reason to re-examine your hygiene around the kitchen. Check that you always:
- Unpack and store frozen and refrigerated food as soon as you return from shopping. Also, cover recently cooked leftovers, then refrigerate or freeze them once they've cooled.
- Store raw and cooked foods separately. Raw meats and poultry should be covered and kept on the bottom shelf of the refrigerator, to prevent their juices from dripping onto other foods.
- Avoid defrosting food outside of the refrigerator.

- Don't refreeze food once it has been defrosted.
- Wash your hands, cooking utensils and work surfaces before and after preparing food.
- Use one board for preparing raw meat and poultry and another for preparing other foods.
- Cook meat, poultry, and eggs thoroughly.
- Make sure reheated food is piping hot all the way through, but don't reheat food more than once.
- Avoid eating honey that is not pasteurized.

AVOIDING INFECTIONS

During pregnancy there are certain foods you should avoid to limit your chances of developing a food-borne infection. The most common infections caught from contaminated food are listeriosis and salmonellosis; less common is toxoplasmosis.

Listeriosis

The bacterium that causes listeriosis is *Listeria monocytogenes*, which is widespread in the environment, especially in soil. A third of all cases of listeriosis occur during pregnancy and severe cases, which are rare, result in miscarriage (see page 278) or preterm labor and newborn infections such as meningitis (see page 363) or a baby being stillborn. Possible sources of listeria, and therefore foods to avoid, include unpasteurized soft cheeses (such as Brie), blue-veined cheeses (such as Stilton), unpasteurized sheep and goat's milk and their products, cooked foods chilled for reheating, ready-prepared coleslaw, hot dogs, and under-cooked poultry. So avoid all these foods during pregnancy.

Salmonellosis

Because salmonella bacteria are hardy and can withstand light cooking, any potential source, such as eggs and poultry, should be thoroughly cooked to destroy all traces of infection. It's sensible during pregnancy to exclude raw and under-cooked eggs and foods that may contain raw eggs, such as home-made mayonnaise, mousses, or ice cream.

Toxoplasmosis

This infection, caused by the organism *Toxoplasma gondii*, can potentially lead to brain damage or blindness in your baby. It is a particular risk in your last trimester. The organism is carried in the feces of animals, particularly outdoor cats, but is present also in soil and in raw and under-cooked meat and poultry. Therefore, make sure that all the meat or poultry you eat is cooked thoroughly: Only eat pork, for example, if it's "well done." In addition, wash all vegetables and fruit thoroughly; wash your hands after stroking pets; avoid dealing with cat litter trays; wear gloves when gardening; and wash your hands before you prepare or eat food.

COMMON AREAS OF CONCERN

Besides the foods that are potential sources of infection, which all experts recommend you should avoid, there are several other foods and drinks that are subjects of debate. With changing notions of what is safe and potentially confusing advice from friends or the press, it can be difficult to know what you can or can't eat or drink. Here are some answers.

Can I drink alcohol?

When deciding whether you should drink alcohol during pregnancy, moderation and common sense must be your guidelines. There is much scientific data to show that daily drinking or heavy binge drinking can lead to serious complications. Moderate drinking—having one or two drinks a day or binging occasionally—has been associated with an increased risk of miscarriage, complications during labor, and low birth weights. Pregnant women who heavily abuse alcohol—drinking five or more alcoholic drinks a day—put their babies at risk of a condition known as fetal alcohol syndrome (FAS), a term which covers a wide range of birth defects, including heart defects, mental retardation, or structural abnormalities of the face and limbs, as well as the risk of growth problems or death.

Although there is little evidence that the occasional alcoholic drink will harm your baby, some experts say that the safest course is to avoid alcohol completely throughout pregnancy—this is the advice offered by Health Canada. Other healthcare providers agree that it is best to avoid alcohol during the first trimester, when the baby's major organs are forming. But if you want to drink alcohol after that, keep in mind that whatever you drink will pass to your baby through your bloodstream. Limit yourself to one to two alcoholic drinks a week at most, preferably taken with meals, as food reduces the absorption of alcohol. Within these guidelines, no one type of alcohol is better than another: A small can or bottle of beer, a small glass of wine, or one measure of hard liquor all contain roughly the same amounts of alcohol.

HEALTH FIRST

Foods to avoid It can be confusing to keep track of everything you can and can't eat during pregnancy, so here's a list of the foods that you should avoid:

- All unpasteurized cheese; feta cheese; mold-ripened cheese such as Brie and Camembert; and blue-veined cheese such as Stilton and Danish Blue, even if they're pasteurized.
- Sheep and goats' milk and their products.
- All fresh pâtés, whether meat, fish, or vegetable; canned pâtés are fine.
- Unheated cooked-chilled meals and precooked poultry foods that can't be reheated safely.
- Raw or under-cooked eggs or products containing them, including some desserts, and home-made mayonnaise or hollandaise sauce.
- Raw meat dishes such as steak tartare or Parma ham.
- Raw fish, including sushi.
- Raw or under-cooked shellfish such as oysters, mussels, cold prawns, and crab.

Is it okay to drink caffeine?

Consuming caffeine in large enough amounts—over 300 mg a day—can increase the risk of low birth weight and miscarriage. An average cup of coffee has between 100 and 150 mg of caffeine. So drinking one to two cups of coffee a day is usually okay during pregnancy—but remember, this is an average cup, not the larger coffees you get in many coffee shops. Also, keep in mind that caffeine is found in tea, many cola-type drinks, cocoa, and chocolate.

Consider, too, that caffeine is a diuretic, so drinking it will increase your trips to the bathroom. If you're already bothered by having to go a lot, you may want to cut your caffeine intake further.

Do I need to restrict my salt intake?

Many women are casually advised by friends or family to restrict their salt intake to prevent "swelling" of feet and ankles. However, this is not a current medical recommendation. Edema (swelling) is actually the result of water retention, caused by hormonal activity. Pregnancy hormones also increase the amount of sodium you lose in your urine. So don't overuse salt, but don't limit your intake either.

Are fish and shellfish safe?

Fish are good sources of nutrients, so aim to include them in your diet. However, you should take care with some types. It's best to cut out raw fish and uncooked shellfish altogether. Also, limit your intake of large fish—like swordfish, tilefish, kingfish, and king mackerel—to once a month. These fish can contain high levels of methyl mercury, a chemical that can harm a baby's developing nervous system.

Will eating nuts give my baby an allergy?

There have been suggestions in recent years that if a woman consumes peanut products while she's pregnant, her baby may become predisposed to developing a peanut allergy. For these reasons, women with food allergies or strong family histories of food allergies might want to avoid nuts and peanuts during pregnancy and while nursing. For women without these histories, there is no need to eliminate peanuts and other nuts from your diet.

CHAPTER

KEEPING FIT

Pregnancy makes demands on both your mind and
your body. Exercising and using relaxation
techniques can help you maintain your health and
sense of well-being throughout pregnancy, during
labor, and beyond.

PREPARING FOR EXERCISE

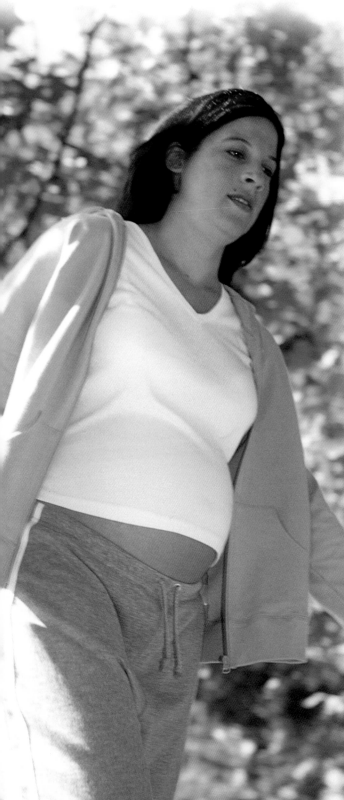

Regular exercise keeps your body in great shape for the physical challenges of pregnancy, but it's vital to learn how much or how little is best for you and the precious cargo you're carrying inside.

Exercising during your pregnancy will improve your heart and lung fitness, improve your posture, boost your circulation, help control excessive weight gain, reduce digestive discomfort, relieve muscle aches and cramps, and strengthen muscles.

Physical activity also causes the brain to release chemicals such as serotonin, dopamine, and endorphins, which help balance mood swings, reduce stress, and promote a positive outlook. At a time when your body is changing dramatically, exercising can give you a much-needed sense of control over your body image. Studies show, too, that a fitter body gives you more stamina to get through the lengthy hours of labor, and helps you recover faster afterward—you'll suffer less muscle soreness and will be up and about more quickly. Moreover, you'll be able to get back in shape sooner, and will have more energy to cope with the demands of your new baby.

EXERCISE SAFELY

Whatever your fitness level, you need to take extra care when you exercise. Working out in pregnancy may carry certain risks, so check with your doctor or midwife before you begin or continue with an existing exercise program. Some women have, or develop, medical conditions that warrant caution in relation to exercise (see box, opposite). In some cases, you'll be able to exercise if the condition is controlled. However, some medical conditions prohibit exercise altogether.

Once you have the go-ahead, keep your healthcare provider updated with your progress. Learn to listen and respond to your body—pregnancy isn't a time to push yourself. Always err on the side of caution—if you're in doubt, don't do it. Remember, too, that pregnancy is a time to maintain, rather than improve, fitness, and you should never work out with the intention of losing weight. Regular exercise can, however, help you keep weight gain within sensible limits. Get the most from your workout with these safety guidelines.

Choose your exercise carefully

Pick an activity that you can do with your partner or a friend. You'll feel more motivated and are more likely to keep active if you are enjoying what you do. Do not perform activities in which you're in danger of falling, losing your balance, or getting hit in the abdomen, such as horseback riding, in-line skating, downhill skiing, or team sports such as basketball or volleyball. Avoid scuba diving throughout pregnancy, as it could cause gas bubbles to form in your baby's bloodstream.

Keep to a moderate level

Try to avoid or limit any strenuous activities, and always go at your own pace. Rest frequently, and take care not to overdo it, particularly in the first trimester. Check your heart rate to gauge how hard you're working (see page 121).

In late pregnancy you may notice a shortness of breath, even when you're just sitting down. This is normal and may be because your resting heart rate is higher than normal—an average rise is about 15 to 20 beats per minute. When exercising, however, try to keep your breathing even and regular. Don't hold your breath at any point, as this increases pressure in your chest and can make you feel dizzy or faint.

Maintain a healthy body temperature

Your overall body temperature is raised by your baby's, and your body releases this extra heat through the skin, resulting in the healthy, "rosy glow" of pregnancy. This raise in temperature means also that when you exercise, you're susceptible to overheating, may tire easily, and can become dehydrated. It's vital, therefore, to stop if you feel too hot and to drink plenty of water—you should drink a minimum of 4 pints (2 liters) of fluid a day anyway (see page 103) and then take frequent sips of water before, during, and after exercise.

Make sure, also, that you dress appropriately. Don't overdress on warm days, as it may exacerbate overheating, and exercise at cool times of the day. If it's cold outside, dress in layers so that you can peel off clothes if you get too hot. Also invest in a good sports bra and quality sneakers that support your feet and ankles.

HEALTH FIRST

Signs that you shouldn't exercise Some women have conditions that warrant caution in relation to exercise. If any of the following apply to you or develop during your pregnancy, do not exercise again until you speak to your healthcare provider—you may need to adapt your routine or stop exercising altogether:

- Persistent uterine contractions—more than six to eight per hour—or a history of spontaneous miscarriage or premature labor in previous pregnancies (see page 278).
- Absence of usual fetal movement once it has been detected initially.
- Respiratory disorders or cardiovascular disease, such as hypertension (high blood pressure) (see page 253) or pre-eclampsia (see page 254).
- Anemia (see page 252).
- Spotting or bleeding (see page 275).
- Twins, triplets, or another multiple pregnancy.
- Your baby is small for your dates.
- Placenta previa (see page 276).
- An incompetent cervix (see page 279).

Stretch safely

During pregnancy your body produces the hormone relaxin, which is thought to soften the connective tissue around your joints, making them more flexible in preparation for the birth, but also more susceptible to injury. Stretching before and after exercise can help prevent injuries, but stretch gently to protect your extra-supple body and take care not to overstretch. Also avoid exercises that jar your joints, such as jogging or high-impact aerobics.

Adapt your position

Don't exercise on your back past your fourth month, as the weight of your uterus presses on blood vessels and can restrict blood flow to your heart and baby. From the fourth month on, adapt any exercises that you would normally do lying flat so that you are sitting, standing, or lying on one side. Also check that you maintain good posture during other activities. As your pregnancy progresses, you'll be carrying extra weight in front, so you may experience a shift in your center of gravity, which can make you feel slightly unbalanced.

Eat right for exercise

Boost your energy by eating a light meal based on complex carbohydrates, such as wholewheat bread, pasta, rice, and potatoes, at least 30 minutes to 1 hour before exercising.

HOW TO maintain great posture

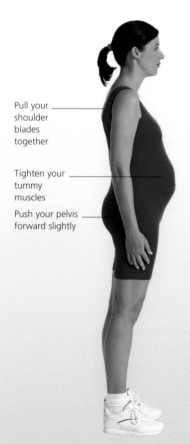

Pull your shoulder blades together

Tighten your tummy muscles

Push your pelvis forward slightly

As your pregnancy progresses, the forward shift in your center of gravity can result in bad posture, upper back and shoulder pain, and lower back discomfort. Maintaining good posture in your everyday activities may help eliminate these stresses and strains. Initially, you'll find you have to make a conscious effort to correct and keep a balanced posture, but after a while you'll find it more natural.

To find a good posture, stand with your feet hip-width apart and your arms by your side. Check that your weight is evenly distributed between your feet. Stand tall and lengthen your neck—it can help to imagine a string pulling you up through the top of your head. Try to look straight ahead and keep your chin parallel to the floor.

Relax your shoulders. If you find that your shoulders are slumping forward, push your shoulder blades together until you find a comfortable—but not rigid—position. This will help open out your chest.

A common mistake many pregnant women make is to let the weight of their abdomens pull their spines forward, which puts strain on the lower back. To keep your lower back strong and to support your baby, tighten your abdominals. Once you have found a comfortable position, try to maintain it. Never adopt the two extremes of pushing your pelvis all the way forward or all the way backward.

PLANNING YOUR PROGRAM

Find an exercise that you enjoy and try to build it into your schedule. Once you start to feel the benefits of your workouts, you'll soon want to exercise regularly.

Your best source of information about exercise during pregnancy will be your healthcare provider. He or she will probably advise that if you were exercising regularly before you became pregnant and currently feel healthy and well, then simply carry on. However, keep in mind that you'll probably have to adapt your current level and the length of your sessions (see page 115).

If you haven't previously done much exercise, seek advice from your healthcare provider before embarking upon an exercise program. You may be advised against starting a new regime until your second trimester, when the risk of miscarriage and overheating has decreased, and you're likely to have more energy. Once you have approval and you feel up to it, you can gradually build up the amount of exercise you do. However, whatever your level of fitness, always be aware of warning signs while you are doing your workouts (see box, right).

WHAT MAKES A GOOD WORKOUT?
The ideal workout components are: a warm-up; aerobic activity; muscle strengthening; and a cool-down. A good warm-up prepares you for your workout. Doing some aerobic exercise works your heart and lungs. You can improve your muscular strength and endurance by performing conditioning exercises, in which groups of muscles are isolated and worked through repetitions. Careful stretching and breathing exercises are excellent ways of returning your body to normal at the finish.

Warming up and cooling down
These two stages are important before and after every activity—even gentle exercise, such as walking—as they prevent muscle soreness and

stiffness. So be sure to include short sessions—between 5 and 15 minutes—of warming-up and cooling-down activities with any exercise routine.

The best warm-up consists of low-intensity, rhythmic activity, such as walking in place or stationary cycling, followed by slow, controlled stretches (see page 118). The initial gentle activity increases blood flow to your arms and legs. This warms your muscles, meaning that when you stretch them, they'll be less liable to damage.

Just as you should start slowly, a gentle cool-down is the best way to end your session. To cool down effectively, stretch each muscle group in turn. Gentle toning exercises are also safe if you want to include them here (see page 122). Also, consider including relaxation or deep-breathing exercises (see page 125) in your cool-down.

SAFETY FIRST
Signs you should stop If any of the following problems occur while you're exercising, stop immediately and seek medical advice:
- Bloody discharge from the vagina.
- Any gush of fluid from the vagina—a possible sign of rupture of the membranes.
- Unexplained pain in the abdomen.
- Persistent headache or changes in vision.
- Unexplained faintness or dizziness.
- Marked fatigue, heart palpitations, or chest pain.
- Sudden swelling of ankles, face, or hands.
- Swelling, pain, and redness in one calf.

Stretches for pregnancy

Stretching is an integral part of good warm-up and cool-down routines. These stretches also can help relieve some common pregnancy complaints such as cramps in the legs and feet. However, always warm your muscles with gentle exercise before you stretch, and take care not to overstretch (see page 116).

Calf stretch Stand with your feet slightly apart. Take a step back with your right foot **1**. Bend your left knee until it's over your left ankle, and press your right heel into the floor. Lean slightly forward **2**. Hold until you feel the stretch in your right calf, then release. If you can't feel it, move your right foot back. Repeat with the other leg.

Front-of-thigh stretch Stand with your feet hip-width apart and rest your hand on the back of a chair. Flex your left knee slightly. Lift your right knee in front of you and hold your shin **1**. Move your right knee back until it's directly under your hip and next to your left knee. Tilt your pelvis forward slightly **2**. Hold until you feel the stretch, then release. Repeat with your left leg.

Side stretch Stand with your feet shoulder-width apart and your knees slightly bent. Place your hands on your hips. Stand tall and stretch your right arm up to the ceiling just in front of your head. Bend directly to the left, reaching your arm up and over to the side. Hold until you feel the stretch, then release. Repeat on the other side.

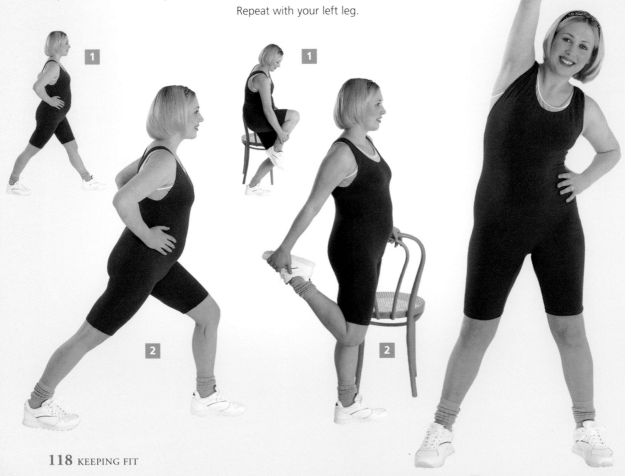

Upper-arm stretch Stand with your feet shoulder-width apart. Keeping your stomach pulled in, lift your right arm toward the ceiling **1**. Bend your right elbow and reach your fingers down between your shoulder blades. Place your left hand on your right elbow and gently pull the elbow behind your head **2**. Hold until you feel the stretch in the back of your right arm, then release. Repeat with your left arm.

Seated buttock and thigh stretch Sit on the floor with your legs in front of you. Place your right foot on your left thigh just above the knee **1**. Gently bend your left knee, sliding your left foot toward you. Keep your tummy muscles tight **2**. Hold until you feel a stretch in your right thigh and buttock, then release. Repeat on the other side.

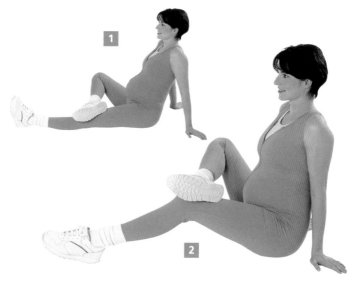

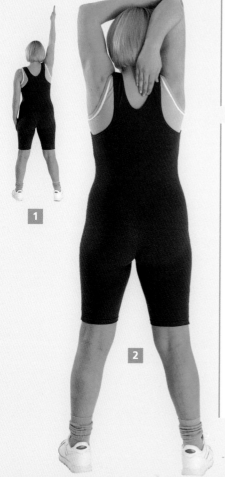

Seated chest stretch Sit on the floor with your legs loosely crossed. Rest your hands on your buttocks. Keeping your stomach muscles tight, lengthen your spine and draw your elbows back, squeezing your shoulder blades together. Hold until you feel the stretch across your chest. Repeat if required.

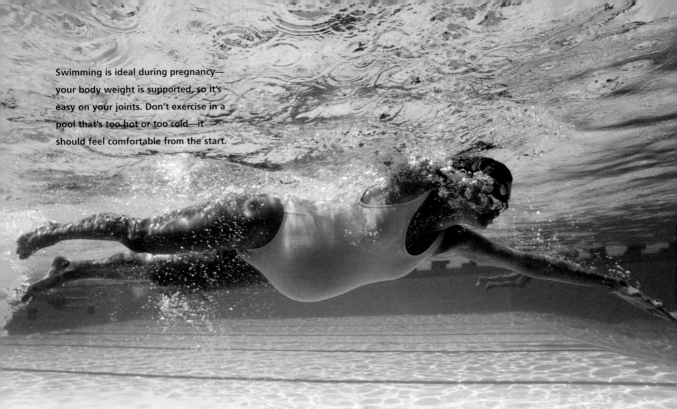

Swimming is ideal during pregnancy—your body weight is supported, so it's easy on your joints. Don't exercise in a pool that's too hot or too cold—it should feel comfortable from the start.

Exercising your heart and lungs

Regular aerobic exercise boosts your circulation and improves the performance of your lungs. Also known as cardiovascular exercise, aerobic activities are those that involve moving large muscle groups—basically your arms and your legs—for a sustained period of around 15 to 30 minutes. To work effectively during this time, your muscles require a higher oxygen supply than when at rest, and to meet these extra demands, your heart rate and breathing rate have to increase. With repeated exercise, your heart and lungs begin to function more efficiently.

Whether you choose to walk briskly around your local park, swim, or join a local prenatal fitness class, incorporating some form of aerobic exercise into your routine is essential to your all-around well-being—it will help you get through the physical exertion of labor and delivery and will speed your recovery afterward.

Strengthening and conditioning your muscles

Pregnancy is almost a weightlifting exercise in itself, and because you're carrying those extra pounds, it's more important than ever to keep your muscles strong and toned. To promote muscular strength and endurance (your muscles' ability to perform an exercise repeatedly), you need to isolate groups of muscles and work them against a form of resistance, such as lifting weights at the gym or pushing against water in a water aerobics class. Before you begin this type of workout, consider the following precautions:

- *Use correct techniques* Make sure that you know how to perform exercises in a class or use free weights and weight machines correctly. If you're unsure, ask a qualified instructor to show you how—lifting a weight incorrectly is worse than not doing the exercise at all.

- *Never lift heavy weights during pregnancy* The general rule to follow is to use a weight that you can comfortably lift 12 to 15 times. If you can't manage this many repetitions, use a lighter weight until you can. Aim to do two to three sets (12 to 15 repetitions comprise a set) on each muscle. But don't get too tired.

- *Work within your limits* If you take part in a class using weights or resistance tools, don't push yourself above your target heart-rate zone (see opposite). Modify exercises that are normally performed on your back so you do them standing, sitting, or on your side.

- *Keep breathing* When using weights or resistance tools, it's important not to hold your breath. Learn to use your breathing to help you carry out the exercise—exhale when you exert and inhale when you relax your muscles.

HOW MUCH EXERCISE SHOULD I DO?

An easy way to decide how often and how much exercise you should do, particularly with regard to aerobic exercise, is to follow the FITT principle—FITT stands for frequency, intensity, time, and type.

Frequency

According to new guidelines issued by the American College of Obstetricians and Gynecologists, unless there are medical reasons not to, pregnant women should try to exercise moderately for at least 30 minutes on most, if not all, days. But with your enthusiasm at a peak, don't immediately start to run

5 miles or play tennis every day if you're not used to it—build up gradually. If you were already exercising regularly before you became pregnant, you can keep it up as long as there are no complications, but adjust the level of effort you put in (see below).

A good benchmark when starting out is to do a workout three times a week—less than this and you won't see any improvement in your heart and lung fitness. Then try to progressively increase your number of workouts. If you find that you get too tired at this level, cut back to three times a week.

Intensity

The amount of effort you use to perform an activity is called the intensity. Throughout your pregnancy, moderation is the key—too little effort isn't effective and too much can be exhausting or even dangerous. Intensity must be monitored carefully, so that you don't overexert yourself (see box, below). Because

HOW TO monitor your intensity levels

A good indication of whether you're working too hard or not hard enough is your heart rate, which is measured in beats per minute (bpm). Your ideal effort levels are indicated on the chart right. Look for your age along the bottom, then look at the highlighted band above it. When exercising, try to keep your heart rate within the minimum and maximum bpms. If you work out regularly, you can keep toward the higher limit of this zone; if you're unused to exercise, work at the lower limit. But always listen to your body: If you get too tired, slow down.

If you exercise at the gym, you may find it helpful to use cardiovascular machines, such as stationary bikes and cross

trainers, that measure your heart rate through metallic pads or a clip on your thumb. Portable heart-rate monitors, which fit around your chest, are also available in fitness stores.

If you don't have access to these, you can take your pulse as you're exercising. To find your pulse on your wrist, place the index and middle fingers of one hand on the inside of the other wrist, just below the thumb. If you have trouble finding a pulse there, try the stronger pulse in your neck. To find this, place your index and middle fingers on the side of your neck about three finger-widths below your jaw.

When you have a pulse, count how many beats you feel in 10 seconds. Multiply this figure by six to get your heart rate in bpm.

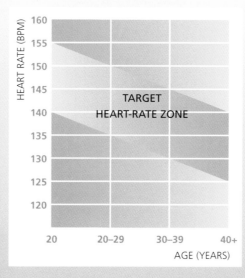

TARGET HEART-RATE ZONE

HEART RATE (BPM): 160, 155, 150, 145, 140, 135, 130, 125, 120

AGE (YEARS): 20, 20–29, 30–39, 40+

your heart is already pumping about 15 to 20 beats per minute faster than normal, it's essential that you don't push yourself too hard. Learn how to take your pulse and make sure that you exercise within your target heart-rate zone.

Another easy check to make sure that you're not overexerting yourself is known as the "talk test." As you're exercising, if you can continue a conversation without getting out of breath, then your intensity should be fine—as long as you stay within your target heart-rate zone. If you find that it's difficult to talk and that you're gasping for breath, however, reduce your effort levels until you feel more comfortable, even if it means dropping below your target heart-rate zone.

Time

Start exercising in short sessions; pushing yourself too soon will only lead to sore muscles and exhaustion. For the first few weeks of your program, doing 15-minute sessions of aerobic activity at your target heart-rate zone is a great start. Once you're happy at this level, you should be able to increase your aerobic sessions in 2-minute steps, until you reach a maximum of 30 minutes. Experienced and regular exercisers can aim for a maximum of 30 minutes each session, again within their target zones.

However, even if you were exercising before pregnancy, it's not a good idea to increase the amount of exercise you do prior to week 14. The best time to start increasing the length of your

Daily super-strengtheners

As well as doing a good all-over workout, strengthening your pelvic floor and your abdominal muscles can be helpful for a healthy pregnancy and delivery.

Perfect pelvic push-ups Your pelvic-floor muscles form a supportive "hammock" within your pelvis, encircling the urethra, vagina, and rectum. Pelvic-floor

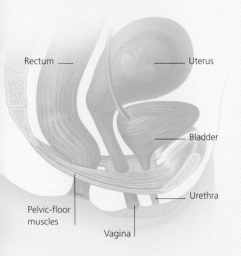

Rectum

Uterus

Bladder

Urethra

Pelvic-floor muscles

Vagina

exercises—also called Kegels after Arnold Kegel, the doctor who introduced them—will help tone these hard-working muscles, enabling them to support the weight of your growing baby and to help push your baby out during delivery. Also, keeping these muscles toned will help them recover more quickly after the birth, preventing problems such as stress incontinence (see page 68).

To practice Kegels you first have to identify the correct muscles. Next time you urinate, try to break the flow of urine briefly but without dribbling. Remember how this feels—the muscles you use to stop the flow are your pelvic-floor muscles. Once you have identified these muscles, don't repeat this exercise during urination. If your bladder isn't emptied completely each time, you may get a urinary tract infection.

You can carry out your pelvic-floor exercises literally anywhere— sitting in the car, watching TV, even standing in the checkout line. Simply tighten your pelvic-floor muscles, hold for a count of five, then slowly release them. It can help to imagine your pelvic floor as an elevator. As it ascends to each floor, try to pull up your muscles a little more until they're completely tight. Then, as the elevator descends floor by floor, gradually relax the muscles until it reaches the ground floor. Repeat this exercise five times.

Initially, it may seem like hard work even reaching a count of five because these muscles tire easily, but repeat the exercise several times a day and you'll soon be able to build up your repetitions.

sessions is in the second trimester, when you're likely to have lots of energy. In the third trimester, you may want to cut down again, if you tire easily.

Listen to your body and cut back sessions if you find that you're overly tired or your muscles are aching. Try to follow your aerobic sessions with muscle-strengthening exercises and always remember to include a good warm-up and an easy cool-down.

Type

Whether you prefer to exercise on your own or in a group, activities that are excellent during pregnancy—for both aerobic exercise and muscle strengthening—include swimming, walking, stair-climbing, stationary cycling, and special prenatal aerobics and aquafit classes. Walking and swimming are so safe that most women are able to carry them out until the day of their delivery. T'ai chi and yoga are other good choices, as they help you relax and improve your body awareness. Some yoga poses, however, should be avoided during pregnancy, so always check with your instructor or choose a special prenatal class. If you find that your choice of exercise strains your weight-bearing joints, such as your hips, knees, or ankles, try switching to one in which your weight is supported, such as cycling or a water-based activity.

SAFETY FIRST

Diastasis recti Before you start abdominal exercises, check that you aren't suffering this condition, in which the vertical muscles of the abdomen begin to separate:

- Lie on your side with your knees bent.
- With your chin tucked in, reach for your knees with outstretched arms.
- If your abdominal muscles have parted, a bulge will appear down the central line of your stomach.

If you think you may have this condition consult your healthcare provider, as you may need to adapt your abdominal exercises.

Tummy tighteners Several groups of muscles run from your rib cage to your pelvis. Strong muscles here help you maintain good posture and push your baby during delivery.

Although you would normally lie flat on your back to perform abdominal strengtheners, you should not do so after the fourth month of pregnancy (see page 116). Instead, perform this exercise when sitting, standing, or lying on your side. Place your hands by your side or behind your head and slowly curl your body toward your knees, contracting your abdominal muscles. Relax and repeat. Do as many times as you can without tiring yourself.

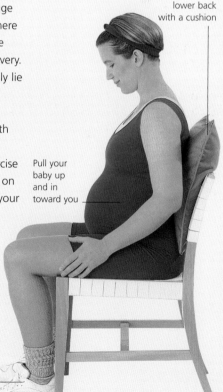

Support your lower back with a cushion

Pull your baby up and in toward you

Keep your feet flat

USING RELAXATION TECHNIQUES

If you've never practiced any relaxation techniques before, pregnancy is an ideal time to begin. Learning how to relax will help you stay healthy while you are pregnant, cope well with labor, and enjoy your baby after he is born.

Pregnancy is a wonderful time to learn how to make space in your day for relaxation. Get into the habit of prioritizing tasks you have to accomplish. What has to be done today? What can wait until tomorrow? And what doesn't really need to be done at all? Acquire the art of saying "no" if people ask you to do something that's going to put you under strain. Plan a little time for yourself each day and time for you and your partner to spend together. Learn not to feel guilty because you're relaxing.

HOW TO HANDLE STRESS

A certain amount of stress is essential in life—it gives you the edge that helps you rise to challenges and cope with any minor crises you encounter. Too little stress can mean that you function below your capacity, but too much can make you irritable, tired, and ill. It is probably good for your baby to encounter stress hormones while he is developing in the uterus—it can prepare him for the stress he'll experience during the birth. But if your blood is continually flooded with these chemicals, your baby may be adversely affected. To handle stress well, it can help to raise your body awareness.

In this time of physical and emotional upheaval, every system in your body is affected: the respiratory, cardiovascular, nervous, excretory, endocrine, and, of course, the reproductive. The prospect of being pregnant can be quite daunting and worrying, and you may suffer from unexpected headaches, stomachaches, and muscular pains—messages that your body sends out to tell you that your muscles are tense. If you take some time to get to know your body better, you'll be able to reduce the daily wear and tear of stress and provide the best growing environment for the baby inside you. Set aside some time today to do the exercise *10 Steps to Stress-Relief* (see box, opposite). It will make you aware of how your muscles feel when they are tense and how they feel when you are really relaxed.

Learn how to breathe

You might not be aware of just how much space your lungs take up in your body. There is lung tissue above your collarbones, stretching right down to your diaphragm. If you use only part of your lungs' capacity for breathing, you're denying your body,

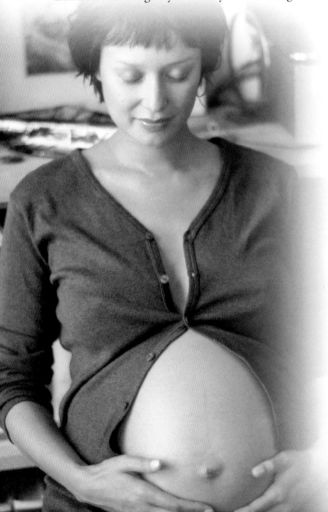

Breathe deeply. Feel your belly push against your hands as you breathe in and then fall back as you breathe out.

and particularly your brain, the oxygen it needs to perform at its peak, and you'll find that your resources for coping with stress are reduced.

Take a few moments to find out whether you have a healthy breathing pattern. Sit down, and put your hands on your belly. When you breathe in, you should feel your abdomen expanding to draw air into your lungs and when you breathe out, your abdomen should flatten again. Many people have an inverted breathing pattern and suck their abdomens in when inhaling.

Relaxed shoulders mean relaxed breathing. Try tensing your shoulders by pulling them up toward your ears. Notice how tight your breathing becomes; pulling your shoulders too far downward or backward has the same effect. When your shoulders are loose, your breathing is easy. Get in the habit of checking your shoulders regularly throughout the day, especially when you're feeling tense. Let your arms hang down and roll your shoulders backward and forward slowly, making sure they're relaxed so that you can breathe well.

Beat stress instantly
When you feel stressed, use this quick exercise for on-the-spot relaxation. Breathe in deeply. When your lungs are full, sigh out gently through your mouth and let the out-breath carry the tension away from the top of your body right down to your toes. When your lungs are ready, let them fill again. Then sigh out gently, relaxing your forehead, jaws, shoulders, hands, stomach, and legs. The out-breath is the breath that cleanses your body of stress. If you feel tense at any time remember: Sigh out slowly.

10 steps to stress-relief

Set aside 20 minutes in your day to find out the difference between muscles that are stressed and those that are relaxed.

1 Put the answering machine on, dim the lights, and sit in a comfortable chair or lie down—don't lie on your back after your fourth month, try lying on your side with your belly supported by a cushion.

2 Spend a few moments settling down and trying to calm your thoughts.

3 Now stretch your toes and feel the tension. Let your toes gently relax, wiggling them a little.

4 Tighten your knees and your thigh muscles, feeling the effort. Hold for a few seconds and then relax, letting your thighs roll slightly apart.

5 Tighten your tummy muscles to give your baby a big hug. Relax, giving baby as much room as possible.

6 Make fists with your hands, hold, and then let your fingers gently unfurl.

7 Pull your shoulders up toward your ears and let them drop. Shrug them a little and let them drop again. They should feel loose and easy.

8 Screw up every muscle in your face—don't worry, nobody's watching. Now relax so that there's no expression at all on your face. Your mouth should feel very soft; it may be slightly open.

9 Take a few minutes to become aware of how your body feels now that it's relaxed. Your baby will enjoy the extra oxygen he's receiving while your breathing is deep and your body is calm.

10 When you're ready, yawn, stretch, sit up gently, and prepare to get on with whatever it is you have to do.

SOOTHE WITH MASSAGE

In pregnancy, massage is an ideal way to help you relax, as it stimulates the release of endorphins—nature's own opiates—which give you a sense of well-being. In addition, massage has beneficial effects on your circulation, digestion, and excretory system, all of which come under particular stress when you're pregnant.

Although massage is largely risk-free, it's wise to check with your healthcare provider before you have any kind of massage, and always advise anyone giving you a massage that you're pregnant. Avoid massages of the abdomen and lower back during the first trimester. Also, if you find any techniques uncomfortable, immediately tell your masseur.

It's an excellent idea for the person who is going to be your companion during labor to practice massaging you throughout your pregnancy so that he or she understands which parts of your body are particularly prone to stress and what kinds of massage you find relaxing. The box below gives some simple techniques. Here, too, are some guidelines for the masseur:

- Try to relax.
- Tell your partner when you're going to start.
- Keep your strokes firm, rhythmical, and slow.
- Always keep at least one of your hands in contact with the person you're massaging.
- Ask her if the pressure and the pace are right.
- Try to be aware of her body—what is it telling you? Can you feel where she's tense, and what helps her relax?
- Tell her when you're going to stop.

The important thing is to experiment with different techniques and for your partner to build up a repertoire of strokes that enable you to relax. Keep

Stroking away your aches

Massage can ease some of the discomforts of pregnancy and help your partner get to know your body before labor. Set aside at least 10 minutes for each technique.

Back massage Kneel on a bed or the floor and relax into a large pile of pillows so that your abdomen and head are comfortably supported. Place a pillow between your calves and buttocks to assist with your circulation.

Placing the flat of his left hand on your left shoulder, your massage partner strokes firmly and slowly down the side of your spine to your buttocks. Before removing his hand, he places his right hand on your right shoulder and strokes firmly down that side of your spine. He continues to alternate between each side. Tell him if the pressure is right.

Next, he uses his thumbs to make small circles in the grooves on either side of your spine, gradually working down, vertebra to vertebra. At the bottom of your back, he makes larger circles using his palms to circle down over your hips.

in mind, however, that the kinds of massage you find enjoyable during pregnancy may not be the most effective in labor.

Which oils are safe?

Essential oils can provide wonderful aromas during massage and some are thought to have beneficial properties, such as relieving headaches and aiding sleep. However, you should use an essential oil for massage only if a qualified aromatherapist has recommended it to you. Some aromatherapists don't use any essential oils during pregnancy, and all experts agree that there are some—such as clary sage, rosemary, peppermint, and pennyroyal—that should definitely be avoided.

A base oil, however, such as almond or olive oil, is always safe and will help the masseur's hands glide smoothly over your skin. Your masseur should pour a little of the oil into his cupped hands and hold it there for a minute to warm it before spreading it lightly onto your body. He should position himself so that he can massage you without having to bend down or twist his back. It's important that he should be relaxed while he's massaging; otherwise, his hands will communicate tension to you and your baby.

FIND PEACE WITH MEDITATION

During pregnancy, you're in a state of heightened mental awareness. You may find yourself bursting into tears over something on the news that normally wouldn't have affected you. You may be very conscious of the changing seasons and of the different moods of nature. Certain objects in your home, perhaps from your childhood, may take on extra meaning and your thoughts may dwell on many memories as you make the transition

Foot massage Women often enjoy having their feet massaged during labor, so it's a good idea to practice early.

Sit in a chair with one leg supported on a pillow placed on a stool. Your massage partner kneels in front of you. Gently resting your heel in his hand—without squeezing it—he uses his other hand to stroke firmly from your ankle to your toes. This movement is repeated slowly and regularly for several minutes.

Using his finger, your partner next strokes between each toe. He then flexes your toes upward, supporting your heel on the pillow, and makes small circles with his thumbs across the sole. Provided that the pressure is firm, this shouldn't tickle you.

Gently lifting your foot by the ankle again, your partner then strokes you several more times from the ankle to the toes. The whole process is then repeated on your other foot.

to motherhood. You're very conscious of your body and of the changes it's going through. Meditation, which involves focusing on your thoughts and emotions, can help you make maximum use of this self-awareness, while enabling you to achieve profound states of relaxation.

However, if you feel at all depressed, and certainly if you're being treated for depression, it's best to avoid meditation. The deep introspection it encourages may be distressing to you if your view of yourself and your life is unbalanced.

Meditation can't be learned in a single session, so it should be practiced regularly. But there are two simple ways of focusing your mind: mantras and visualization. Try alternating them day by day. As your mind learns how to still itself using the mantra, you'll find that visualization stimulates an ever richer exploration of your thoughts and feelings.

Meditate with mantras

Find a peaceful room in which you won't be disturbed by harsh lights or sudden noises. Sit comfortably and start your meditation by focusing on your breathing. Breathe in deeply and, as you sigh out gently, let your whole body relax. Repeat until you feel fully relaxed.

Your mantra should be a word that you can match with your breathing, such as "baby" or "relax." When you breathe in, say silently to yourself "ba…" and as you breathe out, say "by…" Or you could think "re…" on the in-breath and "lax…" on the out-breath. Or simply hold the word "peace" in your mind as you breathe out.

Focus your mind exclusively on the word you're repeating. Whenever your mind wanders, bring it back gently to your chosen mantra. Continue repeating the mantra so that it drowns out all other thoughts. With practice, you'll find a vast space in your mind where you can know yourself and be at peace with yourself.

Join a class. Many centers offer basic courses that will help you learn different techniques.

Visualize your baby

Meditation is an excellent technique for clearing away jumbled thoughts, and practicing visualization can teach you how to focus your mind—a useful technique during labor. Try the following exercise, which focuses on a candle. In subsequent sessions, choose other items that have special meaning, such as toys you have bought for your baby, things relating to your childhood, or photos of important people in your life.

Settle into a comfortable chair. Place a lighted candle in front of you and let your eyes rest on the flame. Keep your gaze focused. You'll become aware of different colors and intensities of light in the flame, from the white-hot core, to the yellows and oranges that flicker along the outer edges. When your eyes start to feel heavy, let them close gently, but continue to see the candle in your mind's eye. Place your baby in the flame image, surrounded by light, and let him stir thoughts in your mind.

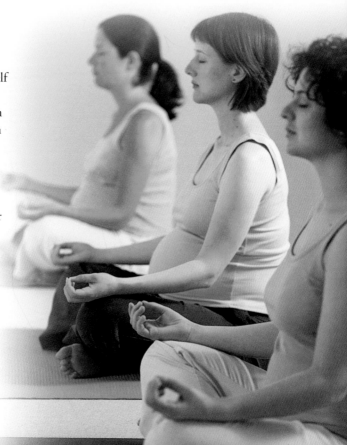

CHAPTER

LOOKING GREAT

Pregnancy is a great excuse to really lavish attention

on yourself—particularly as it will be hard to find

time for pampering once your baby is here. Also,

this is a time to pay special attention to your hair,

skin, teeth, breasts, and feet.

TOP-TO-TOE CARE

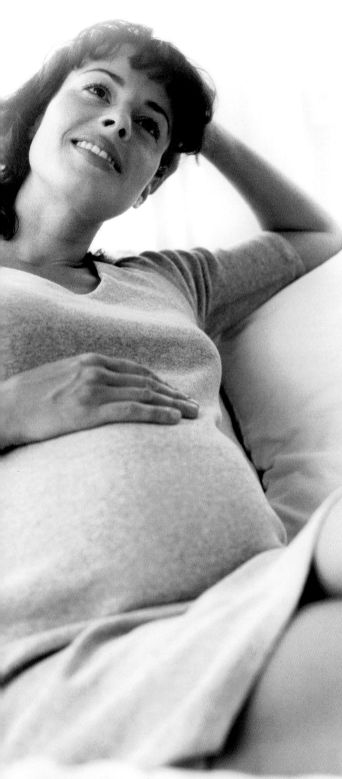

Coping with all the physical changes of pregnancy can sometimes be challenging, but focusing on the positive effects—rounded curves, shiny hair, and glowing skin—can make a huge difference to the way that you feel.

Everyone talks about the bloom of pregnancy—the radiant complexion and lustrous hair—but they don't often mention the less flattering aspects—the painful breasts, swollen feet, and flaky skin. While it can help to understand that such changes are just part and parcel of being pregnant, they can be demoralizing. That's why it's important to take proper care of yourself and your changing body.

Expensive products aren't essential to good skin—a thorough, consistent daily routine is the basis of a healthy complexion and will keep you looking your best. Beauty products targeted specifically at pregnant women don't contain any magic ingredients, despite what they may claim, so use them only if you're really impressed with their results. Buying yourself the occasional luxury item as a treat, however, can give you a real boost.

HEALTHY HAIR
Your increased metabolism and boosted circulation may mean that your hair grows faster, while hair loss slows down. This vigorous growth means that your hair will look thicker and more lustrous than usual. Some pregnant women, however, are less lucky and find that their hair becomes greasy or unusually dry or lifeless. Don't worry if this happens to you: Any changes you experience will be short-lived and your hair will soon return to normal.

Hair care tips
Be gentle with your hair during pregnancy. You should make the most of thicker, vibrant hair while you can, as, unfortunately, the extra hair will disappear within six months of your baby's birth. You may find the following useful:

- *Use special shampoos* If greasiness is a problem, wash hair frequently with a specially formulated shampoo and try not to brush your hair too vigorously, as this will encourage the sebaceous glands in the scalp to produce even more oil.
- *Condition it well* If your hair becomes dry and fly-away, invest in a hot oil treatment or deep conditioner to use once a week. Mousse can add volume, improve "bad-hair days," and keep your style in place. Again, don't brush your hair too much as this will encourage the hair to split.
- *Invest in a good cut* As your pregnancy progresses, and certainly once your baby is born, you probably won't want to bother with a complicated hairstyle, so go for an easily managed style. This will keep your hair looking and feeling healthy throughout your pregnancy and beyond.

Hair treatments

Although some health professionals are cautious about dyeing or highlighting hair during pregnancy, there's no evidence that these pose any risk to your baby. Many years ago, hair dyes contained some potentially worrying substances such as formaldehyde, but today most dyes don't contain such chemicals. The only ingredient of dyes that you might want to avoid is coal tar, which some experts suspect could be carcinogenic. If you're at all concerned, use vegetable-based products. One proviso—be aware that pregnancy hormones may make your hair react differently so that you could end up with a color you weren't expecting.

There's also no evidence to suggest that the chemicals in permanents are harmful to you or your developing baby. However, your hair may react unpredictably to them and you could end up with frizzy rather than wavy hair.

Hair relaxers contain strong chemicals and although there is no evidence that they are dangerous during pregnancy, there is no proof that they are completely safe, so their use is best avoided.

A RADIANT COMPLEXION

The greater volume of blood circulating in your body—50 percent more by the time your baby is ready to be born—combined with the slight rise in your body temperature, may give your skin the characteristic pregnancy "glow" and a soft, velvety texture as it plumps out and retains more moisture. Don't be surprised, however, if your skin becomes a bit unpredictable—it may get unusually dry or greasy, and you may even develop pimples or acne.

You also may notice some other changes, such as spider veins (tiny broken blood vessels) on your cheeks, and chloasma, known as the mask of pregnancy, across your nose and cheeks (see page 66). Most of these marks will fade after delivery and your skin type will return to normal, but if you wish to even out your skin color, use a good quality concealer rather than lightening fluids, which contain bleach and could damage your skin.

Sun protection

Hormones make your skin more susceptible to the effects of the sun, so that it may burn much more quickly than before. Apply a foundation or moisturizing cream containing sunscreen daily, and cover all exposed skin with sun cream with a sun protection factor (SPF) of at least 15 before you leave the house. Don't forget to take care of your lips, too. They may seem drier than usual, so use a moisturizing lip balm regularly—on its own or under lipstick—to stop them from cracking.

Your facial care

Adapt your daily skincare routine to accommodate any changes to your complexion and be prepared to keep making minor adjustments as your pregnancy progresses. In all cases, follow these guidelines for a healthy-looking complexion:
- *Cleanse your face at least once a day* Use a non-soap product suitable for your current skin type. Soap can be too harsh for your face and strip

your skin of its natural oils. If you develop pimples, scrupulous attention to hygiene is even more important, to keep the pores clear.

- *Use a mild astringent* This will tone greasy skin and clean out clogged pores.
- *Lavish moisturizer on dry skin* Allow it to sink in and rehydrate your complexion. If your skin becomes dry only in patches, treat it like combination skin: Apply more moisturizer to the drier areas.

If you have regular facials as part of your skincare routine there's no reason to stop while pregnant. And they are a great way to relax. Facials won't worsen any pregnancy-related skin changes, but your skin may be more sensitive than usual, so always check that any products being used are suitable.

Anti-wrinkle creams

Although anti-wrinkle creams containing vitamin A don't seem to pose a problem, it may be best to avoid using them during pregnancy, as it's possible that the nutrient can be absorbed through the skin and enter the bloodstream. There is strong evidence to suggest that vitamin supplements or medications containing vitamin A can cause birth defects (see page 106). If you're at all in doubt about what's safe to use, discuss it first with your healthcare provider.

STRONG TEETH AND GUMS

It's even more important than usual to maintain good dental hygiene throughout pregnancy. The pregnancy hormones circulating in your body will probably cause your gums to swell slightly, making them more susceptible to bleeding during brushing and flossing. They also will make the gums more susceptible to plaque and bacteria.

Daily dental care

If you don't do so already, start to brush your teeth at least twice a day, and ideally after every meal. This may mean taking a toothbrush to work with you.

- *Use a soft-bristled brush* This is less likely to cause your gums to bleed. Massage your gums gently with your fingertips after brushing to encourage blood circulation.

SAFETY FIRST

Fillings Although research is inconclusive, many experts believe that amalgam fillings should not be inserted or removed during pregnancy. This is because they contain mercury, which poses a slight risk to an unborn baby. If removal is unavoidable, ask your dentist's advice, and if you need a new filling, opt for a non-amalgam one. You could have a temporary filling now and the permanent amalgam inserted later. There's no evidence to suggest that amalgam fillings that are already in place will affect the baby.

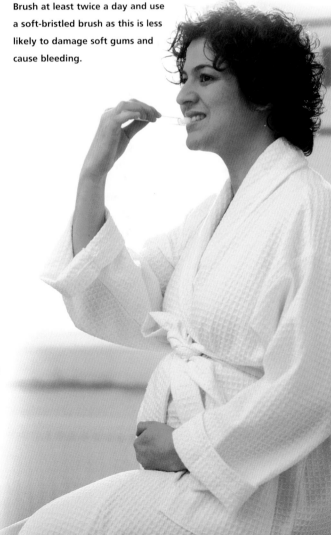

Brush at least twice a day and use a soft-bristled brush as this is less likely to damage soft gums and cause bleeding.

- *Floss daily* But floss gently, and throw out your toothbrush as soon as it shows signs of wear.
- *Chew gum* When you can't brush after eating, chew a stick of sugar-free gum as this will help prevent plaque building up on your teeth.
- *Visit your dentist regularly* You'll need to see him or her more regularly than normal during pregnancy—once every six months is advisable. Tell your dentist that you're pregnant, as he or she will want to avoid using X-rays at this time and may advise that any extensive treatment should wait until after your baby is born.

Teeth whitening

Although no major studies have been done on the effects of using whitening systems—many of which use peroxide or ultraviolet light—until more is known, it's recommended that teeth whitening should be avoided during pregnancy.

TAKING CARE OF YOUR SKIN

Your increased blood flow will probably make you feel warmer than usual and, as a result, you'll sweat more easily than you usually do. Make time for a daily, or even twice daily, bath or shower—use warm water rather than hot, as hot water will open your pores and make you even more likely to sweat. If your skin is feeling dry, a light aqueous cream can be used as a soap substitute or as a moisturizing skin cream, which should be applied after washing, while your skin is still wet.

You also can help prevent sweating by choosing cotton rather than synthetic underwear, and if you wear pantyhose, opt for types with cotton-lined gussets. Wear clothes made of natural rather than synthetic fibers to help stay cooler.

Keeping skin soft and supple

You probably won't need reminding to pay particular attention to your abdomen and breasts. The skin in these areas is being stretched considerably and, as a result, may feel particularly dry and itchy. Massage your belly with a moisturizing cream or oil—a nice way to communicate with your developing baby as well as supplying a well-earned period of relaxation. If your breasts are dry, apply moisturizer here also. However, avoid over-moisturizing your nipples—if they become too soft and damp they may feel sore. If you do experience any discomfort from sore nipples, expose your breasts to the air occasionally while you're relaxing at home.

5 ways to minimize stretch marks

1   Eat sensibly and avoid gaining too much weight. If you gain a great deal of weight in a short space of time, your skin won't have a chance to adapt and will have to stretch to accommodate your new shape.

2   Wear a well-fitting bra throughout your pregnancy. Keep your growing breasts adequately supported as they become heavier.

3   Wear a sleep bra if your breasts are large. Looking after your breasts during the day isn't enough—they need 24-hour care.

4   Keep your skin supple and itch-free. Massage cream into your breasts and belly to elasticize the skin. Cocoa butter or almond oil extract—available from pharmacists—have proved effective for some women.

5   Apply pure vitamin-E oil locally to moisturize your skin.

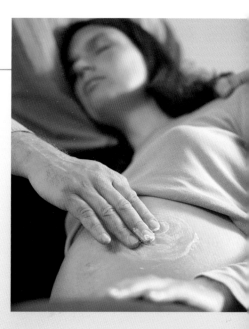

Along with your thighs, your abdomen and breasts are the most likely places to develop stretch marks. There's no surefire way of preventing them, nor any miracle cure for them once they have arrived, but there are some things you can do to make their appearance less likely (see page 133).

Like many women, you may enjoy massages, and during pregnancy these are fine, as long as care is taken with aromatherapy oils (see page 74). Many massage therapists now offer pregnancy massages and some use special tables with a cutout center so you can lie face down and rest your belly.

Hair removal

Bikini, leg, or facial waxes, which use a hot wax that is applied to the skin, allowed to cool, then removed from the skin along with the unwanted hair, are topical preparations that contain no substances harmful to a developing baby, so there's no reason why you can't have waxing done during pregnancy.

Although there is no known risk of depilatories or bleach harming the baby, your skin may not react well to them, and there is a possibility that their chemicals can get into the bloodstream. Electrolysis is also not recommended, even though there is no proof that it could harm the baby. Shaving and plucking unwanted hair are safer alternatives.

Tattoos and body piercing

Even if you attend a reputable parlor, tattoos and piercings should not be undertaken during pregnancy because of the high risk of infection.

Breast implants

With all the changes that are going on in your body, pregnancy is not the time to get implants for the first time. In any case, most doctors would not be prepared to operate on a pregnant woman. The breasts of women with silicone or saline breast implants may be affected by pregnancy. Some women have increased breast tenderness as their own breast tissue grows, and that growth combined with the increased size present from the implants stretches the overlying skin to an uncomfortable degree.

CARING FOR YOUR HANDS AND FEET

You may find that your fingernails split and break more easily during pregnancy; if so, keep them short and wear rubber gloves for washing dishes and doing housework. You also should use gloves to protect your hands when you're doing yard work and to avoid picking up soil-borne infections (see page 257). Apply hand cream regularly, ideally the type with nail strengthener.

Pregnancy places additional strain on your feet, both through the extra weight they have to bear and through potential swelling (see page 73). You may find it helps to soak your feet in a bowl of water in the evening and to massage with peppermint foot cream after a bath or shower. Keep toenails short, but not so short that they may ingrow, and cut them straight across. If you can't reach your toes in the later stages of pregnancy, you may need to ask for some help or have a professional pedicure. It makes sense to go to a reputable salon where the equipment is properly cleaned.

HEALTH FIRST

Semi-surgical procedures Because they use concentrated chemicals whose effects on the unborn baby are not known, chemical peels and botox and collagen injections are not recommended during pregnancy, and possibly not during breastfeeding.

YOUR MATERNITY WARDROBE

In recent years, glossy images of sexy, heavily pregnant celebrities have turned pregnancy into a fashion statement. This glamor and chic has filtered down to the woman on the street, so, from a fashion point of view, there has never been a better time to be pregnant.

You may feel the urge to buy a whole new wardrobe once your pregnancy is confirmed, but try to resist until your own clothes become uncomfortable. Your pregnant state probably won't become obvious until about week 20 with a first baby and week 14 in a subsequent or multiple pregnancy. If you wait until you really have to wear proper maternity clothes, you're less likely to be sick of them by the time that your baby is born.

As your belly grows, your clothes will start to feel tight around your middle and you'll feel very uncomfortable if your belly is squeezed. Tops also may start to feel tight as your breasts grow. You can adapt many of your existing clothes for a while with a few simple adjustments. Try covering open zippers on pants with long, loose shirts or use suspenders to keep your pants up. This is a good time to start "borrowing" from your partner's wardrobe. You can replace the elastic in sweat pants with cord to give you room for expansion—sewing buttons on with elastic thread also can give valuable extra space. But if you want to wear any clothes again after your baby is born, don't wear them for so long that they're permanently stretched out of shape.

TIME FOR A CHANGE

Inevitably, you'll need to add to your wardrobe at some stage in your pregnancy. If you choose carefully from regular fashion stores, the clothes you buy will have a second lease of life in the first few weeks, or even months, after your baby's birth while your figure gradually reverts to something like its pre-pregnancy state. If you plan to breastfeed, make sure that you choose tops, dresses, and nightgowns that give easy and discreet access to your breasts—those with ample material or ties or buttons down the front are ideal.

5 useful pregnancy accessories

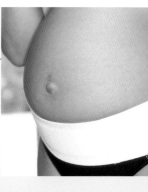

1   Bra extenders may be useful in the early stages if your chest size has increased but your cup size hasn't. The extra fastening attaches to the hooks and eyes on your existing bra to create more space.

2   Maternity pantyhose have extra material in front to accommodate your belly and the waistband sits high enough to keep your pantyhose up. If you have problems with aching feet or varicose veins (see page 73), maternity support pantyhose—available in light, medium, or firm—can be helpful. Slip them on in the morning, even before you get out of bed.

3   Mini maternity briefs fit snugly under your belly, while full briefs have ample material to fit over it. If you suffer from backache, maternity support briefs incorporate a semirigid back panel.

4   Support belts are special belts that fit just below your belly to provide support, relieving aching legs and a strained back. They are especially helpful if you are carrying larger or multiple babies. If you do buy such a belt, avoid wearing it all the time, as it can weaken your abdominal muscles.

5   Swimming is one of the safest and most effective forms of exercise for a pregnant woman. Maternity swimsuits grow with you and your baby.

Styles to suit you

There's no need to change your image just because you're pregnant—if you didn't like flowery prints or big bows before, why should you now? Equally, if you didn't flaunt your figure before, pregnancy may not be the best time to start.

Long, loose tops and dresses will drape your belly gracefully, while jogging suits can make comfortable everyday wear. Check that, as well as being loose around the waist, your clothes have enough material around your buttocks. If not, your growing belly will pull the fabric forward, causing it to bunch rather unattractively at the back. If you prefer more figure-hugging clothes, choose those containing plenty of stretchy fabric so that they grow with you.

Throughout pregnancy, avoid skirts, pants, underpants, or pantyhose that have tight elastic waistbands. Apart from being uncomfortable, the elastic may restrict your blood flow. Similarly, hold-up stockings, garters, or tight knee socks may affect blood flow in your legs and could lead to varicose veins (see page 73).

Choosing maternity clothes

When you're choosing your maternity clothes, ask yourself when you'll be wearing them. If you're working in an environment where you need to look smart, a suit with a selection of tops may be the best answer, plus some weekend wear. Simple, elegant items that can be dressed up or down, depending on the occasion, offer great flexibility. Easy-care, minimum-iron fabrics will save time if you're tired.

The main advantage of maternity clothes is that they have been designed specifically for pregnant women. Skirts and dresses are usually longer at the front than the back so that your growing belly does not cause a wavy hemline. Tucks and darts are positioned to ensure that clothes continue to hang well as your belly grows. Ribbed panels and special stretch material can accommodate your expanding belly without distorting more fitted styles. Fastenings are usually adjustable, often with several holes and buttons sewn on with elastic thread. As a result, the clothes will grow with you and continue to look good until the end of your pregnancy.

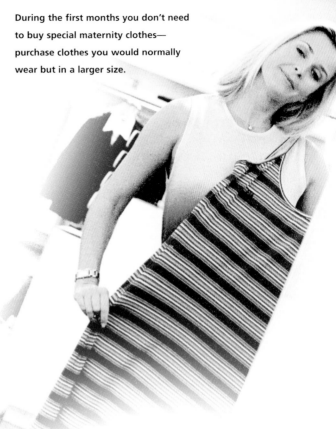

During the first months you don't need to buy special maternity clothes—purchase clothes you would normally wear but in a larger size.

As well as specialized maternity wear stores, many department stores sell maternity clothes, and you'll find a wide variety of mail-order catalogs available. The often bewildering choice makes it all the more important to shop wisely, but you needn't buy hundreds of new outfits—just a few carefully chosen items will keep you looking stylish during pregnancy and beyond. Some mail-order companies offer "wardrobes-in-a-box," consisting of a selection of mix-and-match items, often a dress, skirt, top, and slacks or sweat pants, which can be combined in various ways. It's also worth looking out for stores that sell good-quality, secondhand maternity wear as these often have tremendous bargains. However, never buy secondhand bras, as your bra needs to be well-fitting to give you support. Once your baby is born, clean and properly store any special maternity clothes for your next baby or for a good friend.

WELL-SUPPORTED BREASTS

It's vitally important to look after your breasts as an expectant mother. Breasts themselves contain no muscles and so are supported by the muscles on the chest wall. Unsupported or badly supported breasts are more likely to develop stretch marks or to sag, so even if you have never felt the need for a bra before, you should wear one now.

Invest in good fit

Check the fit of your existing bras or bra tops, and if they don't offer good support or if they squeeze your breasts in any way, measure yourself and invest in some new, well-fitting ones. By the end of nine months, your breasts may be up to two cup sizes larger than before, and your bra size (the measurement around your chest, below your breasts) will probably increase as your ribs expand to accommodate your growing baby. After the birth—and once you have stopped breastfeeding—your breasts will reduce in size, but probably won't be the same size and shape as they were before pregnancy.

You won't need special maternity bras for most of your pregnancy, but you should buy a new bra each time your breast size increases so much that you feel uncomfortable and cramped inside your existing one. Some women find they need new bras around week 8, others don't need to change until about week 24. Most women need a larger size again at about week 36—these bras will also be useful for the first weeks after the birth, so you may want to buy a nursing bra, suitable for breastfeeding. Every woman develops differently, however, so be guided by the changes in your size and shape, not by the calendar. If your breasts become particularly large and heavy, you may find that a sleep bra (a lightweight maternity bra worn through the night) will help make you feel more comfortable. Consider the following points when buying a bra to wear during pregnancy. Choose a bra with:

- *Wide, adjustable shoulder straps* These are more comfortable than narrow shoulder straps—which can dig into your skin—because the weight is distributed more evenly.

HOW TO size up for pregnancy

Keep your breasts comfortable by ensuring that they're properly supported at every stage of your pregnancy. You may find it easiest to be measured professionally when you buy a new bra, but there is a good range available by mail-order, for which you'll need to know your size.

First, take a tape measure around your rib cage directly below your breasts **1**. This is your bra size.

Next, put the tape around the fullest part of your breasts while wearing a lightweight bra **2**. The difference between this figure and your bra size will help you determine your cup size. Use the box right to see how this difference translates to the sizes you see in stores.

FINDING YOUR CUP SIZE		
0 inch	=	A
1 inch	=	B
2 inches	=	C
3 inches	=	D
4 inches	=	DD
5 inches	=	E
6 inches	=	F
7 inches	=	G
8 inches	=	H

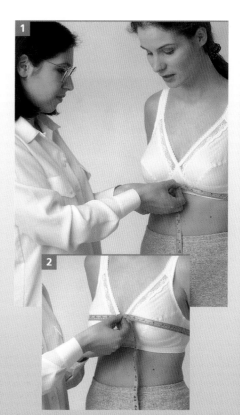

- *A high proportion of cotton* Natural fibers allow your skin to breathe.
- *A broad band of elastic under the cups* This will support your breasts as they become heavier.
- *An adjustable back* The ideal is to have four hook-and-eye fastenings so that you can loosen your bra as your rib cage expands.
- *No underwiring* The stiff wire can pinch and damage your breast tissues, so go for a softer fit.

Choosing a nursing bra

If you're planning to breastfeed, the bras you buy around week 36 should be specially designed nursing bras. A good nursing bra has all the features listed above, and also allows you to expose one breast at a time to feed your baby.

Several types are available, including: drop-cup, where each cup unhooks from the shoulder strap; zip-cup, where the bra unzips under the breast; and front opening, where each cup is attached to the center of the bra by a hook-and-eye fastening. If you prefer bra tops, these are also available with all the maternity features. Try on different types to discover the one you find most comfortable. Whichever you choose, make sure that you can open and close it easily with one hand—the other will be occupied holding your baby.

SHOES FOR COMFORT

It's not unusual for your feet to swell, so you may need shoes in a larger size than usual. Some women find that their feet remain slightly larger after the birth. Whether or not you buy new shoes, always bear the following in mind:

- *Avoid shoes with high heels* Apart from being uncomfortable, they'll also throw your posture out, making you thrust your belly forward and possibly leading to backache.
- *Wear comfortable, low-heeled shoes* These should be in a material that allows your skin to breathe. Avoid completely flat styles, as these don't help your balance either.
- *Avoid wearing lace-up or buckle styles* In the later stages of pregnancy you won't be able to bend easily to do them up.

- *Alternate your shoes* As a rule, it's best not to wear the same pair of shoes two days in a row, but to swap between at least two pairs to allow each pair time to breathe and dry out.
- *Choose cotton socks and pantyhose* Cotton or cotton-rich materials are preferable to synthetic, as they allow your skin to breathe. Make sure also they aren't too tight for your feet. Shorter socks, such as ankle socks, ensure that the veins in your legs aren't compressed but, ideally, you should go barefoot in the house as much as you can, to exercise the muscles in your feet and improve your circulation.

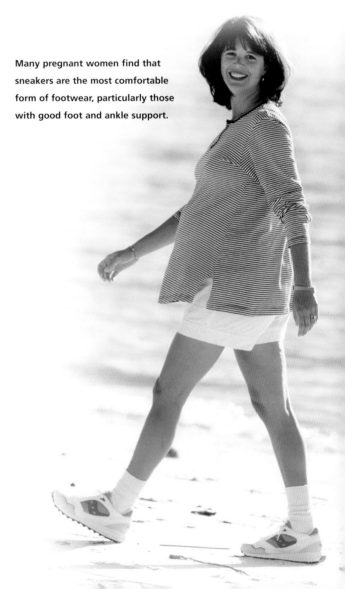

Many pregnant women find that sneakers are the most comfortable form of footwear, particularly those with good foot and ankle support.

THE SECRET LIFE OF YOUR UNBORN BABY

It takes nine months for a baby to grow—and these

nine months are a period of intense activity for your

baby, as he masters all the skills he needs to survive

in the outside world.

THE SAFETY OF THE UTERUS

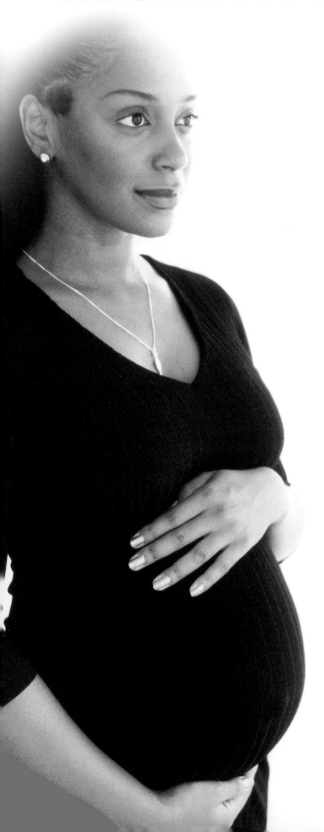

Protected by the amniotic sac, and supplied with oxygen and nutrients from the placenta, your baby is in the ideal environment for growth.

Advances in research have greatly increased our understanding of life in the uterus. As early as 8 weeks, when she's about the size of a grape, your baby's starting to move; from about 9 weeks she's practicing how to breathe; and by 12 weeks, she's showing off her acrobatic skills with somersaults and back flips. In later pregnancy this movement will be in response to sounds—and possibly even smells and tastes—she begins to experience via her senses.

YOUR BABY'S LIFE SUPPORT SYSTEM

From the moment your baby's conceived, your body provides her with everything she needs for complete and normal development. Initially, the uterine lining, where nutrients have been stored for nourishment, supports the developing embryo. Meanwhile, your body is hard at work preparing a more efficient life support system: the placenta.

Chorionic villi

During the first few weeks, spongelike protrusions sprout from the wall of the fertilized egg. From these, capillary-filled tissue called chorionic villi grow. By the 8th week the chorionic villi have developed blood vessels, which carry nutrients and oxygen to the fetus. These blood vessels gradually join to form a system of blood vessels and finally the umbilical cord. At the site where the embryo implanted itself, the chorionic villi multiply to form the placenta. At about week 14 the placenta takes over the job of helping your baby survive and grow.

The placenta

Responsible for nourishing your baby, supplying her with oxygen, and removing waste products, the placenta is an incredibly efficient organ. The placenta is also responsible for generating vital

THE STRUCTURE OF THE PLACENTA

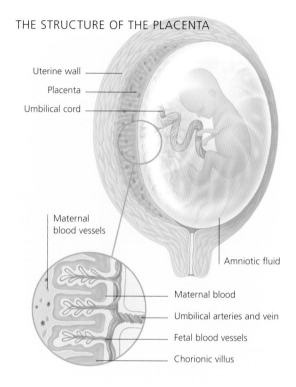

Uterine wall

Placenta

Umbilical cord

Maternal blood vessels

Amniotic fluid

Maternal blood

Umbilical arteries and vein

Fetal blood vessels

Chorionic villus

pregnancy hormones such as progesterone so it plays a key role in stimulating your body to adapt to and maintain pregnancy (see page 60).

Attached to your uterine wall, the placenta contains blood vessels that belong to both you and your baby. In the event of identical twins, the placenta may be shared; nonidentical twins or triplets will each have their own placenta. Your baby is connected to the placenta via the umbilical cord, which is made up of a vein and two arteries. The blood vessels in the placenta intertwine but remain separate, so your blood and that of your baby never actually mixes. Everything that needs to be exchanged between the two bloodstreams is carried out by a process of diffusion. The nutrients, antibodies, and oxygen that your baby needs are passed from your bloodstream into your baby's and flow into her body along the umbilical vein. Waste products and blood that's low in oxygen are removed from her body along the umbilical arteries. These waste products pass into your bloodstream and are excreted via your kidneys.

The diffusion process means that your baby's growth and development are totally dependent on you—everything you take in, your baby takes in as well, which is why it's so important to eat a healthy, balanced diet and to avoid any substances that could harm your baby. Some research suggests that even flavors and smells from food you eat may be transferred across the placenta (see page 142).

The placenta reaches its prime at about 34 weeks, after which it begins to age. Two or three weeks later it has become less efficient in transferring nutrition to your baby. It also becomes fibrous instead of spongy, and blood clots and calcified patches appear—a sign that the blood vessels are aging. After 40 weeks, the placenta begins to deteriorate and there's a risk that it won't produce an adequate supply of nutrients and oxygen for the baby.

MORE **ABOUT** | the amniotic sac

During her time in the uterus, your baby grows inside the amniotic sac. This is filled with amniotic fluid, which cushions and protects her while also providing room for growth and movement within the uterus. The amniotic fluid is made up of fluid from the placenta, as well as fetal urine and lung fluid from your baby. At 40 weeks, your baby is surrounded by between 1 and 3 pints (0.5 and 1.5 liters) of amniotic fluid.

YOUR BABY'S SENSES

Far from floating dreamily in a watery world unaware of what's happening around him, your baby is hard at work developing his senses—and, surprisingly, there's plenty to stimulate them.

Your unborn baby's senses of touch, taste, smell, hearing, and sight are stimulated by what is going on in your body as well as by sensations that filter through from the world outside. And learning to recognize your voice or smelling and tasting the foods that you eat may give him a sense of familiarity and security after he's born.

TOUCH

Your baby's sense of touch is the first to develop. About the same time he starts to move—at about 7 to 8 weeks—he becomes responsive to touch. At first, only his lips are sensitive, but soon he'll show a response in his cheeks and forehead. By about 10 to 11 weeks, the palms of your baby's hands become touch-sensitive and he'll start to feel his face, perhaps beginning to explore what he looks like. By 14 weeks, your unborn baby's whole body, with the exception of the back and top of his head, responds to touch in a similar way to newborn babies.

Plenty to explore

As your baby grows bigger, parts of his body will also touch the wall of your uterus and he'll have to curl up to fit inside you. In addition, your unborn baby is constantly brushing against his umbilical cord, and ultrasound often shows babies holding onto their cords or "playing" with them.

Interestingly, your baby's initial response to a touch on the cheek is to move away from the stimulus; if his hand touches his right cheek he'll turn his head to the left. This early response to touch is a result of the immaturity of his central nervous system. Later on in pregnancy, this response changes so that your baby turns his head toward the touch. This is possibly the start of the rooting reflex, which will be important in breastfeeding.

A sensitive mouth

Your baby may suck his thumb in the uterus, although he hasn't yet connected sucking with satisfying hunger. In a baby's immature body, the tongue, with its hundreds of nerve endings, is one of his most sensitive parts, and sucking is an excellent way of getting a feel for things. This can be seen in the behavior of young children who put unfamiliar objects in their mouths to get an idea of proportions and textures, rather than feeling them in their clumsy hands. As your baby sucks his thumb in the uterus, he discovers the feel of his skin and the shape of his thumb and may receive the same sense of comfort from sucking that babies do after birth.

TASTE AND SMELL

Your baby starts to swallow amniotic fluid—the fluid surrounding him in the amniotic sac—from about 12 weeks and continues to do so throughout pregnancy. Some experts have suggested that it is through this swallowing that your baby begins to learn about taste and smell, because the amniotic fluid contains the flavor and odor of the foods you eat.

DID YOU KNOW...

Twins react to each other As well as being in close physical proximity, twins often jostle for position. If one twin reaches out and touches the other, his brother or sister reacts to the touch and often reciprocates. This may be the beginning of the affinity that most twins have throughout life. Often one twin is more active than the other and reacts to a stimulus more readily with a faster heartbeat or harder kicking; again, this difference seems to continue in later life.

When you eat garlic, for example, your baby may taste and smell it through several routes: From your bloodstream the garlic enters your baby's, where it could stimulate the sensory receptors within your baby's nose. Second, the garlic disperses directly into the amniotic fluid and, as your baby "breathes" and swallows, he may smell and taste the garlic. Third, as the garlic is "expelled" from your baby's body when he urinates into the amniotic fluid, he might get a second chance to experience taste by swallowing the amniotic fluid. So while the taste of a garlic meal may be with you for a few hours, it may last some 24 hours or longer for your baby.

Developing likes and dislikes

Research has shown that unborn babies seem to be able to tell the difference between sweet and sour tastes, swallowing more when they taste a sweet substance, but less when they taste something bitter. So it may not take long before your baby starts to recognize your diet. As your breast milk is flavored in much the same way, a radical change in diet after the birth could mean that your baby may take longer to get used to breastfeeding.

HEARING

The way your baby responds to sounds has been extensively studied, largely because hearing is the easiest sense to stimulate in the uterus. Your baby starts reacting to sound at around 24 weeks and the louder the sound, the stronger the reaction.

Your baby's environment is full of rich and varied sounds: Your heartbeat and the blood pulsing through your arteries and veins form a sound backdrop, and he also can hear intermittent gurgles from your stomach and intestines. Sounds from the world outside your body, such as voices, music, and TV, also carry through your abdomen and are heard by your baby. These sounds, however, are much quieter for your baby than they are for you. This is because as a noise travels toward you, many of the

sound waves are bounced back or absorbed by your clothes and skin—only a small amount of noise penetrates through the wall of your abdomen to reach your baby's ears. Sounds with a high frequency are reflected more easily, so your baby hears mostly low-frequency sounds.

His favorite sounds

Of all the sounds your unborn baby will hear, your voice is the one that will stand out most. This is because your baby hears you in two ways: first, through the sound waves that come out of your mouth and travel through the air; and second, from the vibrations that travel through your body when you speak. This is similar to the way that you hear yourself speak, which is why your voice sounds different when you hear a recording of it—you're listening to only the airborne sounds and not the

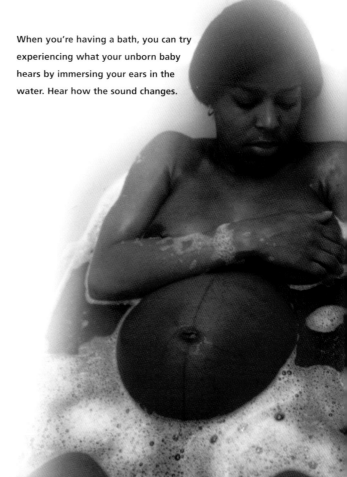

When you're having a bath, you can try experiencing what your unborn baby hears by immersing your ears in the water. Hear how the sound changes.

internal vibrations. Your body's vibrations transmit your voice to your baby very efficiently, so whenever you speak, sing, or shout, your baby hears you. It's not surprising, then, that at birth your baby will know your voice better than anyone else's. Babies don't usually recognize their father's voice at birth, although they usually can tell the difference between male and female voices.

Your voice isn't the only sound that your baby learns before he's born. Researchers have used ultrasound to observe how babies react to familiar and unfamiliar tunes played through headphones placed on their mothers' abdomens. At about 26 to 27 weeks, babies tend to increase their movements on hearing a familiar tune, almost as if they're dancing to their favorite tracks. But when they hear music that they don't recognize, they tend to stop. In some cases, familiar music may have a soothing effect on your baby after he's born, calming him down when he is crying. But use this tactic sparingly or its effects could wear off.

SIGHT

Your baby's sight is the least stimulated sense in his watery world and the last to develop. His eyelids remain closed until about 27 weeks, at which stage his eyes open and begin to blink, possibly practicing for this reflex that he'll need after his birth.

However, inside the uterus, your baby's world is essentially a dark one. This is because the skin of your abdomen and the material of your clothes prevent any light from reaching him. If you were to sunbathe on a bright sunny day wearing a bikini, he might experience a diffuse, orange glow through your skin—similar to what you see when you put your hand over a flashlight. Studies have shown that babies' pupils can constrict and dilate from week 33 onward and they can perhaps even distinguish dim shapes at this stage.

5 ways to stimulate your unborn baby

1   Give your baby a gentle nudge and see if he gives a nudge in response. Praise him if he does—he may learn to do it again.

2   Place some headphones on your abdomen and play some music just for your baby. Feel him moving or "dancing" inside you.

3   Talk and sing to your baby. He loves the sound of your voice, so read him a story or sing him a lullaby. Get your partner to join in, too—he may react differently to his voice.

4   Open up an inner dialog with your baby. Lie down in a quiet, darkened room, and visualize your baby inside you. Communicate your love for him through your thoughts.

5   Go swimming. Both you and your baby will enjoy the feeling of weightlessness that it gives you.

YOUR ACTIVE BABY

Your baby is a regular little acrobat in the uterus and, by the time of birth, she's mastered a range of movements essential for her new life.

Your baby's movements play an important part in the normal development of her joints and muscles. The continual movement of her developing joints molds the surfaces to each other's contours, so the bones can move together smoothly and easily. Moreover, just as you exercise to keep your body in shape, so does your baby; her movements are a kind of keep-fit program to ensure the full development of her muscles. She needs to be in good shape to get down the birth canal on her birth day.

FIRST MOVEMENTS

Your baby first starts to move when you're about 7 to 8 weeks pregnant. At this stage, she's only about 1 inch (2.5 cm) in length, but she already has muscles along the length of her spine. As she's so small, you won't be able to feel anything yet, but these movements are just discernible on ultrasound, and researchers have described them as looking like "twitches" or "rippling."

By the 12th week your baby is rolling and flipping over, even frowning, and, over the next few weeks, she'll develop an amazing range of movements. Over 20 different types have been identified in the early part of pregnancy, including sucking, yawns, and hiccups. Between 13 and 17 weeks your baby is hard at work practicing her full range of movements.

Patterns of activity

Your baby's movements may occur in bursts that continue for as long as 7 minutes, but more commonly these activities last for 1 to 2 minutes, from the age of about 9 weeks. Your baby is likely to have a favorite resting place, too, where she will always return after a bout of activity. Usually this is at the lowest part of the amniotic sac.

Gaining control

Your baby's first movements are produced solely by electrical activity in her muscles: Her brain is not instructing her muscles as yet. In this early part of pregnancy, her movements may be continuous and vigorous. However, as your baby's nervous system develops, her spinal cord, brain stem, and then the higher centers of her brain, take over the control of her movements. The bigger movements such as back flips and rolls make way for finer movements such as moving her eyes or stretching one leg. Moving her arm, for example, is a more complex action than a somersault, because each joint in the arm has muscles that allow it to extend and flex. Your baby must learn how to master both of these sets of muscles before her movements can become more graceful and controlled.

Will your baby be left-handed or right-handed?

Some of your baby's earliest movements are single, independent arm movements, which appear around week 10. At this time, about 90 percent of babies

DID YOU KNOW...

Your baby practices breathing Your baby can't breathe air in her fluid-filled uterine environment— the oxygen that she needs for life is transferred from your bloodstream into hers via the placenta. However, she'll make regular and rhythmic breathing movements with her diaphragm and rib cage from around 9 weeks; by around 30 weeks, she is "breathing" about 30 percent of the time. These movements are essential for developing the physical structure of your baby's lungs, and they are the beginnings of the automatic reflex that will be essential for survival in an air environment.

move their right arms more, while the remaining 10 percent prefer to move their left arms—the same proportion as for adults. This preference remains throughout pregnancy—right-handed babies at 10 weeks are still right-handed at 36 weeks—and statistics suggest that this preference lasts for life.

It used to be thought that the differences in structure between the left and right halves of the brain caused the individual to be left or right handed, but this preference in your baby's movements occurs before the two halves of her brain develop any differences. It may well be that by choosing to move her left or right arm, your baby actually causes the differences in brain structure between the two halves of the brain. In other words her physical movement could be shaping her brain.

WHAT YOU FEEL

Feeling your baby move for the first time is one of those unforgettable pregnancy milestones. If this is your first pregnancy, you may not feel any movement until 18 to 20 weeks, possibly as late as 24 weeks. These early movements will feel like flutterings or butterflies in your belly and you might even wonder if it's gas at first. If you've been pregnant before, you may be able to identify movements slightly earlier, as you'll have learned the signs from your first pregnancy.

A lot of what you feel depends on how quickly your baby grows, and, to make you aware of her presence, she needs to be big enough to nudge and poke at your insides. When you do feel movement, you're not actually feeling it on the lining of your

Patterns of sleep and dreaming

By 36 to 38 weeks your unborn baby's activity is well coordinated, with definite periods of activity and rest, and, just like a newborn, she spends much of the time asleep.

Research has shown that during some of this sleep, unborn babies exhibit rapid eye movement (REM), which in adults is an indication of dreaming. This has led some scientists to believe that babies could be dreaming in the uterus, consolidating their experiences of

the day. Perhaps your baby might be dreaming of stretching out her limbs, listening to your voice, or playing with her cord.

Research has indicated that your baby may spend much of her time in the following states:

Quiet sleep For about 40 percent of the time, your baby's almost inactive, moving only occasionally, as if she's sleeping.

Active sleep For about 42 percent of the time your baby seems to be

sleeping but also moving and making some random, sweeping gestures with her limbs, perhaps while she's dreaming.

Active awake Your baby moves around most vigorously in this active awake state—and you'll notice it. Although it occurs only about 10 percent of the time, it usually happens at night when you're trying to sleep.

Quiet awake For about 2 to 3 percent of the time, your unborn baby doesn't move her body much, but her eyes move constantly. This is similar to the way that newborns behave when they're quiet but appear to be paying attention to what's going on.

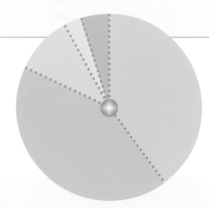

- QUIET SLEEP
- QUIET AWAKE
- ACTIVE SLEEP
- ACTIVE AWAKE
- CHANGING STATE

uterus, as the uterus doesn't contain the necessary sensory receptors. But when your baby kicks, the uterus is knocked against muscles or organs such as the abdominal wall or bladder, and this is what provides the sensation of movement. The position of your placenta can influence this sensation. If your placenta is on the front of your uterus rather than at the back, you probably won't feel the movements of your baby as much.

MORE **ABOUT** | shared emotions

Recent studies have looked at whether your emotions affect your baby's behavior. Researchers in Italy observed mothers who had been shocked by an earthquake and found that their unborn babies were more active. An Australian study found that unborn babies were much more active while their mothers were watching an emotional movie than when they were watching a more neutral one. The greater the mothers' emotional reactions, the greater the babies' responses. This isn't a "psychic" link, however, it's simply a reaction to the chemicals that your body releases into your bloodstream as your moods change. These mood swings won't harm your baby, but you might like to try some relaxation techniques (see page 124) to keep your own emotions calm and your baby's world steady.

LATER MOVEMENTS

As your baby gets larger, she won't move so often, but you'll feel it more distinctly when she does. In late pregnancy, you may feel quite strong kicks to the ribs and bladder as your baby makes her presence felt. Although this reduction in activity is partly due to your baby's increasing size, it also occurs because more refined movements are required to strengthen and develop the nerve connections in your baby's neurological system.

Patterns of activity

You might notice that your baby becomes more active in response to food you've eaten—sugary food will give your baby a hit of energy resulting in a burst of movement—or to your emotions (see box, above), or simply to get comfortable when you change position. You'll probably feel her moving more at night when you're free from the distractions of the day and you're lying down, relaxed and quiet. Research has shown that unborn babies' level of activity tends to peak around midnight, possibly foreshadowing the periods of sleep and wakefulness they will exhibit as a newborn.

Learning a sense of self

Movement also teaches your baby a sense of self, an understanding of herself as a separate entity. Through her own movements—and yours as well— plus the restrictions of her uterine environment, your baby gains a sense of what the various parts of her body are, how they're connected, and where her body starts and finishes.

We all need to know where our limbs are at any particular time. To pick up a cup, for example, we need to know the position of our arm and hand, the position of the cup and how to move our hand from its current position to the cup. For your baby, the very act of brushing a leg against the walls of the uterus, for instance, floods her system with vital information. Every movement activates sensory pathways and fuels a growing sense of self.

It's also believed that babies learn a sense of where they are in space. By about 25 weeks, most babies show a "righting reflex," which enables them to adopt a head-down position in the uterus. Your baby will also experience gravity in her watery world. As you move around, your baby experiences this motion, so she goes through something of a roller-coaster ride as you go about your business in the world. Sitting, lying down, walking, running, and bending over—everything you do will be experienced by your baby.

THE BIRTH INSTIGATOR

The processes leading up to the birth are a carefully choreographed set of interactions between you and your baby. Almost like the most graceful of waltzes, your and your baby's bodies respond to each other to ensure that each step carefully follows the preceding one.

A variety of studies on animals and humans have found that it's your baby who first indicates that he's ready to be born, probably about three to four weeks before labor begins. Exactly how your baby "knows" when it's time is a mystery, but the events that follow are better understood.

GETTING READY FOR BIRTH

Before he's born your baby needs to be sufficiently mature to be able to survive outside his uterine environment. In the uterus, he has relied on you to provide oxygen and nutrients, and to deal with waste, but as soon as he's born, his own body will have to take control of these vital functions. So, once your baby's body is mature enough, his brain sends hormone signals to the placenta to produce enzymes that will help his vital organs mature and then stimulate labor.

A chemical reaction

Research has shown that as the time of birth approaches, your baby's brain stimulates his pituitary gland to release the chemical adrenocorticotrophin (ACTH), which, in turn, stimulates the release of another chemical, cortisol. These chemicals are passed from your baby's body to the placenta, which reacts by converting progesterone into estrogen. This is a significant stage, because progesterone is the hormone that keeps your powerful uterine muscles from contracting during earlier pregnancy, whereas estrogen is responsible for triggering birth contractions. You may notice this change in hormone levels as a tightening in your uterus in the days before you go into labor.

As your baby's head presses against your cervix, a signal is sent to your brain to stimulate your pituitary gland to release the hormone oxytocin. Oxytocin stimulates the muscles of your uterus to contract, forcing your baby's head farther into your cervix and so continuing the cycle of contractions. Moreover, oxytocin stimulates the release of chemicals called prostaglandins into the bloodstream, and these intensify uterine muscle contractions. This self-perpetuating process escalates during labor, becoming more forceful and eventually resulting in the birth of your baby. It's an astounding, incredible process, with you and your baby working in perfect harmony with each other.

Preparing the birth canal

Your cervix also has to undergo changes in order to facilitate your baby's birth. Up until birth, the fibrous, tendon-like tissues of the cervix have kept your uterus tightly closed. For birth to happen according to plan, the cervix must soften and dilate, enabling the muscle contractions of the uterus to propel your baby down the birth canal.

Approximately three to four weeks before birth, as the placenta produces more estrogen, your cervix begins to loosen and soften in preparation for birth. Finally, when labor begins, your cervix changes dramatically, becoming much thinner and shorter and dilating (opening out) to enable your baby to be born. Again, the chemical signals sent out by your baby seem to be responsible for starting this process.

These hormonal changes also stimulate your breasts to prepare for the production of milk to feed your newborn baby—a process rounded off when your baby begins to suck at your breast.

8

CHAPTER

MANAGING YOUR EMOTIONS AND INTIMACY

If you have mixed feelings about your changing

body, are worried about the impending birth, or feel

overwhelmed with the idea of becoming a parent,

then you're certainly not alone—these are natural

responses to pregnancy. Don't worry though. You'll

be able to cope.

YOUR RESPONSE TO PREGNANCY

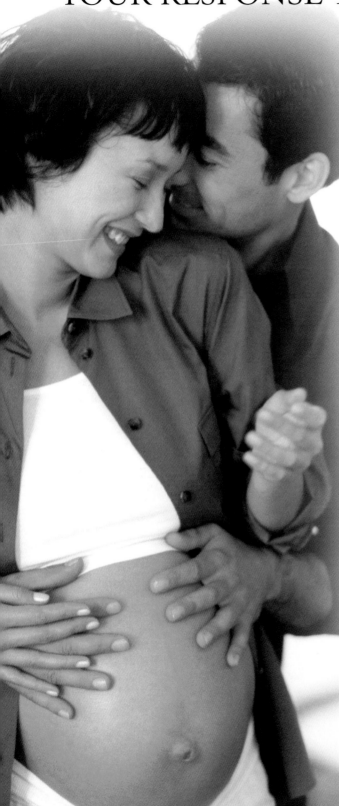

It's partly due to your hormones, partly to the huge physical and emotional adjustment you need to make, but your emotions can run riot during pregnancy, affecting every aspect of your life.

When you first discover that you're pregnant, you might feel sheer delight that you're having a longed-for baby, a sense of triumph that you're fertile, or tender closeness with your partner, since it was your physical union that created this baby. Alternatively, pregnancy may loom as an enormous problem; if you don't feel ready for a baby, your natural response may be anxiety or even panic.

EARLY REACTIONS

Even if you've known for a while that you wanted a baby, it's absolutely natural for some less positive feelings to creep into the picture: You may feel that it's happening too quickly; you may feel trapped; you may wonder how your body will cope with being pregnant, and feel frightened about the birth; or you may be overwhelmed by the sense of lifelong responsibility for another human being.

Initially, your emotions may be working overtime to process all the changes that are taking place, but over the following weeks, some of this turbulence simmers down. Like many women, you may gain a new respect for your body, and even if early discomfort threatens to undermine this satisfaction, you'll probably be amazed by the work your body is doing to grow a new life. If this is your first pregnancy, you might be feeling grown up in a new way—you're joining the community of mothers.

ADAPTING TO CHANGES

The waiting period before your baby's arrival can sometimes seem like forever, but these nine months provide time for you to adjust to the huge changes that are taking place—not only will you be getting used to the effects on your body (see page 151), but also adapting to an altered lifestyle. Suddenly you might feel that it's more important to take care of your safety in order to protect the tiny human being within you. You may find that you drive more cautiously and take greater care to avoid accidents. You'll probably make changes in your eating habits, limit your alcohol, or give up smoking. Even your social life might alter.

Such changes in the way you think and act can make you feel like quite a different person—a sensation that's intensified if you give up work and can no longer define yourself by your career but don't yet consider yourself to be a mother. You may find it easier to take on this new aspect of your identity if you spend time daydreaming and visualizing yourself with your new baby. Also, consider keeping a diary to help you work out your changing moods.

Respect your body

Pregnancy is a time of continuous physical changes. Some of these changes are expected and visible to the outside world, such as the enlargement of your breasts and the filling out of your abdomen, while others are less visible and may be unexpected, such as your hair becoming a little greasy or your feet swelling.

Emotional reactions to pregnancy are highly individual and unpredictable, but it's almost impossible not to have a strong reaction to your changing appearance—you may love your new look or hate feeling bulky.

Some women who are conscious of their figures feel disturbed by their increasing size during pregnancy. If you begin to feel like this, try not to feel embarrassed about your abdomen: You aren't getting fat, you're growing a baby—a physical task that draws continuously on your energy and on every system of your body.

Accept your new image

As the months go by, you'll come to terms with your changing shape. At first, you may feel frustrated that there's nothing to see. In the second or third month, as your clothes begin to feel tight, you may experience impatience, because you're no longer the

MORE **ABOUT** | the effect of hormones

The hormones estrogen and progesterone play a vital role in orchestrating all the physical changes needed to initiate and maintain a pregnancy (see page 60), but they also have a profound effect on your emotions. Hormones can cause some women to experience a newfound serenity, their focus turning inward to form a protective cocoon around their babies. Other women experience a roller coaster of emotions: sadness turning into floods of tears; a new sensitivity to the sufferings of others; and joy so intense that it, too, spills over into tears. It can be difficult to judge whether these ups and downs are due to your hormones or simply an emotional response to your new lifestyle. But whatever happens, accept that for the next nine months, you may be less in control of your emotions than usual. It's as if your hormones are opening up the emotional part of your psyche and preparing you to be receptive to your newborn baby.

shape you were, but neither are you recognizably pregnant. Around the fourth month, you'll probably be relieved that your protruding abdomen is clearly visible. With your pregnancy public knowledge, you may find that people openly scrutinize your shape or even want to touch your belly. Some women resent the invasion of their personal space; others enjoy people's involvement. In the later months, you may hardly believe that your body can go on growing and that your abdomen is so firm. You may feel unwieldy and be inwardly shocked by the struggle of getting out of an armchair. This is the time to take it easy and to look forward to meeting your new baby.

Acknowledge your worries

It's difficult to be completely relaxed all the time about the well-being of your baby, even if you have no rational reason for concern. You may worry about miscarriage during the early months (see page 278), particularly if you have miscarried before. In these instances, it's perfectly natural to feel anxious until you're safely past the date at which your other baby was lost. Hard though it might be, try to stay relaxed and trust your body.

It can be tremendously exciting to see your tiny but complete baby moving around or sucking his thumb during an ultrasound scan, but prenatal testing (see page 236) is a common source of worry for expectant parents. Even though it's designed to provide reassuring information, testing can prompt new anxieties. Keep in mind that testing is designed to detect problems early so that your baby has the best chance of being born healthy. But if you feel pressured about taking a particular test, make sure you discuss your need for it with your doctor.

If any problems are picked up during testing, try to stay positive. If you are told, for example, that your baby has a one-in-ten chance of developing Down syndrome (see page 249), turn the statistic around—your baby has a nine-in-ten chance of not being born with Down syndrome.

You may have concerns, too, about the impact of your lifestyle on your unborn baby. The damaging effects of smoking, alcohol, and exposure to other hazards (see page 75) are widely publicized. The best way to limit your anxiety is to adjust your lifestyle so that it provides a healthier environment for your growing baby. If you think that you've taken any risks—for example, if, like many women, you believe you were drinking too much before you discovered that you were pregnant, tell your healthcare provider; he or she will probably be able to discuss any possible risks and provide reassurance.

5 ways to quell anxiety

1   Talk to other expectant parents. Most are keen to share their feelings and experiences with others, and many join prenatal classes primarily for this reason (see page 172).

2   Try to find a prenatal teacher who puts a high priority on discussion and support. You shouldn't feel that you have to know everything, nor should you be afraid to ask questions—that's what your teacher is there for.

3   Read up as much as you can about pregnancy. The more informed you are, the more in control you'll feel and, consequently, less worried.

4   Visit your healthcare provider. If you have any symptoms that worry you, don't put off going for fear that something is really wrong. It will probably be nothing, but it's best to put your mind at rest.

5   Remember, while our awareness of potential problems is greater than ever, there's never been a safer time to have a baby. Medicine and society haven't eliminated all problems, but for healthy women who receive good prenatal care the outlook for their babies is excellent.

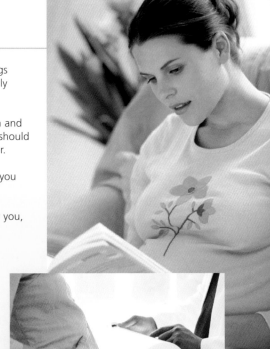

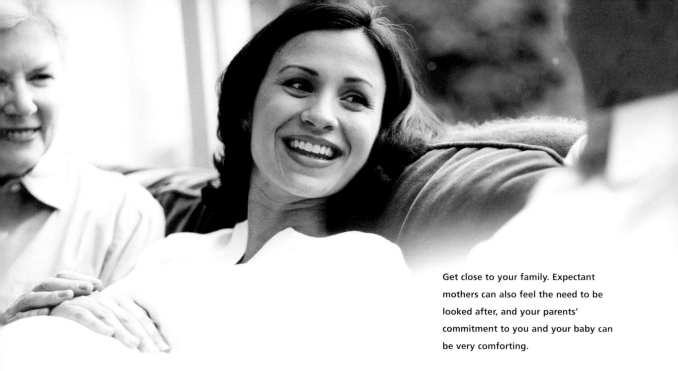

Get close to your family. Expectant mothers can also feel the need to be looked after, and your parents' commitment to you and your baby can be very comforting.

THINKING ABOUT PARENTING

You may anticipate parenthood with confidence, or you may feel distinctly nervous about this untried role. If marriage or moving in with your partner seemed a huge step, the addition of a baby is an even more momentous change.

It takes time for an individual to grow into a parent. Being a good mother or father certainly doesn't happen as soon as your baby is born. Pregnancy, besides being a period of waiting, is a time of preparation for parenthood. Talk to other parents, and use every opportunity to get close to newborns. The best way to learn is by hands-on experience, so ask to babysit for a friend and practice holding, changing, and playing with a baby. Your friend may be kind enough to return the favor after your baby is born, when you need a break.

Look to your relatives and friends

Pregnancy often brings women closer to their parents, in-laws, and siblings. You may feel a need to ask your mother how you were born or to look through baby photos of your partner for clues as to how your baby will look. Families often give much needed support during pregnancy, particularly if you don't have a partner around to help (see page 154).

However, if you're going through pregnancy without the support of your own mother, you may find yourself feeling a particular kind of loneliness. If this leaves a gap in your life, an aunt or a friend who is a mother will probably be happy to be there for you. In addition, you may be able to find a self-help organization in your area or on the Internet.

At this time, you also might find yourself thinking back to your upbringing: Which aspects of your childhood do you want to replicate for your child and which would you rather not repeat? Experts believe that open and trusting discussion with your partner about how you were each brought up helps replace negative patterns with positive ones. Consider how the expectations you and your partner bring from your family backgrounds can be meshed into a cohesive philosophy of parenting. But, keep in mind that it's impossible to work out a complete strategy before your baby puts in his appearance—part of the fulfillment of parenthood is learning from new situations and from your child himself.

Expecting a second baby

If this is your second pregnancy you will have learned a lot. However, there are extra considerations when having a second child. Most mothers find that

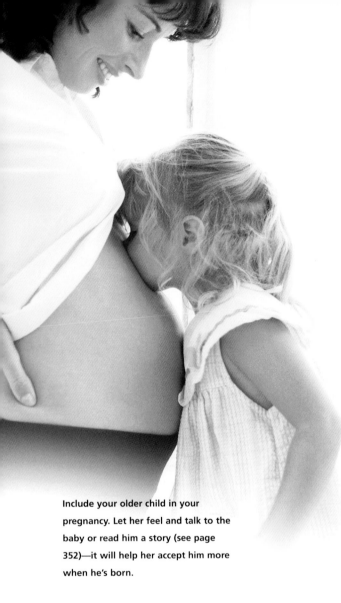

they're a lot more tired during the second pregnancy, as they have a child to look after at the same time. There are also the practicalities of caring for two children—two require extra work and extra expense.

Some parents expecting their second child worry about whether they'll love their new baby as much as their first. It can seem almost like a betrayal to bring another baby onto the scene. However, once the baby is born, parents are surprised to discover in themselves a new fount of love for the youngest member of the family.

Your older child may feel insecure when she realizes that there's another child on the way, so make time to prepare her for the new arrival. She might, for example, be secretly afraid that you'll have less time for her, that you might not love her as much, or even that the baby might have to sleep in her bed. These fears are very real in the mind of a child, so talk to her as soon as your pregnancy is noticeable. Calmly explain that she'll soon have a new baby brother or sister who will love her very much. Give her lots of cuddles and smiles so that she adopts a positive attitude, too.

Include your older child in your pregnancy. Let her feel and talk to the baby or read him a story (see page 352)—it will help her accept him more when he's born.

HOW TO face pregnancy alone

Whether or not your pregnancy was planned, facing pregnancy on your own can be very hard—and the prospect of having sole responsibility for a baby overwhelming. The absence of a partner to share in the care and decision-making can leave you feeling isolated and lonely. This is why it's vital to enlist as much support as you can. Many single mothers find that their families prove to be enormously supportive. Indeed, a baby can positively benefit from growing up in the protective, loving environment of an extended family.

If you don't have a family to fall back on, local or Internet-based self-help organizations can put you in touch with other single parents and provide emotional and practical support. You'll probably need to draw on other people not only for friendship, but also to be with you throughout labor and, later on, to provide you with some adult company and occasional time off from caring for your baby.

YOU AND YOUR PARTNER

Pregnancy should be seen as a great opportunity to strengthen the bond between you and your partner. Adjusting to the changes that pregnancy makes to your life together will prepare you for the challenges of parenthood.

The arrival of a first child is a major milestone in the life of any couple. Until this time, your partner has probably been the person you put first in your life, and you no doubt spend a lot of time solely in each other's company. At the moment, you may lead roughly parallel existences—both going out to work, contributing to the income, sharing the tasks, and decorating your home together. Evenings are times for unwinding, talking over your day, and enjoying the support you get from each other. It's easy to go out for a meal on the spur of the moment or to meet up with friends in a bar.

Nearly every aspect of this lifestyle is likely to be affected by the arrival of your baby, and some of the changes begin during pregnancy. You may already have noticed that your roles are diverging—perhaps, to your surprise, developing into male and female stereotypes. As pregnancy advances, a woman is less able to do heavy physical work, so it falls to her partner. She stops work, becomes more home-based, and may take over more of the cooking or household chores. You may both enjoy this change, but equally, you might find it difficult to adjust to some aspects of this development.

Other changes are on the horizon or nudging their way into view. Does your baby make you and your partner feel closer together than ever, or does she seem an intruder on your intimacy as a couple? Is becoming a parent going to involve some losses as well as gains? It's easy to share happy thoughts about pregnancy, but are you also making time to explore your negative feelings? By discussing these things, you'll enhance your mutual understanding and develop the trust and openness that will help you cope with being parents together.

CHANGES TO YOUR SEX LIFE

Pregnancy almost inevitably affects the sex life of a couple—changes that can be both negative and positive. There are physical and psychological factors at play, and a woman's responses can be very different to those of her partner.

Is it safe?

A lot of couples worry that making love during pregnancy will harm the baby. Some parents fear that sex might cause an infection in the uterus or their baby, but unless one partner has a sexually transmitted disease, there is no possibility of this happening—the baby is protected by the mucous plug sealing the cervix as well as by the amniotic sac. In most cases, there is no risk to the unborn baby when her parents make love. The few exceptions are listed in the box, below.

You can, however, make sex more comfortable and manageable with a few precautions. After the fourth month of pregnancy it's not a good idea to spend too much time lying on your back and you

---

SAFETY FIRST

Miscarriage and preterm delivery Although there is no evidence that sexual activity is a cause of miscarriage, if you have a history of miscarriages, you may be advised to avoid penetrative sex until you are beyond the danger period (see page 278). Likewise, if you've previously had a premature delivery, or are experiencing signs of early labor, it may be suggested that you avoid sex in the last trimester, as it could trigger the onset of labor (see page 208). You should also avoid sex in late pregnancy if your membranes have broken or if you have any bleeding (see page 275).

may well find this position uncomfortable when making love. But this shouldn't be a problem, as the process of finding alternatives can be fun (see box, below). You may want also to make love gently so consider using a lubricant to avoid the possibility of abrasions and soreness in your extra-sensitive vagina.

Sex can be better

In the early weeks of pregnancy, nausea and extreme tiredness can mean that sex is the last thing on your mind. Bed is for one thing only: sleep. As this stage wears off, however, you may enjoy a new liberation in your lovemaking, as there's no longer pressure to become pregnant or any need for birth control. What's more, the emotional closeness that you feel can lead to particularly tender, loving sex.

The physical changes associated with pregnancy also can intensify the sensations of sex: Your breasts and nipples may become more sensitive; the extra blood and fluids circulating in your body suffuse the vaginal tissues, making them more sensitive; and the pregnancy hormones promote extra lubrication to the vagina. These changes in your body also can enhance your partner's enjoyment of sex; for example, the engorged tissues of your vagina will grip his penis more tightly.

Some pregnant women describe being in an almost constant state of arousal, particularly in the middle three months (see page 27), and many women experience more intense orgasms than before they became pregnant, with the vaginal tissues remaining swollen long after orgasm. This may mean, however, that you can feel somewhat unsatisfied after sex—a sensation that can be eased with masturbation.

It's possible that your unborn baby benefits from your lovemaking, although this theory is difficult to prove. What is more certain is that such activity is likely to make you feel happy, loved, and relaxed—feelings that are passed onto your baby. You may

Comfortable lovemaking

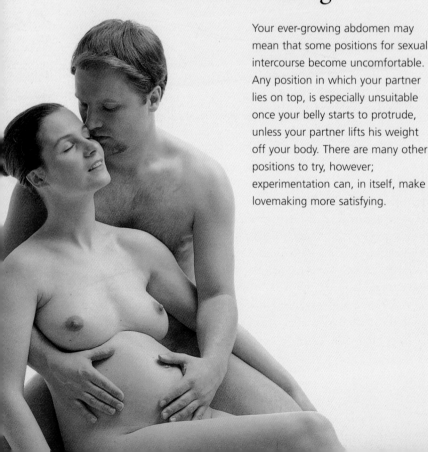

Your ever-growing abdomen may mean that some positions for sexual intercourse become uncomfortable. Any position in which your partner lies on top, is especially unsuitable once your belly starts to protrude, unless your partner lifts his weight off your body. There are many other positions to try, however; experimentation can, in itself, make lovemaking more satisfying.

Woman on top This involves you positioning yourself astride your partner either on your knees or squatting. Take your weight on your arms rather than your belly. As your abdomen grows, you might find squatting rather than lying on your partner more comfortable.

Sitting down Your partner sits on a sturdy chair or on the side of the bed and you sit astride him, either facing him or facing the other way. In this position, you can control the depth of penetration, while his arms are free to caress you.

notice that she seems to respond to your lovemaking, either by becoming more lively or by calming down. But your baby's reactions are nothing to do with your lovemaking, they are responses solely to hormonal and uterine activity.

Sex can be worse

Pregnancy doesn't always mean satisfying and carefree sex, however. You might feel uncomfortable, tired, or so dislike your new shape, that you don't feel at all sexy. If your breasts are tender, particularly in early and late pregnancy, you might prefer that your partner doesn't touch them. Be prepared also that, late in pregnancy, your breasts may leak colostrum (see page 298) if they are stimulated, which you or your partner might find off-putting.

In turn, your partner may feel daunted by your changing shape or anxious about hurting you or your baby. He also might start to see you more as a mother figure than a lover, and this could disturb

his usual response. Some men are put off sex by the very proximity of their babies, who seem to be "witnessing" the whole performance. Be assured, however, that your baby will have no memory of you making love while she's in the uterus.

It's all too possible in pregnancy for one partner to feel rejected by the other—not because there's less love between you, but because the usual patterns of expressing it are disturbed. If you feel turned off sex for any reason, it's important to talk about it, to be specific about what has changed for you, but also to express all the positive feelings that are unchanged. It may be that what you both need is simply reassurance of each other's love and commitment.

Other ways of showing affection

Sex doesn't have to mean full intercourse. If you prefer to avoid penetrative sex, then you could try extended foreplay. If your partner is masturbating you, he should use a lubricant—saliva, if nothing

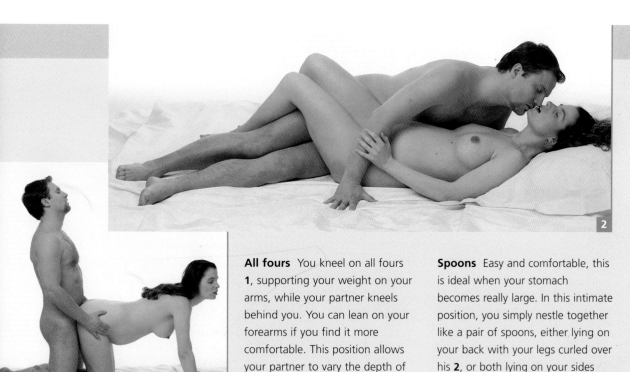

All fours You kneel on all fours **1**, supporting your weight on your arms, while your partner kneels behind you. You can lean on your forearms if you find it more comfortable. This position allows your partner to vary the depth of penetration and gives him great freedom of movement.

Spoons Easy and comfortable, this is ideal when your stomach becomes really large. In this intimate position, you simply nestle together like a pair of spoons, either lying on your back with your legs curled over his **2**, or both lying on your sides with your legs bent. Your partner enters your vagina from behind.

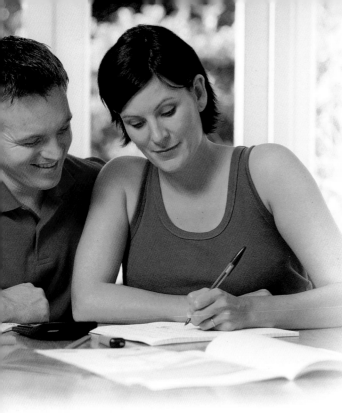

Sit down with your partner and work out your budget. If you haven't done so already, start cutting down on luxuries and putting away the money you save.

else—to avoid causing abrasion. Your partner should be aware, too, that your vaginal secretions may taste stronger during oral sex. He should also take care not to blow into your vagina, as there is a small risk that this can lead to an embolism (a small air bubble in a blood vessel).

Pregnancy is a great opportunity to explore other ways of enjoying intimacy; you can express your feelings with simple kisses, cuddles, and stroking, or you might decide to share a bath together. Massage is a welcome luxury when you're pregnant, especially if you're feeling uncomfortable and finding it difficult to relax (see page 126).

CHANGES TO FINANCES

Apart from sex, another area of potential change can be in your family income. The impending arrival of a new baby might mean a reduction in money coming in—you or your partner may have to give up work, and it will inevitably entail some new expenses. It's worth thinking ahead about the impact of these financial changes before they hit home.

Consider your income

One of the important things to think about is how early or late you plan to leave work, but keep in mind this might be affected by health circumstances beyond your control. Also, you might want to weigh up a loss of income during your maternity leave against any benefits you might receive.

Although it's a long way off, there's no harm in researching your options for returning to work—when the time comes, you'll be able to make an informed decision. You could compare the costs of childcare to the money you'll get from working or think about possible alternatives to full-time work (see page 193).

Be creative with your savings

You don't need to spend a fortune on your new baby. Decorating her room may be a labor of love, but you don't have to break your back or your bank account to do it. Your baby's needs in this respect are modest. While she does need love, attention, and stimulation, she's not too bothered about a super-smart nursery. If you have the time and can resist the temptations of catalogs and shops, consider the secondhand market in baby clothes and equipment (see page 195). Most items are outgrown rather than worn out, so it's quite possible to set up your baby's nursery and wardrobe with almost-new items. Contact local parenting organizations to find out if they run any sales in your area. However, certain items, such as car seats and crib mattresses, you should always buy new (see page 197).

MINIMIZING LABOR WORRIES

At some stage in your pregnancy, the inevitability of giving birth will suddenly strike you, and you may well have qualms about how you will cope with the challenge.

Excitement, fear, anticipation, bewilderment, and uncertainty about recognizing the start of labor—all these emotions and more will probably fill your mind in your last trimester, as your due date looms. Childbirth is always a journey into the unknown and this is particularly true of first births. But, however many babies you have, there is always an element of unpredictability about how this particular delivery will go.

All women experience a mixture of feelings when approaching labor and delivery, but some women can draw on a lot more confidence in the face of this challenge than others. Your confidence will be influenced by a number of factors:

- Your past experience of coping with any particularly stressful events.
- Your trust in your own body and the process of childbirth itself.
- The extent of your knowledge about what childbirth involves.
- The love and support of those close to you.
- The respect and encouragement of all your healthcare providers.

Dreaming your fears

Many women experience unusually vivid dreams during pregnancy and it's possible that these are caused by hormone changes. Dreams often feature the forthcoming labor or the baby himself, and can be so vivid that they disturb your sleep patterns and are difficult to forget about.

The following common dreams bring certain fears to light. You may dream that:

- The pregnancy isn't real and that you will give birth to nothing, or simply deflate.
- You give birth to a baby animal, or even some mundane household object.
- Your baby is damaged or deformed in some way.

Such nightmare-like dreams can be disconcerting, if not plain upsetting. They do, however, allow you to express anxieties that are normally suppressed during waking hours. Such fears may stem from the fact that, despite prenatal scans and examinations, the human being growing inside you is a shadowy figure, not fully seen or known.

If you're prone to disturbing dreams, try to spend some time daydreaming about your baby in a positive way, imagining yourself holding him, thinking about names, or picturing him in his crib. Experts agree that this is an excellent way to "practice" relating to your baby. Compare your dreams with those of other pregnant women—discussing what they may mean might help relieve your anxieties.

THE KEY TO DREAMS
Some common themes and what they might refer to:

- Sex in a positive or negative light: normal sexual confusion during pregnancy.
- Loss and forgetfulness: fear of the responsibility of motherhood.
- Pain and hurt: a sense of vulnerability.
- Being trapped: concerns about loss of freedom.
- Losing your partner: worry about your body image.
- Dramatic changes in weight: concerns about your diet.

WILL YOU MANAGE THE PAIN?

A good prenatal teacher won't have concealed the fact that labor is a physically intense experience, and that it can range from discomfort to excruciating pain. Strong messages about labor come from other sources, too, and these can influence your expectations, for example listening to the birth experiences within your circle of family and friends. However, your prenatal teacher will have provided you also with skills to ease the pain—such as relaxation, breathing, massage, and mobility (see page 218)—and should have helped to reinforce your confidence in your ability to give birth.

If you're worried about the pain, or you are concerned about your ability to cope when the time comes, think now about the pain-relief options that you have (see page 178). The way that you envisage labor will affect your response to it, so you might find it comforting to practice visualization techniques. When you think about contractions, imagine the muscles of your uterus opening up your cervix. See in your mind's eye your baby moving down the birth canal and remind yourself that each contraction will take you a step closer to his birth. Remember, too, that it's easier to cope with pain when it's a sign that the body is simply working naturally and efficiently.

WILL YOU LOSE ALL CONTROL?

Many people feel inhibited about showing strong emotions in public, or even in private, so don't be surprised if you find yourself feeling uneasy about crying, shouting, or simply being helpless in the presence of others. Being in hospital, away from your home environment may add to your anxiety, particularly if this is your first baby, as you may have little real experience of the extent of your strength and inner resources.

It helps if you can accept the probability of some loss of emotional control. Many women find that making a noise during labor—groaning or grunting—helps release tension. You'll work more efficiently through childbirth if you can let yourself go, be in tune with your body, and almost forget about the people around you.

A messy business

Some women say that dignity goes out of the window during birth, and first-time mothers particularly worry about losing physical control. You'll certainly have no control over loss of amniotic fluid. At the height of contractions you may have less control over your bowels and may even vomit. Your genital area is exposed and indeed is the focus of attention. However, keep in mind that all these aspects of birth have been experienced by women throughout the centuries. Your healthcare providers will not only have seen it all before, but they will be too focused on your well-being and that of your baby to think about anything else. Moreover, you'll probably find that any personal embarrassment disappears as you concentrate on the intense physicality of your task, and you'll be filled with wonder at the miracle of bringing your baby into the world. If you're particularly worried about the physical exposure of labor, however, talk to your healthcare providers, who will guide you through the process gently and sensitively.

MAKING THE GRADE

There's a tendency among women in their first pregnancies to perceive labor as a test in which some women meet the standard and others don't—for instance, if a woman had planned for a drug-free delivery, but later decided that she needed an epidural, she may feel that she was weak in some way. But there's nothing standard about childbirth—a woman can't know what cards nature will deal her, nor what the experience is really like for other women. The important thing when you go into labor is that you feel supported by those around you and that you're able to interact positively with every challenge with which you're presented. Aim to allow all the emotions of the birth to sink in, so that you can look back and feel that you made the most of this incredible experience.

9

CHAPTER

PREGNANCY FOR DADS

Pregnancy is a partnership between two parents

working together for a baby. For a dad, this is the

time to support your partner, emotionally,

financially, and physically and to develop a

relationship with the new life you've helped create.

NEW TO FATHERHOOD

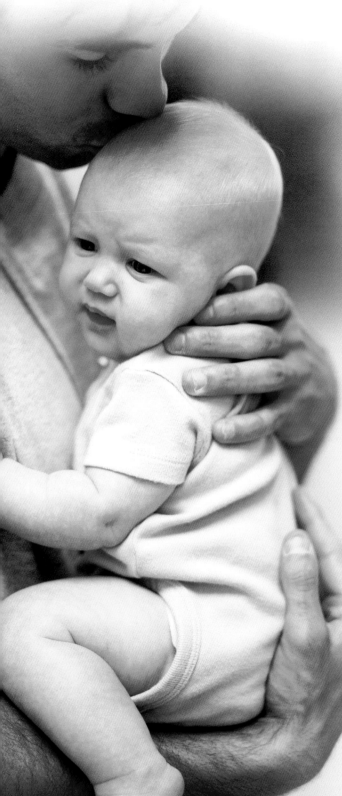

Finding out you're going to become a father can evoke a mixture of emotions. You'll probably feel delight, pride, and a sense of fulfillment, but it is also quite natural for your happiness to be tinged with some uncertainty as you confront the reality that a tiny person, who is part of you, is on her way into the world.

Your feelings about becoming a father may well be influenced by past and present circumstances. If you are in a warm and loving relationship with your partner; if you've had previous good experience with babies; if the pregnancy was planned or desired; if you had a happy childhood yourself; and if your lifestyle and financial status can accommodate a child, you are likely to have a positive outlook on pregnancy and fatherhood. If some of these factors are missing, it is quite natural for you to feel some trepidation about the future. However, you should bear in mind that becoming a father is one of the most momentous events in your life. Whatever your situation, your life will never be the same again, so don't be too surprised if you find yourself feeling ambivalent about fatherhood some of the time and elated at others.

TACKLING YOUR WORRIES

It's always best to acknowledge any concerns you have rather than bottle them up, and if this is your first baby, you're likely to have a few anxieties. As pregnancy advances, your emotions may alter, just as your partner's will, and you'll have to come to terms with changing feelings about your partner and your new baby. If you're finding it difficult to cope with the way you are feeling, discuss your anxiety openly with your partner.

Dealing with unexpected news

If this pregnancy wasn't planned, you might still be reeling from the shock. Contraception, whatever method you use, isn't infallible, and accidents do happen. If you've been taken by surprise, you may feel frustrated or even angry about the situation in which you suddenly find yourself, particularly if you're not in a serious relationship with your baby's mother. But take time to let the news sink in, and trust that you can still have a deep, lifelong relationship with your child, even without a similar commitment to her mother—and the best time for that relationship to begin is during pregnancy.

Feeling left out

Most fathers feel excluded at one time or another during pregnancy, so you're not alone if you find yourself becoming a little jealous of your unborn baby. From early on, you could feel that you're taking second place to an extremely demanding newcomer. You also might feel that your partner's family, friends, and even her doctors are taking over your usual protective role and that there's no space for you. But don't feel pushed out and withdraw into the background. Try explaining what you're going through to your partner. Be careful not to

demand too much of her, though—she's already receiving an emotional crash course in dependency from the baby growing inside her.

If you find it difficult to overcome your sense of alienation, consider discussing your feelings with a close friend, family doctor, or professional therapist. Also, there may be a group for fathers-to-be in your area where you can talk to men in the same position as you—your local doctor or library should be able to provide you with details or you could try searching on the Internet.

Often, the best way to tackle worries about feeling left out is to throw yourself into the idea of becoming a parent. Fathers today have plenty of opportunities to be directly involved in their partner's pregnancy, and there are many things you can do to join in (see box, below). Immerse yourself in this exciting time with your partner—after all, you're both expecting this baby.

5 ways to share your partner's pregnancy

1 Attend prenatal check-ups. You'll learn more about what's happening to your partner and to your baby.

2 See your baby. Ultrasound scans will offer you exhilarating glimpses of your baby. Ask for pictures.

3 Listen to your baby. From about week 30, you can press your ear to your partner's belly and hear your baby's tiny heart beating.

4 Feel your baby moving. From five months into the pregnancy, you'll be able to feel your baby shifting position—you may even be able to identify tiny hands and feet.

5 Talk, read, and sing to your baby. She can hear your voice from within the uterus, so bond with her and entertain your partner in the process.

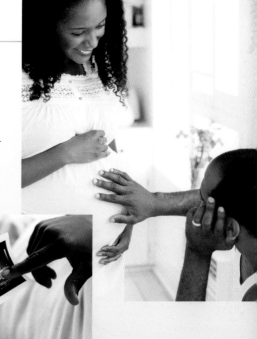

REDEFINING YOUR RELATIONSHIP

Gaining an understanding of your partner's changing body will help you appreciate how she is feeling. Remind yourself that while she's carrying your child, you have a key role to play too, part of which is adapting to her needs.

A sense of security will be vital to your partner at this time, and this will be influenced by the way you communicate. If you avoid intimacy and don't discuss your emotions, she may feel that she's on her own. But if you share your feelings, she is more likely to want to confide in you. Try to be sensitive, and encourage her to discuss her hopes and fears.

EXPECT CHANGES TO YOUR SEX LIFE

It's not uncommon for a man to be turned off by his partner's pregnant body. Often this is not so much due to physical changes, but anxieties the man has about the growing baby inside. If you find yourself losing interest in sex, it can help to find out more about what's happening to your partner physically, so that you become more at ease with the changes. Don't lose sight of the fact that after the birth, her body will begin to return to normal.

It's more likely, however, that you'll be turned on by your partner's softer curves and find the voluptuousness of pregnancy extremely sexy. This

Everyday help

Your relationship with your partner will be affected profoundly by how you handle these crucial nine months. It certainly will be a challenging experience, but if all goes well, you'll be closer than ever.

There is also ample evidence to suggest that if your partner is happy, relaxed, and relatively stress-free during pregnancy, your baby will experience long-term emotional and even physical benefits. What's

more, a supportive relationship between parents may make delivery less stressful, postpartum depression less likely (see page 328), and breastfeeding easier—and it should enable you both to bond with your baby more readily.

Aside from attending scans and medical check-ups, there is a wide range of everyday "services" you can provide to make your partner's life more comfortable.

Exercise together Join your partner in the pool or go for a brisk walk—getting in shape is a great way to spend time together and tone up both of your bodies.

Massage her As your baby grows, your partner may experience discomfort in her back, feet, and legs. A gentle massage can ease the

POSITIVE REINFORCEMENT

Just as you can help your partner by doing a few thoughtful things, you also can do a lot of good by avoiding some things:

- Cut down on smoking or smoke away from your partner. If she's a smoker, it helps her quit (see page 75), and it avoids the possibility of cigarette fumes "passively" filtering through to your baby.
- Reduce your alcohol intake. It will show your support at a time when your partner shouldn't drink in high quantities (see page 111).
- Avoid junk food, and eat healthily together. Choose from a selection of mouthwatering ideas on page 104.
- Resist pressure to go away on business or with friends during the last month of the pregnancy—some babies decide to arrive early.

may increase your desire for intercourse at a time when your partner's sexual drive is erratic. In this case, you will need to adapt to her needs and desires, which could mean finding new ways to express your feelings, such as through cuddling, kissing, massage, and non-penetrative sex (see page 155).

ENCOURAGE FAMILY SUPPORT

During the pregnancy, it's possible that you'll see more of your partner's mother than ever before. This is a time when the bond between mother and daughter is stronger than ever. Try to encourage this closeness, as your partner will need that special support. When your baby is born, your in-laws, as well as your own parents, will be anxious, no doubt, to get involved with the new family member. Try not to see their enthusiasm as interference—it's important that your child gets to know all his grandparents. By including them in your family life, you'll be doing far more than acquiring willing babysitters: You'll be offering your child the experience of another generation and encouraging him to develop a sense of respect for older people.

tension and it's a great way of showing you care. See page 126 for ideas on how to give her a relaxing massage.

Do the shopping Your partner should avoid lugging around heavy grocery bags, particularly in late pregnancy. She also may find walking supermarket aisles tiring, so, if you're not already doing the shopping, now's the time to start. Of course, if you do the cooking some of the time, that's something else she'll appreciate.

Get your baby's room ready
Your partner shouldn't be climbing ladders, so decorating your baby's room could be your job. Discuss color schemes together and then start painting. You also could help shop for baby clothes and

equipment (see page 195) so that the room is 100 percent ready for its new occupant.

Let your partner sleep late She needs more rest than before, so encourage her to get a few extra hours in the mornings. You could serve her breakfast in bed also—a thoughtful gesture that can ease morning sickness (see page 67).

Make time for prenatal classes
You'll not only be supporting your partner, but you will also learn a good deal yourself, particularly about the physical side of labor. Both you and your partner will gain a lot of confidence through meeting other parents-to-be.

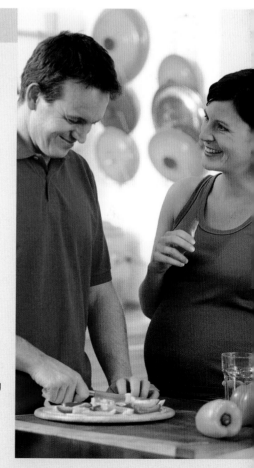

YOUR ROLE AT THE BIRTH

It's likely that you'll play the role of primary birth partner, which means that you'll need to be ready, alert, and, most important, available when her water breaks or contractions begin.

Until the 1970s, fathers were routinely banned from most delivery rooms, so they didn't have the opportunity to see their children's arrival into the world unless they opted for home births. Today, about 90 percent of fathers in the Western world are present at the births of their children.

PREPARE YOURSELF

If you and your partner decide that you'll be present at your baby's birth, you should have a clear idea of what to expect—although there are bound to be a few surprises. During the course of the pregnancy, you may have attended prenatal classes, had a tour of the hospital, and read a book or two on the subject, but when it comes down to the birth you may still find yourself shocked by the blood, mucus, excreta, moaning, and screaming involved. While most labors aren't particularly complicated, things

often don't go precisely as expected: The onset of labor seldom happens on the due date; there may be false alarms; it may be over within an hour, or last through the day, the night, and beyond. Events may not proceed in the order you anticipated, but keep a cool head, try to remain sensitive to your partner's needs and, if possible, retain your sense of humor—you're not her instructor but you're there to help her and share an unforgettable experience. There are few events in life that approach the joy of seeing your own child being born. Don't be surprised if you burst into tears when your baby finally arrives—and be sure to hold her as soon as possible.

Help create the birth plan

Fear, pain, and anxiety don't create the ideal environment for rational decisions, so it's a good idea to get to know your partner's birth plan (see page 185) well before the due date. You may eventually discard it, but the sense that things have been worked out beforehand will reassure you both as you prepare for labor. The birth plan should include details of how your partner hopes to handle her labor through to delivery. It will answer questions such as: Is she happy with a "normal" hospital birth or does she want a water birth or a form of active birthing (see page 174); what is her preferred birthing posture—perhaps on her back, squatting, or kneeling? It will also include details of what sort of pain relief she wants, if any. It should stress whether you both have objections to any methods of delivery, such as the use of forceps. You'll need to be fully versed in the details of the plan and make sure the birth attendants are familiar with it. You may have to adapt your birth

---

MORE **ABOUT** | sympathetic pregnancies

Some men become so emotionally involved in their partner's pregnancies and labors that they share certain physical symptoms. This is known as couvade—from the French word couver, *meaning "to hatch"—and is usually a sympathetic response that emerges from a man's extremely close identification with his partner. Men who experience couvade may gain weight, become constipated, and suffer from morning sickness. Occasionally a difficulty arises during labor when the father finds himself becoming more than usually distressed at the pain of childbirth, and even experiencing labor-type pains himself. If you find yourself suffering from such symptoms, you should seek professional advice.*

plan and make some on-the-spot decisions should anything unusual occur during labor or delivery—so listen to the professionals and heed their advice.

YOUR ROLE IN LABOR

There's plenty you can do to assist your partner during labor: holding and supporting her; massaging her lower back, neck, inner thighs, and feet; and reminding her of relaxation and breathing techniques. See page 182 for specific advice on how to help. Prenatal classes will provide further ideas.

Be prepared, however, that when the moment comes you may find that your partner wants something quite different. For instance, you may have been practicing patterned breathing together, only to find that all she really wants is for you to hold her hand or wipe her forehead with a cool cloth. Or, after the first contraction, you may find that she no longer wants to go natural and asks for an epidural injection instead. Don't discourage her if she does ask for pain relief—she's the one going through the pain and it's better for her and the baby if she's not distressed.

Be prepared, too, for the unexpected in your partner's emotional response. During the transition phase, for example, (see page 216) it's not uncommon for the surge of adrenalin and pain to prompt her into outbursts of the "get out—I never want to see you again" variety. In most cases, the best option is to ride it out without leaving her side. As the moment of the birth draws closer, you may find her suddenly expressing terror, and she will need you there for comfort and to reassure her about the options available. Try to be clearheaded, flexible, and sensitive to your partner's needs.

Will I be able to cope?

It's not at all unusual for men to worry that they'll feel faint or sick in the delivery room. Be reassured, however, that it's highly unlikely that either of these

7 things to remember

1   Book time off work. Four to six weeks before the due date, alert your employer to the impending birth and negotiate your parental leave (see page 170).

2   List your contacts. Compile a list of emergency telephone numbers, including your partner's caregivers and the hospital. Don't forget to list family and friends you'll want to call with the good news.

3   Within the final month, get to know the home birth midwife or visit the hospital so that you understand the techniques and machines used in labor and delivery rooms.

4   Keep talking. In the final three weeks before the birth, keep in regular contact with your partner when you're at work—it will reassure you both.

5   Secure the transportation arrangements. If you're using your own car, make sure that you keep the gas tank full and work out the most reliable route to the hospital. If you're using a cab, contact a reliable company and ensure that it is expecting your call.

6   Check, check, and recheck. Before leaving for the hospital, make sure that you have everything you need: your partner's hospital bags (see page 206), snacks for both of you, the birth plan, your list of phone numbers, and perhaps a cell phone.

7   Take charge. When you reach the hospital hand the birth plan to the birth attendants and explain it to them if they don't know it already.

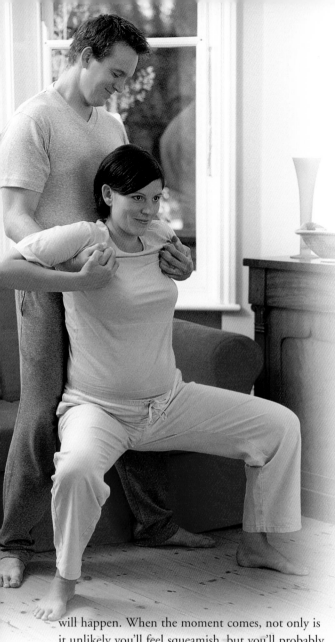

Practice birth positions together. If your partner wants to squat, for example, you will need to support her weight with your arms. Remember to try several alternatives (see page 220).

fathers. Remember, if there's anything you're unsure of during the birth, you can talk to the doctor or midwife. The more you understand, the better you'll be able to play your vital supporting role. However, if you're still concerned about how you'll cope, talk to your partner about the possibility of having a doula at the birth (see page 184). The doula will be able to support your partner, explain procedures to you both, and take some of the pressure off you.

If you're not planning to be at the birth

You may prefer not to be present at the birth: You may simply have no desire to be involved in the process, or there may be cultural reasons—men in some societies, for example, are traditionally excluded from the delivery room. Some men worry that witnessing a bloody vaginal delivery will make it difficult for them to see their partners in a sexual light afterward; others fear that the pain and mess will make them fall apart. If you don't want to be there when your baby physically arrives, you may consider being present to support your partner during labor, but withdrawing from the process during the birth. Not being at the birth shouldn't make any difference to the bond you have with your baby—you'll still experience the feeling of delight and fulfillment when you first set eyes on her.

On the other hand, some women prefer that their partners don't attend the birth, perhaps because they think they will feel inhibited by them. If your partner feels like this talk to her about her feelings and respect her wishes—it's not a reflection on you.

will happen. When the moment comes, not only is it unlikely you'll feel squeamish, but you'll probably be fascinated by the miracle of your baby's birth.

If you do feel you have to look away at any stage, focus on your partner's face and help her with her breathing—you'll probably find, however, that you can't resist watching. And don't worry if you need to step outside to get some air. Sit with your head between your knees until you're ready to return.

The best way to combat your fears is to find out as much as you can before the birth. Read all the books, visit the hospital labor and delivery rooms, attend prenatal classes together, and talk to other

How to deal with an emergency birth

It's extremely unlikely that your partner would have to give birth in the back of the car. Even if she does go into labor quickly, there's usually time to get help. However, for your peace of mind, here's how you can help your partner should medical help be unavailable:

Don't panic Call an ambulance, making sure that you tell the dispatcher the expected due date, the name of the hospital and any special medical needs.

Help her get comfortable
Reassure your partner and help her lie down on a bed or the floor, with her knees bent and apart.

Scrub up Wash your hands with soap and water—don't use disinfectant. Cover the area where she's going to have your baby with clean sheets or towels.

Tell her when to push Don't let your partner bear down until you can see your baby's head. Get her to pant or blow if she wants to push too soon. Only when your baby's head "crowns" (when it can be seen at the entrance of the vagina) should you tell your partner to push during each contraction for a count of ten.

Support your baby's head Rest your hand very gently on your baby's head so that it doesn't come out too quickly. Don't pull on her head; it will come out naturally.

Help your baby breathe As the head is delivered, hold it with your hands. Once it's free, ask your partner to stop pushing. If the umbilical cord is around your baby's neck, check that it's loose and gently hook it over her head. Clear any mucus from your baby's nose and mouth with the corner of a clean towel.

Deliver the rest of your baby
Put your hands either side of your baby's head and very gently direct it down toward the ground. Ask your partner to push at the same time, until the top shoulder comes out. Now direct your baby upward and support her head and shoulders as the rest of her body emerges, which should happen quite quickly. If your baby's shoulders are stuck at any stage, ask your partner to push hard—don't pull.

Drain any fluids Immediately after the birth, lay your baby across her mother's stomach, with her feet higher than her head, to drain any fluids from her mouth and nose.

Wrap up your baby Use clean towels or blankets to wrap her and lay her back on her mother's stomach. Don't wash her at all, and don't cut or pull the umbilical cord.

Deliver the placenta If an ambulance still hasn't arrived, your partner may have to push out the placenta. Once it's out, put it in a plastic bag. Gently massage your partner's stomach, just below the navel, to encourage the uterus to contract and stem the bleeding from the site of the placenta.

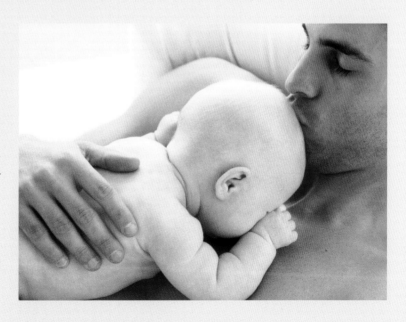

THINKING ABOUT THE FUTURE

Your baby will change you in ways that you could never anticipate. Not only will he depend on you for love, companionship, learning, discipline, life skills, and financial support, but for the rest of your life, you'll never stop caring about his well-being and trying to do your best for him. So it's worth thinking now about the kind of relationship you would like to have with your child.

CONSIDER PARENTAL LEAVE
A lot of fathers today take time off to develop a loving relationship with their child from the start. Many fathers in the United States are entitled to 12 weeks of unpaid paternity leave on the birth of a child, and some companies offer a period of paid leave. However, not all companies are covered by this law and employees need to meet certain requirements to be eligible. For full details, contact the US Department of Labor. In Canada, fathers who are eligible may take unpaid parental leave ranging from 12 to 52 weeks, but in some jurisdictions this period is shared between both parents. Again, some companies offer a period of paid leave. For full details, contact Human Resources Development Canada.

DID YOU KNOW...

Father-baby bonds are strong The Aka pygmy men, from the northern Congo in Central Africa, remain within arm's reach of their infants about 47 percent of the day, hold their babies close to their bodies for up to two hours a day, and sometimes provide their own nipples as pacifiers. And like most fathers, the more time they spend with their babies, the stronger the bond between them.

If you have the option of paid leave, take it; not only will it help you form a lasting relationship with your child, it will be a very good way of offering support to your partner in the crucial first weeks.

CHANGING NOTIONS OF FATHERHOOD
Nurturing was once considered the terrain of mothers, but today there is far more flexibility in the way men relate to their children and the kind of families into which children are born. For example, over one-third of children in the United States and around 10 percent in Canada are born to unmarried parents, and the proportion of single parents is growing rapidly—single fathers now represent 17 percent of US single parents and almost a quarter of Canadian single parents. Mothers are earning increasing proportions of the family income, while fathers are increasing the amount of time they spend with their children. If it's financially viable and you and your partner agree, then why not consider becoming a stay-at-home dad?

Making the most of your time
If you're planning to continue working full time there are still plenty of things you can do to make the most of your time with your baby. Help out with evening and nighttime feeds, give him a bath, or sing him a lullaby at bedtime—you can enjoy time with your baby and give your partner a break. If you usually work long hours, you may want to consider cutting down when the baby's born. The more time you spend caring for your baby, the better you will get to know each other.

Remember, however, that you're not just a parent but part of a couple. It's important for you and your partner to set aside time alone together, perhaps in the evenings, when your baby is asleep—your mutual support will be invaluable.

CHAPTER

CHOICES IN CHILDBIRTH

What sort of childbirth class should you attend?
Where's the best place to have your baby? How do
you make a birth plan and what, if any, pain relief is
best for you? These are all important considerations
that will help give you and your baby the best
possible birth outcome.

CHILDBIRTH CLASSES

Birth is such a natural part of life that it may seem unusual that you need to prepare for it, but childbirth classes have an important role to play in helping you understand and make informed decisions about the type of birth you want.

The growing use of complex medical equipment and the variety of pain relief available are both good reasons to know the benefits and risks of all the available procedures. You may find yourself having to make a quick decision during labor, and you'll want to be able to make an informed choice.

WHAT A CLASS CAN DO FOR YOU

First and foremost, a childbirth class gives a great opportunity for you to discover more about your pregnancy. Visits to your healthcare providers rarely include leisurely chats—they're over before you know it—and questions you meant to ask can remain unanswered. Childbirth classes provide an environment in which you can ask almost anything,

and if you forget to ask, the woman next to you will remember. The central goal of childbirth education is to prepare you for the experience of birth. Your instructor will outline what happens physically and emotionally, and there will be demonstrations and practice sessions for specific coping mechanisms.

Meeting in a group can be very supportive. The other women in the class are in the same situation, so they fully appreciate everything that's going on in your life. A prenatal class is also a great place to make new friends who share a common interest in babies and children. Many "graduates" go on to form new-parent support groups or play groups.

If you have a partner, a prenatal class will be good for him, too, helping him understand his role in the birth and involving him more fully in the pregnancy and preparations for childbirth. Becoming a new parent is a period of intense emotional growth, for you, your partner, and your relationship—a good class instructor will recognize this and suggest ways to help you make the most of these changes.

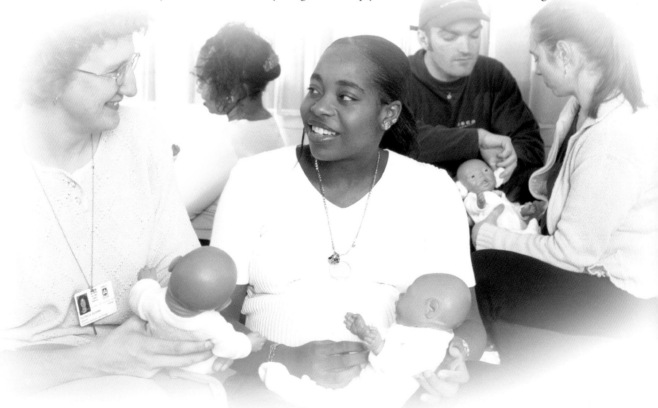

WHAT YOU'LL LEARN

Childbirth classes usually begin at around 28 to 32 weeks. Depending on what you feel you need, you can attend classes spanning a number of weeks, or brush up your knowledge at a one-off refresher session. Classes are often held in the evenings and on weekends and are conducted by a childbirth instructor. Although the emphasis can vary, all classes cover the basics: what happens during labor and birth; when to call your healthcare providers; relaxation and breathing techniques; medical pain relief; cesareans; and care of your newborn.

CHOOSING A CLASS

Many childbirth classes approach the subject from a specific angle or philosophy, so it's important to find a course that shares your views on childbirth. At the same time, approaching classes with an open mind will help you learn about the variety of possible birthing methods, so that you can make informed choices that really suit you.

Ask doctors, midwives, friends, or family for recommendations and seek out the classes in your neighborhood. Classes may be offered by hospitals, birth centers, county health units, doctors' offices, or private childbirth educators, and some will allow you to sit in on a session so that you can decide if it's right for you. An ideal class size is around five to seven couples—large enough to provide good discussion but small enough for everyone to get individual attention during sessions.

Finding the right teacher

Keep in mind that childbirth educators are usually trained and certified by specific organizations, although they may also be nurses or midwives:

◆ *Lamaze International Inc* Childbirth educators with Lamaze certification encourage active birth—in which you move during labor to help progress—and specific breathing patterns to distract from the pain of labor.

DID YOU KNOW...

Childbirth education can make the birth easier
Surveys show that, on average, mothers who attend childbirth classes have easier and healthier births than those who don't. They tend to have shorter labors, use less medication, and, later, are more likely to breastfeed.

◆ *International Childbirth Education Association (ICEA)* This certification reflects extensive training in techniques for coping with labor, focusing on imagery and natural breathing patterns. This qualification is more common among independent childbirth educators.
◆ *Bradley certification* These classes focus on husband-coached, "natural" childbirth with emphasis on diet, prenatal exercise, and inner focus to cope with the pain of labor. The courses run for eight to ten weeks and are very intense.
◆ *County Health Units* In Canada, classes are given by prenatal or public health nurses in these units.

OTHER CLASSES

There are classes for almost every month of pregnancy and beyond. In the early stages, you can attend exercise and nutrition classes, while breastfeeding classes, which are well worth going to, are usually offered just before birth. Before or after your baby arrives, you might want to try baby-care and infant-massage classes. Some hospitals also provide classes for other family members: for siblings, with tours round the birth facilities; and for grandparents. Afterward, there are postpartum exercise classes and new-parent support groups.

DECIDING WHERE TO GIVE BIRTH

You may want to have your baby in the hospital to take full advantage of medical technology. Or you may want to give birth in a more relaxed, less medical setting, such as a birth center or your own home. But it's important to know all the options so you can make the decision that's right for you.

Research has shown that women achieve the greatest satisfaction in childbirth by having a good relationship with their healthcare provider and by being involved in decisions. Start these early on and you're laying the foundations for a positive delivery.

HOSPITAL CARE
In the United States and Canada, 99 percent of babies are born in hospital. A hospital birth means you have instant access to potentially life-saving technology, which can be very reassuring, particularly if you are a first-time mother. Specialists are available to address any complications; you can have partial or total pain relief; and a cesarean can be performed, if necessary. If you want all the benefits of a hospital birth yet prefer as little medical intervention as possible, you could consider a certified nurse midwife (CNM) or certified midwife (CM) as your birth attendant (see page 177).

Choosing a hospital
If you have an established relationship with an obstetrician, doctor, or midwife, you'll be more inclined to have your baby in the hospital with which they are affiliated. Some healthcare providers have privileges at several hospitals, which may give you more choice.

Alternative ways to give birth

Recent years have seen a move away from hospital births with pain relief, and women now have greater choice about the circumstances in which they give birth.

Natural birth
Those who favor giving birth without drugs believe that birth is a natural, healthy process, which women's bodies are equipped to deal with on their own. Natural childbirth gives a woman a great deal of control over the events surrounding labor and delivery. You can choose: how mobile to be; which birthing positions to try; and which labor aids, such as meditation or a warm shower, you want to use.

You can have a natural birth at a birth center or at home, and, while it's perfectly possible to have a natural birth in a hospital, it's important to find out your healthcare provider's views on this. Some are happy to let women dictate certain practices, such as leaving membranes unruptured or not inducing labor, while others feel that while it's important to consider a woman's feelings, medically they need to do what they think is right.

Homebirth
Until the 20th century, most babies were born at home. But then a change in medical philosophy meant that birth moved to hospital and changed from being considered a natural experience to a medically managed condition. Today fewer than 1 percent of US and Canadian babies are born at home.

Mothers who chose a homebirth tend to do so because they want: continuity of care; a homey environment; and the ability to make their own decisions. In contrast, women who choose a hospital birth may place a higher value on access to drugs for pain relief and not needing to be transported if a problem arises.

Opinion is divided over the safety of homebirths. In one US study, researchers found that mothers who had homebirths had greater risks

When it comes to a hospital, in the United States your choice may be limited by your health insurance. Most plans cover the cost of hospital care, but check the small print and be clear about your coverage. Hospital costs are usually broken down separately, and your bill will include any "extras" such as the cost of pain relief or a private room. In Canada, Provincial Health Insurance covers the cost of your hospital care.

Many hospital deliveries today occur in special birthing rooms. These are rooms where you go through labor, give birth, and recover all in one room. These rooms may be called LDRs—for labor, deliver, and recovery. In some hospitals you may even be able to stay in the same room until you check out. This room is called an LDRP—labor, deliver, recovery, and postpartum.

Questions to ask at the hospital

It's important to find out as much as you can about the hospital where you'll give birth. You should ask about cesarean rates and attitudes toward induction. You'll also need information about parking facilities, maps to the hospital, and phone numbers. It's also worth taking a tour of the hospital's maternity units. Questions you could ask include:

- Is the facility family-centered? Does it have open visiting hours and provide accommodation for fathers or other family members?
- Who can stay with you throughout labor and birth? Can other children be present at the birth? Not all hospitals will accommodate siblings, and a lot depends on their ages and how they've been prepared. Keep in mind that you'll need another adult present to look after your child.

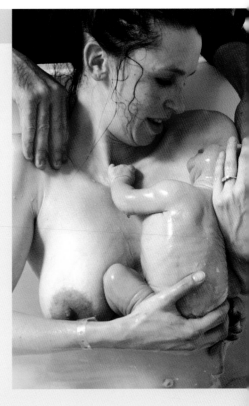

for themselves and their babies than mothers who gave birth in hospitals. On the other hand, studies in both the United States and Britain have shown that homebirths are as safe or even safer than hospital births for healthy women with normal, low-risk pregnancies.

Homebirths are usually overseen by midwives who have obstetricians to consult with or refer patients to if complications arise. Throughout your pregnancy, your midwife will keep a close eye on you and your baby, to keep the birth as risk-free as possible. Keep in mind that in the United States you may have to meet the cost of a homebirth, as it may be difficult to get insurance.

Water birth

This is when you spend part of your labor, and sometimes give birth, in water. The warm water helps your muscles relax, which often speeds up labor. Most water births tend to be carried out by midwives in birthing centers or in the home, but an increasing number of hospitals provide birth pools. However, opinion is divided over the safety of water births; The American College of Obstetricians and Gynecologists and the Society of Obstetricians and Gynecologists of Canada have not yet endorsed the technique.

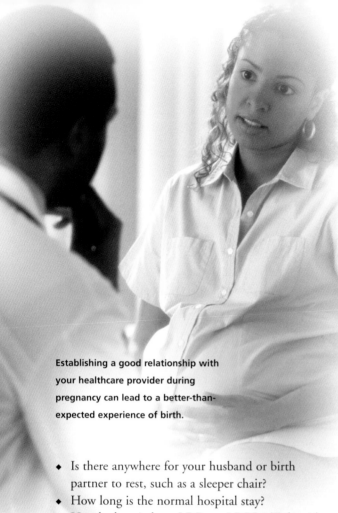

Establishing a good relationship with your healthcare provider during pregnancy can lead to a better-than-expected experience of birth.

- Is there anywhere for your husband or birth partner to rest, such as a sleeper chair?
- How long is the normal hospital stay?
- Has the hospital got LDRs or LDRPs? Today, it's often only women having cesareans or complicated deliveries who give birth in a sterile operating-room environment.
- After the birth, can you keep your baby with you throughout the day and night?
- If you want to breastfeed, does the hospital have lactation consultants (specialists in breastfeeding)? Is the hospital "baby friendly?" (the highest standard a hospital can meet for breastfeeding, awarded by the World Health Organization).
- What security measures are in place? Systems vary, but many hospitals have electronic systems with security tags on the newborns' ankles or umbilical cords that set off an alarm if someone takes the baby out of the building.
- How are newborns identified so that they don't get mixed up? Most hospitals put identification bands on the mother and baby, and often a third

person, such as the baby's father. Hospital staff have to check these bands every time the baby leaves or enters the mother's room or nursery.

BIRTH CENTERS

Available mainly in the United States, birth centers may be independent or part of a larger hospital. Most of them are run by midwives, with emergency backup available. They are designed for women with normal, low-risk pregnancies and births, and usually offer minimum medical intervention. Most birth centers aim to recreate a homelike atmosphere with showers, CD players, and Jacuzzis, and many also provide birthing tubs where you can labor and possibly give birth to your baby in the water.

If you deliver at a birth center, you can expect family-centered care, no routine interventions, and total control over what happens during your birth. You can: choose who you want to have at the birth; move around freely in labor; and deliver in whichever position you find comfortable. You generally return home about 12 hours after the birth. However, if a problem arises, you may have to be transferred during labor to a hospital.

Choosing a birth center

If you're thinking about having your baby at a birth center, ask these important questions:

- Are the birth attendants licensed healthcare providers—for example, physician, nurse-midwife, or licensed midwife?
- Is the birth center approved by the Commission for the Accreditation of Birth Centers?
- What's the procedure if complications arise that require you to be referred to an obstetrician or admitted to hospital?
- What do the charges for care cover, and will your insurance plan pay for these services?

SUPPORT MEASURES FOR LABOR

Although it's impossible to predict what sort of labor and birth you'll experience, there's plenty you can do to turn the experience into a positive one—it's just a question of doing your homework.

This is the time to be deciding who you want to deliver your baby—obstetrician, family physician, or midwife—what sort of pain relief you might like, and who's the best person to be with you and support you through the birth.

CHOOSING YOUR BIRTH ATTENDANT

When it comes to deciding who you want to attend your labor and birth, it's important to choose a healthcare provider who's in tune with your ideas and personality.

Obstetrician-gynecologist

The branch of medicine that deals with birth is known as obstetrics. In contrast, gynecology deals with the female reproductive organs in the non-pregnant woman. An obstetrician-gynecologist has completed a four-year postgraduate training program. Depending on the hospital you choose, there may be residents—doctors training to become ob-gyn specialists—assisting your obstetrician.

If you choose an obstetrician-gynecologist for your healthcare provider, he or she will be able to provide all your obstetric care as well as your non-pregnancy needs such as Pap smears. An obstetrician-gynecologist will care for you during your pregnancy and, when it's time to give birth, he or she will: see you at the hospital; deliver your baby; and perform any necessary interventions. After the birth, he or she will continue to see you until you go home from the hospital.

Your obstetrician also can care for you if your pregnancy becomes high-risk, for example, if you develop diabetes. Or you may be referred to a perinatologist (an expert in high-risk pregnancies)—also known as a maternal-fetal medical specialist.

Family or general practitioner

These terms refer to doctors who have completed training in general medicine after graduation from medical school. Their training includes obstetrics, so your family doctor should be qualified to attend you during the birth of your baby. However, family practitioners aren't usually trained in surgery, so if you need a cesarean section or forceps during delivery, your family practitioner will call in an obstetrician or surgeon.

Midwife

The belief that women's bodies were designed for birth is at the core of midwifery, which tends toward the natural rather than the interventionist approach to labor and birth. Often women seek care from a midwife when they want a healthcare provider consistent with their childbirth philosophy. US studies have shown that healthy women with straightforward pregnancies who chose midwifery care had very good outcomes with fewer interventions and lower cesarean rates.

The majority of trained midwives in the United States are certified by the American College of Nurse-Midwives (ACNM), so when you're choosing a midwife, look for the letters CNM, which stands for certified nurse-midwife, or CM, which stands for certified midwife.

Certified nurse-midwives, registered nurses who are also trained in midwifery, are licensed to practice throughout the United States and Canada. As long as your pregnancy and birth are uncomplicated, a certified nurse-midwife can care for you through pregnancy, labor, and birth.

Certified midwives, while not nurses, are graduates of schools of midwifery, often part of university programs. Certified midwives must pass state or provincial licensing exams.

Lay midwives are midwives who are not professionally trained. They usually learn the skills of midwifery through apprenticeship. Many are trained in other countries where lay midwifery is common. It's best to use a certified nurse-midwife or certified midwife, as they have met professional and licensing standards.

As well as taking care of you during labor and delivery, certified nurse-midwives and certified midwives can carry out your gynecology check-ups, family planning services, pre-conception, prenatal, and postpartum care, as well as provide newborn care. They work in hospitals and birth centers and can deliver your baby at home. You may well find that your insurance plan covers the services of certified nurse-midwives. Find out about your midwife's experience and training and what sort of medical backup he or she has in case of emergency.

PAIN RELIEF IN LABOR

It's very important to think about what type of pain relief you might want during labor, as your choice can make a big difference to your birth experience. Keep an open mind, so that you remain flexible and tuned in to your actual labor experience. Among the standard medical therapies are analgesics, which relieve pain, anesthetics, which block sensations, and tranquilizers, which calm you. Local anesthetic can be given at the time of birth. Local anesthetics are commonly used for epidural insertion, episiotomies, and pudendal blocks. Non-medical pain-relief techniques include relaxation and breathing techniques, hot and cold compresses, acupuncture, labor balls, and other labor aids.

Analgesics

Drugs that are injected into a muscle or given intravenously (into the bloodstream), analgesics dull pain and can make you sleepy if they're narcotic based. Demerol is the most common analgesic used in labor, and is given either by injection in the buttocks or intravenously when labor is well established. It can be particularly helpful when early labor is prolonged and uncomfortable, helping you rest and taking the edge off strong sensations. It can make you drowsy, which may help you cope with the passage of time in labor.

5 vital questions about pain relief

1   Does your hospital have a 24-hour anesthesia service? With certain types of pain relief, such as an epidural, a physician anesthesiologist, or a nurse anesthetist, must be present to administer anesthetic medications and perform the necessary procedures. You may wish to ask for an interview with the anesthetist before your labor. It's important to know the department's availability and philosophy of pain relief in childbirth.

2   Will you be given clear and concise written or spoken information regarding the risks versus benefits of pain relief measures?

3   What are the side effects, short- and long-term, for both the mother and the baby, of the different pain-relief measures on offer?

4   Does your healthcare provider's philosophy of care agree with yours? If you prefer a more natural approach to pain relief, does he or she know and support your wishes?

5   Does your healthcare provider have experience in different types of pain-relief techniques such as imaging, massage, or specific childbirth preparation techniques, for example Lamaze?

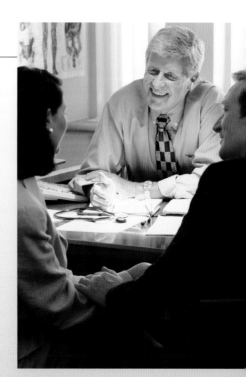

On the negative side, analgesics can hinder your ability to get up and walk about to aid the progression of labor, because they can make you unsteady on your feet. Also, you may dislike feeling drowsy and out of control. If given close to delivery, Demerol can make your baby drowsy and slow to feed and interact. It also may impair his breathing and he may need extra oxygen. The effects on your baby can last longer than they do on you, as his immature liver and kidneys are less capable of clearing the medication from his body. However, medication can be given to the baby after birth to reverse the effects of Demerol.

Regional anesthetics

These medications, which produce a loss of sensation, are given through a tiny tube inserted into the mother's back as an epidural or spinal. They are excellent at taking away pain. There are several different types of regional anesthetics:

◆ *Epidural* The most popular choice in the United States and Canada for pain relief in labor, an epidural blocks most pain sensations in the abdomen, although you can still feel pressure. Only a physician anesthesiologist or a nurse anesthetist, both specialists in anesthesia, can administer an epidural. This is done by placing a small needle into the epidural space, in the lower part of your back. The needle passes between the bones of the lower vertebrae, below the location of the spinal cord. A very tiny, sterile tube is threaded through the needle. The needle is then removed, leaving the tiny tube in place. Medications are given through the tube, and these include: narcotics, such as morphine and fetanyl, which take away pain; and, sometimes, "caine" drugs, such as lidocaine, that block pain but cause numbness. Once the medication is injected into the tube, you may feel relief from pain in ten minutes.

Medication can be injected into the epidural tube by periodic injections, or by connecting the tube to a pump. The pump can provide a continuous low dose of the drug, whereas injections tend to wear off after some time.

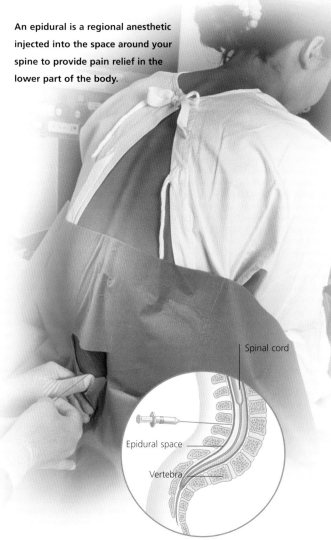

An epidural is a regional anesthetic injected into the space around your spine to provide pain relief in the lower part of the body.

Spinal cord

Epidural space

Vertebra

When epidurals include a "caine" drug, which causes numbness, you may experience little or no feeling, which means that it can be difficult to urinate. A small catheter or tube will be inserted through the urethra, into the bladder so that it can be emptied. An epidural may also make it difficult to push at the end of labor. Sitting in a relatively upright position for delivery—at a 45- to 90-degree angle—and concentrating on pushing can help.

Epidurals can also lower your blood pressure. Since it is essential to keep your circulation going so that your baby gets enough oxygen, your blood pressure will be monitored frequently before and after an epidural is inserted. In addition, you'll be given fluids via an IV to keep your circulating blood volume stable. Your baby will be monitored by an electronic fetal monitor.

While some women complain of backache after birth, it is more likely that this comes from the inability to move around a lot in labor and the passage of the baby through the pelvis. Research has found no link between epidurals and long-term low back pain. Some women do, however, experience headaches after an epidural. This happens if there is a leak of spinal fluid after the epidural is inserted. If the headache persists, it can be treated with a "blood patch," which involves a small amount of blood being taken from a vein on the woman's arm, and injecting it into the epidural space, sealing the leak.

◆ *Walking epidural* The use of narcotics with very little caine drugs, may enable pain to be reduced without the loss of sensation. If you are steady on your feet, your healthcare provider may allow you to get out of bed and possibly walk. If you are not numb, you are more likely to be able to push effectively, as well. The type of epidural you receive depends on the anesthesiologist or anesthetist. You may want to discuss this with him or her before you go into labor.

◆ *Spinal epidural* This is similar to an epidural, but instead of being put into the epidural space, the needle and tube is inserted directly into the spinal fluid, also below the spinal cord. When medication is injected into this area, it causes profound pain relief and numbness. This is desirable if immediate anesthesia is needed, such as for an emergency cesarean. Because it penetrates the dura (the membrane around the spinal fluid) it is possible to get a spinal headache, which can be treated with a blood patch (see above).

◆ *A pudendal block* This less common method is given at the time of delivery, by a needle inserted through the vagina. As these anesthetics numb only this perineal area, you'll feel less pain, but you'll still feel contractions. It's usually given in the case of forceps or vacuum extraction and its effect can last through an episiotomy and subsequent stitching.

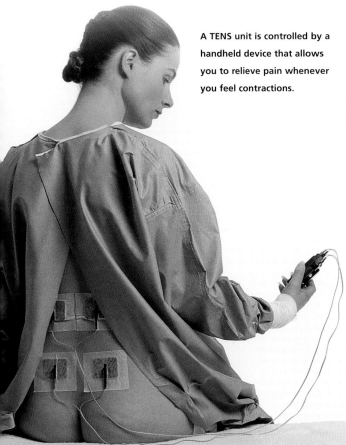

A TENS unit is controlled by a handheld device that allows you to relieve pain whenever you feel contractions.

Tranquilizers

These are muscle relaxants, which can relieve tension. They are usually given with a narcotic to maximize the effect of a small dose of narcotic.

General anesthesia

This is anesthetic gas mixed with oxygen and is only given if medically necessary, in particular during an emergency cesarean. When you awake, you may feel drowsy. It may have the same sedative effect on your baby. Giving a general anesthetic as close to the birth as possible will help to minimize any effect it may have on your baby.

TENS

Transcutaneous Electrical Nerve Stimulation (TENS) is the application of mild electrical pulses, via electrodes, to key nerve areas. A handheld unit delivers tingling levels of electrical stimulation to various points on your body via wires taped to your skin. Its effectiveness depends on where the electrodes are positioned and the intensity and frequency of the electrical pulses. It's thought that it works by blocking the transmission of pain signals to your brain. It also may stimulate the production of endorphins, your body's natural analgesic.

TENS has been proved effective in reducing pain in a variety of medical conditions. In labor, its effect can vary, with some studies showing clear benefits for women and others not, and it doesn't appear to harm the baby. For maximum effect, TENS is begun in early labor, as it may be more helpful in reducing pain such as backache in labor, rather than the on-and-off discomfort of contractions. It can also be used to decrease pain after cesarean birth.

Natural forms of pain relief

If you prefer to have as little medical intervention as possible, you might consider trying more natural forms of pain relief before opting for anesthetics. Support that your partner can give during labor, such as massage and warm compresses (see page 182) can help the body relax and distract you from pain. You might also consider visualization (see page 160).

Alternative therapies such as hypnosis or reflexology are also becoming increasingly popular during labor. For example, acupuncture—practiced in the East for several thousand years—works by balancing the energy of the entire body, using ultra-fine needles inserted into the skin at various points. It can be used during labor to increase or decrease the strength of contractions, for pain control, and to assist the baby's journey along the birth canal. However, as with all such therapies, make sure that you find a qualified practitioner and visit him or her well in advance of your due date to discuss and, if necessary, practice techniques.

CHOOSING YOUR BIRTH PARTNER

Who you want to be present at the birth is a highly personal decision—some people are happy with a large audience and others prefer to keep it private. Keep in mind that you may need more privacy than you expect. Choose carefully—once an invitation is extended, it's hard to take it back—and be sure that you are completely comfortable with those invited and that they are calm and supportive. Children and young people will need to be prepared for this powerful event to avoid misinterpretation, and they will need to be accompanied by an adult. Check

MORE **ABOUT** | water for pain relief

A surprisingly effective form of pain relief, immersing yourself in water during labor, can relax you, making contractions easier to bear and enabling labor to progress more smoothly. It also supports you, so you can move around freely. Several studies have found that water immersion leads to a drop in blood pressure, more rapid dilation, more rapid descent of the baby, and a reduced need for other forms of pain relief. Water therapy seems to work best when labor is fairly advanced. Women have reported that just waiting for the tub to fill up relaxes them, as they anticipate sinking into the warm, supportive water.

with your healthcare provider and the hospital or birth center about visiting policies, some have limits on the number or age of participants. At the same time, find out if there might be students or ancillary personnel present; if you're not comfortable with this, you still have plenty of time to find a solution. Warn your guests that they may be asked to leave at any point during the birth, according to your needs or at the discretion of your healthcare provider.

Ways your partner can help through labor

Keep in mind that the needs of women in labor differ, so tune into what your partner wants. Here are some things you can do that may help her cope better with the process.

According to studies, women in labor have five basic needs: physical care and comfort; pain relief; the constant presence of a supportive person; unconditional acceptance and reassurance; and knowledge of what is happening. The support that a birth partner can offer has numerous positive effects. It has

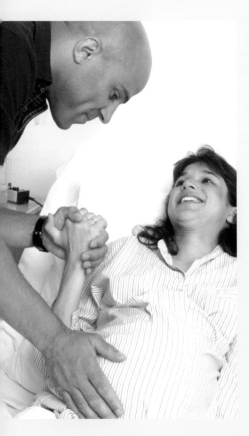

been shown to: decrease the need for medication and intervention; shorten labor; decrease the risk of cesarean birth; and improve outcomes for newborns.

Stay close by Be aware that some women in labor like to be touched and others don't. Physical touch can communicate caring and concern and prevent her feeling isolated.

Consider her position Urge her to change position frequently, as this can help ease backache. Use pillows, rolled blankets, or towels to maximize relaxation. If she's able to get up and walk, encourage and assist her. Some mothers use "birthing balls," large air-filled balls on which they bounce to relieve the pain of a contraction.

Keep her clean and dry Labor may cause a woman to move her bowels or urinate, and at some point her water will break. Help clean her quickly.

Relieve her dry mouth Use of breathing techniques can dry out her mouth, making it feel uncomfortable, so help her drink liquids, or suck on ice chips, if permitted. Use lip balm to lubricate and moisten her lips. Also, help her brush her teeth.

Keep her cool Apply a cool washcloth to her face, throat, or other body parts. Spray her face

gently with water. Alternatively, make a fan from a washcloth, a piece of paper, or gown.

Apply a warm or cold compress Contractions may cause back pain or cramps. Help her out by applying a warm washcloth to her back.

Massage her lower back Ask her to lie on her side so you can give her a back rub, using lotion. This may be particularly helpful if she's having back labor (when the pain of contractions is felt mainly in the back). However, be aware that she might prefer you to stop the massage during a contraction.

Encourage her to pass urine A full bladder may slow down labor, so remind her to go to the bathroom often—she should try at least every hour.

Use relaxation techniques Ideally, practice these before labor begins. One easy technique involves asking her to tighten then relax each muscle in turn, starting with her upper body and progressing slowly down to her toes.

Help with breathing techniques Learn whatever breathing exercise she wishes to use in advance, and help her focus on it during contractions. It may help if you ask her to take a deep breath and sigh after each contraction to help "exhale tension."

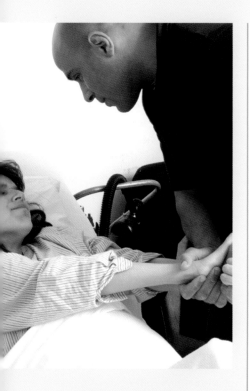

Promote rest Keep her surroundings as peaceful as possible, and encourage her to rest to prevent exhaustion.

Assure her privacy Respect her need—or lack of need—for clothing and draping during labor.

Offer emotional support Whisper words of encouragement. Praise her for her tremendous effort. Tell her "you're doing great!" Compliment her. Use words of endearment, and, if appropriate, express your love for her. As labor progresses, tell her that it's nearly over.

HOW TO STAY FOCUSED ON HER NEEDS

Each woman is unique, responds individually, and has different needs in labor, so it's important to ask her if a particular measure is helpful or desirable. Be prepared to change tactic or give her a bit of space, if that's what she wants. Keep in mind these key points:

Consider your purpose What are you trying to do with your support and comfort measures? Make sure that you focus on what she wants.

Be involved Your constant presence and attention to how she is feeling and the procedures that are being carried out are necessary to enable you to provide meaningful support.

Be prepared Pack necessary items several weeks before the due date, and plan your route to the hospital in advance.

Keep up your energy levels To provide effective support you need to stay energized yourself. Be sure to get something to eat and drink during the labor. It's best to take food and beverages with you. Also, take a break, if possible. Relax in a chair in the labor room or take a short walk on the unit. But don't leave the unit—you could miss the birth.

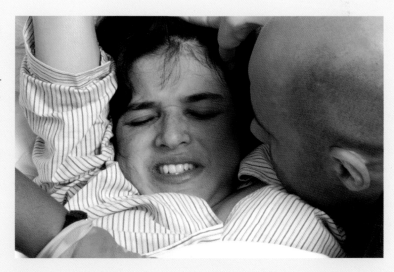

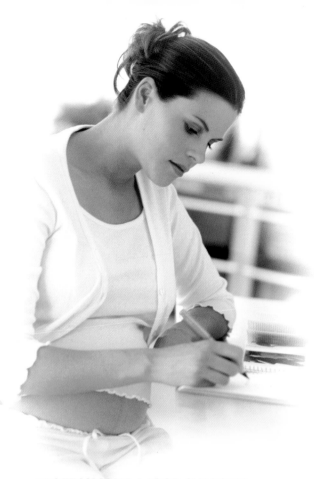

Writing a birth plan can help you
understand your options, and
undergoing childbirth with an educated
but open mind can help your labor.

encourage women to make formal birthing plans, listing their preferences. A sample birth plan is included opposite, but keep in mind that this list is not exhaustive—you can include anything you like. You'll need to bring the plan with you for the birth.

However, it's important to be flexible. Birth isn't a predictable event: Like babies and people, each birth has its own "personality." Even if you have had other children, this birth will be different and special, and you may have to adapt your birth plan accordingly. All sorts of factors influence your decisions about childbirth, including how you feel at the time. For example, if you plan to take very little or no pain relief, you may find that you change your mind during the actual labor. Many women feel that they've somehow failed if things don't go according to their birth plan—maybe an emergency cesarean was necessary because the baby was in distress—but it's no failure to accept the most appropriate medical treatment for the safe delivery of your baby.

PROFESSIONAL LABOR SUPPORT

Hiring a trained or experienced birth helper is another option that can be a great help in some circumstances. If your partner travels away from home on business a lot, you're having a vaginal birth after ceserean (VBAC), or you want to limit medical intervention, it's well worth thinking about professional labor support. For this, you can hire either a doula (Greek for "in service to woman") or a monitrice (from the French, "to watch over"). Their services usually include visits before and after delivery, as well as at-home support during early labor. Ask your healthcare provider for more information and recommendations.

YOUR BIRTH PLAN

After you consider your birth options, it's important to discuss them with your healthcare provider far in advance of your due date. If something is important to you, such as your husband cutting your newborn's cord, discuss this. Some healthcare providers

DID YOU KNOW...

Birth support can shorten labor Studies show that when a doula or other birth partner is present, women have less painful labors, fewer medical interventions, fewer cesareans, and healthier babies. Recent evidence suggests that when a doula provides support, women are more satisfied with their experiences, and the mother-infant interaction is enhanced for as long as two months after the birth. Doula support has been found to have a positive effect on a couple's relationship as well.

Tick all that apply in each section

Birth partners
I would like the following people to be at the birth

- [ ] Partner
- [ ] Friend
- [ ] Relative
- [ ] Doula
- [ ] Other children

Induction

- [ ] I would prefer not to be induced.
- [ ] I would consider induction for medical reasons, only.
- [ ] I would prefer to be induced to control the time/date of my delivery.

Labor

- [ ] I would prefer not to have a routine enema and/or shaving of pubic hair.
- [ ] I want to be able to walk around and be out of bed if possible.
- [ ] I would like to drink fluids and/or eat lightly throughout the first stage.
- [ ] I would like to keep the number of vaginal exams to a minimum.
- [ ] I would like to view the birth using a mirror.

Monitoring

- [ ] I do not wish to have continuous fetal monitoring unless my baby is distressed.

Photography

- [ ] I wish to have my birth photographed/videotaped.

Pain management

- [ ] I wish to have a natural birth and do not want any pain medication offered to me during labor.
- [ ] I would like an epidural as early as possible.
- [ ] I would like an epidural later in labor.
- [ ] I wish to have pain medication available but only given to me if I request it.

Episiotomy

- [ ] I would prefer not to have an episiotomy unless it is required for my baby's safety.
- [ ] I would prefer to have an episiotomy rather than risk tearing.

Cesarean

- [ ] If I need to have an emergency cesarean I would like my partner present at all times during the operation.
- [ ] I wish to have an epidural for anesthesia.
- [ ] If I have to have a full anesthetic, I wish my baby to be handed to (name of person) after the birth.

Post-birth

- [ ] I would like to hold my baby immediately after the birth.
- [ ] I want to wait until the umbilical cord stops pulsing before it is cut.
- [ ] I would like my partner to cut the cord.
- [ ] I would prefer not to have routine pitocin after the birth.
- [ ] I plan to breastfeed my baby.
- [ ] I wish to put my baby to the breast as soon after the birth as possible.

INTERVENTIONS AND PROCEDURES

When considering the type of delivery you want, there may be certain procedures that you want to avoid, if possible. Your healthcare providers should respect your wishes, as long as you and your baby are not at risk.

If you have any concerns about medical procedures, it can help to find out as much as possible about what they involve. Be prepared, however, when the time comes, to allow your healthcare provider a role in judging if intervention is needed.

INDUCTION

When a woman goes into labor naturally, a series of hormonal changes and the pressure of the full-term baby on the muscles of the uterus help initiate the process of labor. But labor also can be started artificially or "induced" by hormones or mechanical pressure on the cervix.

Left to nature, most women will go into labor and deliver their babies within two weeks either side of their due date. Labor is induced when it's better for the baby to be born than remain inside the uterus or when the health of mother or baby is deemed at risk should the pregnancy continue. If a baby isn't growing sufficiently toward the end of a pregnancy or has a serious medical condition, ending a pregnancy by inducing labor may be the best option. Mothers who have high-risk conditions, such as diabetes or pregnancy-induced hypertension (high blood pressure), may be candidates for induction. Even if your labor is not induced, your healthcare provider may help the progress of labor by using oxytocin to make your contractions stronger and more effective.

Oxytocin should be given in such a way as to simulate normal contractions. However, artificially induced contractions are often stronger and more frequent than natural contractions. This, in turn, can lead to abnormal fetal heart readings, so women who are receiving oxytocin are almost always on a fetal monitor to see how the baby is tolerating the contractions. If the frequency of contractions is too high, the dose may be adjusted downward.

Elective induction

Some doctors and women prefer to "plan" delivery and will schedule a date for the mother to be induced at the end of her pregnancy. The American College of Obstetricians and Gynecologists (ACOG) does not support these elective or "social" inductions, but they remain very popular. Before beginning an induction, particularly an elective induction, the healthcare provider must assure that delivery is the best option for the baby, and there are special tests that can be performed to check if the baby is "ready." In cases of elective inductions, the baby should be at full term. Delivering a baby, electively too early—such as three weeks before the due date—may put the newborn at risk.

FETAL MONITORS

These devices are used to check the baby's progress during labor. One of the most common types is the external fetal monitor consisting of electrodes placed on your abdomen. These are hooked up to a machine that displays or prints out readings of your baby's heartbeat and your contractions.

Some hospitals monitor all women in labor with these monitors continuously. But some studies have shown that it can lead to an increase in unnecessary cesareans, because the readings were misinterpreted and the monitors indicated that there was a problem where there wasn't. For this reason, if you have a low-risk pregnancy and birth, you may be checked with a fetal monitor intermittently, or the baby's progress may be measured with a Doppler (a handheld ultrasound device).

If your healthcare providers need a more detailed picture of your baby's condition, they may want to monitor your baby internally by passing an electrode through your vagina and attaching it to your baby's scalp to measure the heartbeat. Internal monitoring is more accurate than external monitoring, but it does have some drawbacks. Your baby may run the risk of contracting an infection from the electrode attached to her scalp; and the use of the monitor restricts your mobility, which may slow down the progress of your labor. Because of these factors, internal monitoring is normally only carried out when there are proven benefits.

EPISIOTOMY

This is a small cut made in the perineum (the skin between the vagina and anus) in order to enlarge the vaginal opening when the baby's head is about to be born.

In many hospitals, episiotomies used to be performed routinely. However, over the last two decades there has been a significant reduction in the percentage of deliveries involving episiotomies—from 64 percent in 1980 to 33 percent in 2000—and the current thinking is that there's no absolute benefit of routine episiotomy. Frequently, the skill and patience of an experienced healthcare provider will stretch the area and allow the baby to be born with minimal or no tears and no episiotomy. Sometimes a small tear is easily repaired and causes less pain than a large and invasive episiotomy.

Episiotomy is still considered valuable in a few situations, for instance, to shorten the pushing stage of birth because of fetal distress or if the mother has a medical problem such as a heart condition and cannot cope with a long labor. An episiotomy may be recommended to protect the delicate skull of a preterm infant or to provide more space for the delivery of breech or very large babies.

FORCEPS AND VACUUM EXTRACTORS

These medical instruments are used to help ease the baby out of the birth canal. Studies show that certain medications and positions in labor may increase the likelihood that these will need to be used. It's wise to talk to your healthcare provider about his or her thoughts on the use of both forceps and vacuum extractors long before you go into labor.

Forceps

Frightening stories about forceps deliveries abound, as they're associated with an increased risk of vaginal or perineal laceration. However, recent studies show that they're no better or worse than other types of delivery. Forceps (metal instruments resembling salad tongs or spoons) may be used if the mother can't push effectively or if the baby has to be born quickly. The use of forceps may prevent the need for a cesarean birth. Forceps also can be used to turn a baby into a different position and, while forceps can cause more damage to the perineum, they can reduce the chances of trauma to the baby.

Opponents of forceps maintain that they can be used out of convenience when labor is slow and the medical team want the baby to be delivered as quickly as possible.

DID YOU KNOW...

The World Health Organization wants fewer cesareans While cesareans have been performed since the 19th century, improved monitoring and surgical procedures have increased their number in the late 20th and early 21st centuries. In 1999, about 22 percent of babies born in the United States were born by cesarean. In Canada, cesareans accounted for 19 percent of births in 2000. Because of the trauma and risk of complications from such a major operation, the World Health Organization is pushing for the rate to be cut to under 15 percent in every country.

Vacuum extractor

This works in a similar way to forceps, but instead of metal tongs, a soft suction cup is placed on the baby's head. Suction helps pull the baby out as the mother pushes. Vacuum extractors can be used higher up the birth canal than forceps and cause less damage to the perineum.

CESAREAN SECTIONS

Only an obstetrician or a surgeon can perform a cesarean, as it involves making an incision in the lower part of the mother's abdomen to deliver the baby. Most cesareans are performed for medical reasons (see box, left.) While some women might prefer to have a cesarean birth to avoid the discomfort of labor, it is not recommended nor acceptable practice. Although surgical techniques have improved vastly in recent years, there are still much greater risks associated with cesareans than with vaginal births. In addition, the recovery period can be considerably longer, and a cesarean may make subsequent vaginal births more difficult.

While cesareans can be a safer means of birth for some babies, there are effects on the baby that may need to be overcome. Sometimes cesarean babies can retain fluid in their lungs—this is normally squeezed out in the birth canal. The newborn also may be drowsy from medication given to the mother.

Vaginal births after a cesarean (VBAC)

In years past, women were told "once a cesarean, always a cesarean." Most cesareans can be accomplished using the low transverse or "bikini" uterine incision (see page 232), which is less likely to rupture in subsequent labors—there is a 0.5 percent risk. Because each repeat cesarean is more difficult due to scar tissue from prior surgery, VBAC after low transverse cesarean section (LTCS) is considered safer for mother and baby. In addition, 70 percent of mothers who attempt labor after cesarean will successfully accomplish VBAC.

However, opponents of VBAC maintain that even with a "bikini cut" there are risks to having a VBAC, including a greater risk of uterine rupture than with a repeat cesarean. Women who have a VBAC induced with medication are at the highest risk for uterine rupture. If you are considering a VBAC, you need to find a healthcare provider who will support your decision.

reasons for a cesarean

1. Ideally, babies are born headfirst, but sometimes the baby is in a difficult position for delivery. Some babies are in a breech position (feet or buttocks first) or transverse (lying sideways in the uterus). Some babies can successfully be born breech. However, many breech babies and all transverse babies are born by cesarean birth.

2. Cesarean rates are often recommended for women with high-risk conditions, such as bleeding, genital herpes, diabetes, and pregnancy-induced hypertension or eclampsia (see page 254).

3. If there's more than one baby in the pregnancy, it's likely that the babies will be born by cesarean, although some twins are successfully delivered vaginally if they're favorably positioned.

4. Poor growth of the baby or a high-risk condition of the mother or baby can make it safer for the pregnancy to end with a planned cesarean rather than an induction.

5. The baby is very large. Some babies are just too big to be born from a mother's birth canal.

6. Fetal distress as result of the stresses and strains of labor. This can be detected by fetal monitoring and special tests.

11

CHAPTER

GETTING READY FOR THE BIRTH OF YOUR BABY

As the last trimester of your pregnancy draws to an

end you'll be feeling excited about the imminent

arrival of your baby and you will want to make final

preparations for labor. Now is a good time to plan

and organize the things you need to do.

DECISIONS ABOUT YOUR BABY

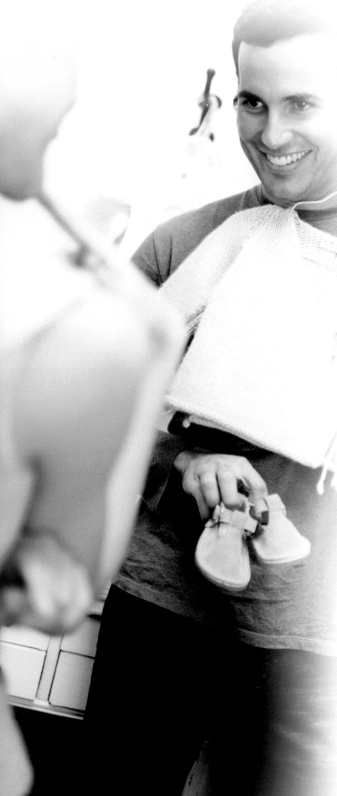

It's well worth spending some time before your baby is born thinking about some of the choices that you'll need to make once she arrives. Of course you may change your mind later but by considering the options now you will be able to make more informed decisions.

Some of the things you will need to consider before your baby arrives include: how you want to feed your baby; which names you want to give her; whether or not you want to return to work after the birth, and if you are returning to work, who will care for your child?

BREAST OR BOTTLE?

Deciding how you will feed your baby is a very personal matter and you should spend some time understanding the benefits and drawbacks of breastfeeding and bottlefeeding so that you can make an informed decision. There's no question that breast milk is best, especially in the initial weeks after birth, but there are many good reasons why women bottlefeed. Ultimately, it's important to make sure that both you and your baby are comfortable, healthy, and happy. See Chapter 14 for more on feeding your baby.

Breastfeeding

Most women can breastfeed, regardless of the size or shape of their breasts. However, if you have flat or inverted nipples you may need a little help in learning to position your baby and may need to use breast shells before birth (see page 202). Breastfeeding may be difficult or painful at first, but most women get used to it within a few weeks with the help of their healthcare providers. Some pregnant women feel uncomfortable about the idea of breastfeeding, but then take to it quite easily after the birth when they are presented with their babies. This is often a result of the natural hormonal changes within their bodies. If you're unsure, you should aim at least to try it—you can always change to bottles if it doesn't work out. It's harder to take up breastfeeding after a baby has started on a bottle, so you may not have another chance if you don't try it from the beginning.

If you're returning to work soon after giving birth, it's definitely worthwhile starting breastfeeding, even if you know that you can't continue; breast milk benefits your baby most during the early weeks by building up her immunity. You also can consider combined feeding—breastfeed your baby when you're at home and rely on formula milk when you are at work. Or you could express your milk before you leave for work so that your baby has a supply of your milk while you're away.

Bottlefeeding

If you have problems with or an antipathy to breastfeeding, you may decide to bottlefeed. There also are some medications and conditions, such as HIV, which aren't compatible with breastfeeding because of the risks to the baby, in which case bottlefeeding is essential. One of the main benefits if you do decide to bottlefeed your baby is that your partner and close family, such as your baby's grandparents, can easily share in the feeding of your baby. Bottlefeeding also allows you to see how much milk your baby is taking at each session.

CHOOSING A NAME

Naming your baby can be a fun and exciting project. Discuss ideas for names with your partner, then write your favorites on a list and attach it to the fridge or put it on a notice board so that you look at the names often and get a good feeling for each one. Some parents prefer to keep the names that they've chosen private until after the birth—a beautiful new baby can help to appease a grandparent who thinks that you have chosen an inappropriate name. Keep in mind that when your

6 benefits of breastfeeding

1   Breast milk is naturally designed to provide all the nutrients your baby needs in the right amounts.

2   Breast milk contains antibodies and other protective factors that help fight infection. Breastfed infants are known to have decreased risks of respiratory and ear infections, gastroenteritis, diabetes, Crohn's disease, autoimmune diseases, SIDS, and obesity, among many other problems.

3   Breast milk is easily digested and is less likely to cause stomach upsets, diarrhea or constipation.

4   Breast milk is cheap, readily available, available at the right temperature, and, naturally, always fresh.

5   Nursing speeds the process of your uterus returning to its normal size and can help you lose the weight you have gained during pregnancy.

6   Nursing can reduce a woman's risk of developing breast cancer.

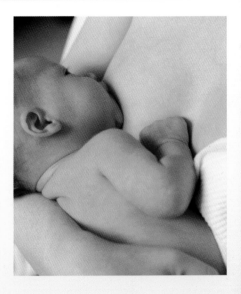

Approximately 65 percent of boys are circumcised in the United States every year. At some stage before your due date, you'll need to decide whether you're going to have your baby boy circumcised and, if so, arrange for the procedure to be carried out soon after the birth. There aren't any medical reasons for early circumcision, and pediatric associations don't recommend its routine use. However, many parents decide on the procedure for religious or other reasons. The procedure is painful, however, and warrants some form of anesthesia; in addition, there are small risks of infection, excess bleeding or scarring. Talk this decision over with your partner and doctor.

shots later. Provide plenty of spare film and batteries and invest in a disposable camera just in case. Check beforehand that you're allowed to take photographs, as some doctors and institutions don't permit them.

Take care that you don't watch the video or pore over the photographs too soon after the event. Giving birth is a very emotional experience and your body copes naturally with this by creating a neurochemical amnesia that softens your birth memories over the following weeks.

baby arrives, you may change your mind about the name you have chosen and decide on a different one that suits her better. Here are some tips:

- *Find out the derivation and meaning* Buy a names book or look on the Internet for all the names you're currently considering.
- *Try to think of possible nicknames* Charles could become Charlie, Alyssa may become shortened to Aly, Samantha to Sam.
- *Avoid difficult names* It's best to avoid names that are very difficult to spell or pronounce.
- *Consider stereotypes* Will you and your child be happy with name stereotypes, such as Clint, Marilyn, Madonna, and so on?
- *Keep it in the family* Is there an important namesake you wish to honor—or avoid?
- *Pay attention to how the name sounds* And with a middle name? If you give your baby a middle name, consider what the initials spell.

PHOTOGRAPHING THE BIRTH

This might seem a trivial thing to think about, but planning how you want to record your baby's birth can save a lot of tension on the day.

Think about whether you want the birth photographed or videotaped. Arrange for someone, preferably other than your partner, to be in charge of the camera. Decide carefully what you want to be filmed, keeping in mind you can always edit the

CHOOSING YOUR BABY'S PEDIATRICIAN

Finding the best doctor for your baby can take some keen detective work. First, get recommendations from your healthcare provider, nurses, friends, and relatives, and then call each suggestion and ask for a telephone interview with the office manager. The following questions will be helpful:

- What is the type of practice? Is it solo or group? It may be better to chose a group practice where there'll always be someone on call.
- Who actually sees your child at a typical visit? Is it a nurse practitioner, pediatrician, or another healthcare provider in the group practice?
- What are the office hours, typical waiting times, and on-call group policy?
- How are after-hours calls handled?
- Does the pediatrician also practice at a hospital?

If you're still interested, make an appointment to interview the pediatrician. At this visit you can obtain the following information:

- What's the doctor's philosophy on issues such as breastfeeding, supplementation, newborn jaundice, circumcision, antibiotic use, immunization, and so on?
- Is the office environment welcoming and clean, and is there plenty to keep children entertained?
- What are your impressions of the staff and how they interact with children?

GOING BACK TO WORK

Another decision that you'll probably need to make before giving birth is when you plan to return to work and how you want your baby to be looked after when this happens. Keep in mind that most daycare facilities have long waiting lists and should be contacted well before the birth to get your baby's name on the list.

You may want to leave it as long as you can before going back to work—most mothers find it harder to leave their babies than they expected. And if the thought of going back to work full-time fills you with dread, consider a more flexible work pattern, such as working part-time—between 20 and 32 hours per week—or flex-time where you fit a full-time job into fewer days with longer hours or more days with shorter hours.

Negotiating different hours

You may be able to change your hours just by talking to your employer, or you may have to make a formal request in writing or negotiate through your human resources department. Either way, here are some tips that will help you get what you want:

- *Test the reaction* Tell your employer you're thinking about working part-time and arrange a meeting to discuss the matter. Ask if he or she would like a written outline of how you think this would work.
- *Prepare your case* Describe exactly how the job would get done if you worked part-time. If you can satisfy your boss that you can work just as efficiently as before, you're almost home.
- *Suggest a trial period* Six to eight weeks will give you enough time to discuss any problems with your boss and find solutions.
- *Explain it to your co-workers* Tell them what you're doing and try and settle any objections before you start. You need them on your side.

Organizing childcare

However, whether you go back full-time or part-time, you'll still need to arrange some form of childcare, and it'll be a lot easier returning to a working life if you feel happy and confident about this. Ask your healthcare provider, family and friends for recommendations, and remember that the most important factor is to ensure the safety and

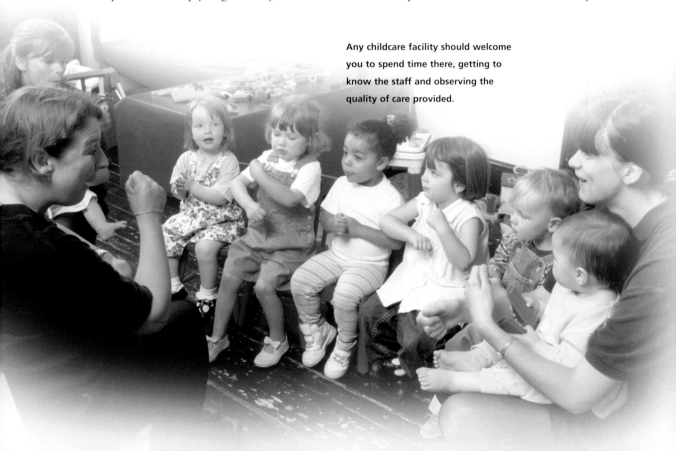

Any childcare facility should welcome you to spend time there, getting to know the staff and observing the quality of care provided.

Daycare can help your children be sociable
Researchers from the US National Institutes of
Health, who followed 3100 families from their
children's births to about second grade, found that
children in daycare with a number of other children
are less likely to have behavior problems than those
cared for in one-on-one situations, or small groups.

well-being of your baby. Licensing, training
certificates, references and any facility you are
considering should always be double-checked.
Finally, the best judge is your child; if you come
home to a happy and healthy baby, you can be sure
that your help arrangement is working well.

Your options

Take time to research your options. Your baby needs
to be with someone that you and your partner both
like and trust, otherwise the arrangement will fall
apart. Your basic choices are:

- *Parent at home* Obviously this is the ideal option.
  One of you stays at home to look after the baby,
  or you both work different hours so that the care
  of your baby can be shared.
- *Family* Having your mother or another relative
  looking after your baby can be an excellent
  childcare solution, providing your baby with
  continuity of care.
- *Nanny* In-home care can be expensive, but if you
  have more than one child it becomes more
  economical. There's no doubt that one-on-one
  care the first year of life is very beneficial, but
  that depends on having a reliable, experienced
  nanny who's in tune with a child's physical and
  emotional needs.

- *Home daycare* This is offered by people who are
  licensed to offer childcare in their homes,
  possibly in combination with looking after their
  own children. This arrangement will provide
  playmates and a family environment for your
  child, and has the advantage of her having the
  same caregiver and being in a small group.
- *Daycare centers* These work well for children of
  any age, as long as they're of a high standard.
  However, not all centers take babies under the
  age of 12 months.

HELP ONCE YOU'RE HOME

Planning ahead for your return home with your
baby is important, since you want to be able to get
to know her and to adjust to your new role in a
relaxed atmosphere. If you've had a difficult or
lengthy birth, you also may be tired and in need of
plenty of rest. Getting help at home for the first few
weeks after the birth can make a huge difference,
but you need to make sure that you choose the right
sort of help—and the right sort of person.

Be clear what you want

Helpers range from full-time professional nurses,
who can train you in childcare and provide
breastfeeding support, to experienced mothers who
are paid to come in for a few hours to help with the
housework and listen to any concerns you may have.
You need to be clear what you want your helper to
do and how long you'll need her. Ask about fees,
training and experience, check references, and make
sure that you're going to get on well.

Some women depend on relatives to help out,
which is ideal, provided that you're on good terms
with your family and are confident in their
knowledge and experience of childcare.

SHOPPING FOR YOUR BABY

Nothing quite beats the thrill of buying your very first items for your baby. However, resist the temptation to buy out the whole store. Stock up on the basics now, and then shop for other items when you require them.

It's easy to be seduced into getting things that look attractive but that you don't actually need. Keep in mind, too, that you will probably receive lots of baby gifts once your baby is born.

FURNISHING THE NURSERY

Your baby won't notice his surroundings for the first few months—all that will matter to him is that he's warm, well-fed, and comfortable. Yet for most parents, preparing the nursery is one of the most enjoyable parts of pregnancy and provides an excellent way for them to feel that they are welcoming their new baby into their home.

Keep in mind that your baby will probably use the same room throughout his childhood and that the decorations should grow with him. Plain background colors and fashionable finishing touches, such as borders, friezes, and stencils, can be quickly updated as he grows up.

Walls should be washable or at least spongeable. Paint is more practical than wallpaper. Choose a natural, water-based rather than a solvent-based paint; these don't give off chemical vapors while the room is being painted.

Your newborn won't need a lot of furniture in his room at first, but make sure that you have enough storage space, especially around the changing area. Unless you plan to replace the furniture as soon as he's crawling and trying to stand up on his own,

Shopping for your baby is fun, and you'll have more time now than after the birth. Try to enlist some help to carry some of the load.

SAFETY FIRST

Decorating There are several things you should watch out for when decorating your baby's room during pregnancy:

- Avoid breathing in paint fumes—get someone else to do the painting.
- If you suspect that old paint may be lead-based, get someone else to sand and paint over it. Lead-based paint can be toxic.
- Remember that your balance will have altered, so be extra careful on stepladders and never attempt to reach too far, even when you are standing on the floor.
- Stop before you become exhausted—you are more likely than usual to have accidents.

furniture you buy should have smooth, rounded edges. You also might like to include a comfortable chair for your own use.

A night-light may help to reassure him as he lies in the dark and a baby alarm will allow you to hear him when you are out of the room and he starts to cry. Thick curtains or blinds will help prevent him being woken by light outside. Fit a dimmer switch to the main light or a side lamp so that you can check on your baby without waking him. At first the temperature needs to be kept at about 75°F (24°C). Many parents use a thermostatically controlled heater in a baby's room so that they don't need to keep the whole home at this temperature.

A PLACE TO SLEEP
You may prefer to put your baby in a bassinet or cradle at first, progressing to a crib when he's about 4 months old; or you could use a crib right away.

5 tips on shopping for baby

1 Consider the practicality of major items before you buy. For example, when choosing a stroller consider whether you could manage it getting on and off public transport, or if it will fit into the trunk of your car.

2 Think about buying some secondhand items; carriers, for example, can be in good condition because newborns outgrow them so quickly. However, items that can be damaged by previous use, such as car seats and mattresses, should always be bought new.

3 Only purchase a few outfits in newborn size; not only will your baby outgrow them very quickly but you'll probably be given a lot of first-sized clothes once he's born.

4 Consider buying nearly-new clothes and equipment from friends.

5 Many mail order and Internet companies specialize in baby clothes and equipment, and their prices can be very competitive.

Bassinets and cradles look gorgeous and create a soft, comforting environment for a tiny baby; however, they can be expensive and are soon outgrown. Cribs are more practical, as your baby can sleep in a crib up until the age of 3 years, but a crib may not be suitable at first if your baby is sleeping in your room and space is a problem.

Choosing a bassinet or cradle
Accommodating a newborn to about a 4-month-old baby, bassinets are light, small, and portable, and come with a stand. Cradles are available in three main types: the rocker cradle that sits on the floor, the pendulum cradle that's suspended from a frame, and the cradle swing with detachable carrier.

Make sure you buy a bassinet that is robust enough to withstand the weight of a healthy, fast-growing infant. But you'll need to move your baby to a crib once he reaches the upper weight limit given by the manufacturer, or if he seems squashed or restless. Consider also the following:

- *Locks on legs/wheels* Make sure that bassinets or cradles with folding legs and/or wheels have locking mechanisms to keep them stable.
- *Hoods that fold back* If hoods won't fold back it can make it tricky to pick up your baby.
- *Rounded edges and corners* Make sure the cradle or bassinet doesn't have any sharp edges that could hurt your baby. This especially applies to woven or wicker bassinets.
- *Avoid quilts, ribbons, and cords* Don't be seduced by cute bedding Remove any ribbons and cords that could strangle your baby. If the bassinet comes with a quilt, discard it—soft bedding has been linked to SIDS (see page 309).
- *A firm mattress that fits snugly* If you can fit two fingers between the mattress and the side of the bassinet, the mattress is too small.
- *A good base* Cradles and bassinets should have strong, wide bases.

Choosing a crib
Whether you intend to put your baby in a crib from birth or later, it's worth shopping around for one now, as you may have to order it in advance. When

making a choice, think about how long you expect your baby to stay in his crib. Buying a big one means your baby won't need his own bed for some time. Some cribs convert into a toddler bed, which can be useful. However, keep in mind that you will need a single bed eventually, and the crib may be needed if you're planning to have another baby.

The more expensive brands of crib tend to offer more features, such as adjustable mattress heights. Some cribs are designed to fit in a corner, while others have sides that can be removed altogether so that the crib can form an extension to the parental bed—an excellent solution if you want your baby as close to you as possible at night without actually being in your bed. Lockable casters make moving and cleaning under the crib easier.

When buying a crib, it's very important that you check for the following safety features:

♦ *Narrow enough gaps in the side rails* The side rail slats should be no farther than 3 inches (8 cm) apart, to prevent your baby from getting stuck between them.

♦ *Dual releases on the side rails* There should be one on each end, to prevent your child lowering them. When lowered, they should also be at least 9 inches (23 cm) above the mattress support to prevent your child falling out. When raised, the top of the side rails should be at least 26 inches (66 cm) above the mattress at its lowest position. Before buying a crib, raise and lower the sides of each model to see which one is easiest to operate. Note that if the release is too easy an older baby may learn to lower the sides himself.

♦ *Well-assembled joints and mechanisms* Check that all the parts of the assembled crib are securely fastened and the crib is sturdy. The moving parts should work smoothly so that fingers or clothing do not become trapped.

♦ *A snug-fitting mattress* There should be no chance that your baby can become stuck between the mattress and the crib. The mattress itself should always be new and needs to be firm, vinyl covered, and with reinforced corners and sides.

♦ *Plain, practical designs* Avoid cut-out designs, as your baby could trap his arm or head in them.

♦ *A clean safety record* Never buy a used or old crib in a garage sale, as you won't know its history. If your crib was made in Canada before 1986, don't use it. Health Canada changed the safety standards in 1986. In the United States, extra voluntary standards were added in 1988.

Choosing a mattress

If you have been given a crib—or you already have one—you will need to purchase a new mattress. Mattresses can be foam or innersprung. Many parents choose foam mattresses, made of either polyester or polyether, because they weigh less and they're cheaper than innersprung mattresses. Always choose a high-density foam mattress—about 1.5 lbs per cubic foot (24 kg per cubic meter)—which has ventilated sections, both at the top and in the middle. An innersprung mattress is likely to keep its shape longer. Look for a mattress with a minimum of 150 coils. For maximum water resistance and durability, choose a mattress covered in vinyl with reinforced corners.

GETTING ABOUT

Your baby will need to be comfortable and safe when you take him out. If you are walking you will need a carriage, stroller, or a carrier; if you are driving, an infant car seat is essential.

Carriages and strollers

One item you will not want to be without is a carriage or stroller. There's a huge range to choose from—traditional carriages with a spring-suspension chassis, lightweight portable strollers, all-terrain strollers, standard-size strollers, and double strollers. To help you decide on the right model, think about your lifestyle. If you're going to use it every day around town, and you are planning on having more than one baby, a traditional carriage offers a comfortable ride and will be long lasting; if you're active and keen to maintain fitness, an all-terrain stroller that you can jog with might be the answer. Check the recommended age range for the carriage or stroller before you buy, to make sure it is suitable for use from birth.

Carriers

A baby sling, which holds your baby close to your chest, can be used indoors as well as out. Some styles leave the legs and arms free; others cover the whole baby. Before you buy, make sure that the sling offers good head and back support, has wide shoulder straps, so that it is comfortable for you, and you can put it on easily without help.

Baby carriers are usually more sturdy and are sold according to your baby's age or with a maximum weight level. They have stiff padding behind the head to give extra support to a young baby who can't yet hold up his head on his own.

Before you buy a carrier, make sure the stitching is free of any faults. Triple stitching gives the most strength and durability. All buckles, zips, and fasteners should work smoothly and the shoulder straps should sit comfortably and be well-padded. Check that the fabric is washable and shrink-proof and that it carries a safety standards logo.

Cotton, padded, and machine-washable baby carriers are the best for transporting a young baby; more substantial backpacks with aluminum frames are better for older, heavier babies.

Infant car seats

This is an essential buy before the birth, as you'll need a car seat when you take your baby home from the hospital. Infant car seats are held in place by the seatbelt, with the baby facing the rear of the car for better protection. These first seats can be used from birth until your baby weighs about 29 lbs (13 kg), usually at around 6 months of age. The most convenient have a three-point, one-pull harness, a one-pull handle, a head-hugger to keep a very young baby's head steady, and deep, padded sides. Infant car seats can be used as comfortable baby seats outside the car—some have rockers, others come with a chassis and can be used as a stroller.

Two-way car seats are fitted into the car and will last your baby for longer, although their design is less suited to a very small baby because they're often too upright. Initially, they're used like a first seat; then they convert to forward-facing seats that take a baby up to 45 lbs (18 kg).

FEEDING

The sort of equipment that you'll need will depend on whether you're planning to nurse or bottlefeed. Even if you want to breastfeed your baby, you'll still need some equipment for expressing milk and bottles for feeding expressed milk or water.

Bottles

Bottles can be standard or wide-necked, hold 4 oz (115 g) or 9 oz (260 g) of liquid, have a standard, wide-necked or a graspable shape, and have a straight or angled top. The angled top means that the baby doesn't swallow so much air, which can lead to gas. Bottles can be glass or plastic. There are also bottles with disposable liners on the market; these are expensive but handy for traveling.

For a new baby, the 4-oz (115-g) size is large enough, but it's more practical to buy larger bottles that will be suitable for when he's older. Most sterilizers take standard and wide-necked shapes, but some travel bags take only standard bottles.

Nipples

There are a variety of shaped nipples available, made from latex or silicone—latex nipples begin to deteriorate after about a month, silicone nipples can last up to a year. Natural or orthodontic shaped nipples mimic sucking at the breast and may be the best choice if you're planning to mix breast- and bottlefeeding. Anti-colic nipples allow air into the bottle as the baby empties it, which minimizes the amount of air he will swallow while feeding. Choose either the smallest hole or variable flow types at first.

Breast pumps

Whether you're a working mom, or you are keen for your partner to be able to feed your baby as well, a breast pump can help you extract milk to be stored for future use. You can choose between electric and manual models depending on your needs.

CHANGING AND BATHING

A purpose-made changing table is well worth having, as it helps prevent back strain; choose one that will hold diapers and cleaning materials.

YOUR BABY'S STARTER KIT

Feeding

Breastfeeding

- ◆ 2 bottles and nipples.
- ◆ Sterilizing tablets or sterilizer.
- ◆ Bottle brush.
- ◆ Breast pads—non-plastic backed.
- ◆ Pump for expressing milk—optional.

Bottlefeeding

- ◆ 6 bottles and nipples.
- ◆ Sterilizer.
- ◆ Bottle brush.
- ◆ Bottle warmer—optional.

Changing

- ◆ Changing mat/table.
- ◆ Baby wipes.
- ◆ Diaper-rash cream.
- ◆ 70 first-size disposable diapers or 24 small-sized cloth diapers.

For cloth diapers

- ◆ Safety pins or clips.
- ◆ Plastic pants.
- ◆ 2 diaper buckets.
- ◆ Sterilizing fluid.
- ◆ Diaper liners.

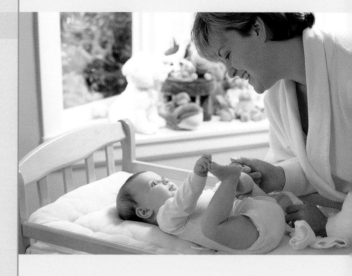

Clothes

- ◆ 4 stretch suits.
- ◆ 2 nightdresses or sleep suits or 2 extra stretch suits.
- ◆ 4 cotton undershirts.
- ◆ 3 open-fronted sweaters.
- ◆ 2 bibs.
- ◆ 4 receiving blankets.
- ◆ Hat—type depending on season.
- ◆ Mittens.

Bedtime

- ◆ Bassinet or cradle or crib and crib mattress.
- ◆ 3 fitted bottom sheets.
- ◆ 3 top sheets—optional.
- ◆ 2 or 3 lightweight blankets.

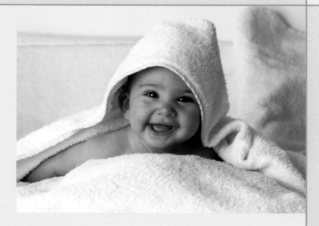

Bathing

- ◆ Baby bathtub.
- ◆ Cotton balls.
- ◆ Baby toiletries.
- ◆ 2 large soft towels.
- ◆ Wash cloth or sponge.
- ◆ Baby hairbrush.
- ◆ Blunt-ended scissors.

However, you can just use a changing mat on a waist-high surface. Changing mats should be wipe-clean and slightly padded to keep your baby comfortable. When you're out with your baby, a smaller travel changing mat will be invaluable—fold-up mats are inexpensive and fit easily into a baby's travel bag.

A special baby bathtub isn't essential but can make it easier to bath your baby. You may want to consider a sling-type insert for the tub that holds your baby in a lying position with his head above water, leaving both your hands free to wash him.

Baby products

Until your baby is around 3 months old, it's best not to use any soaps or bath products for bathing. Plain water is sufficient. However, baby oil or moisturizer may be useful for dry, flaky skin. Avoid baby powder, as there is evidence to suggest that it can choke a baby if inhaled. Always make sure that your baby's skin is protected from the sun with total UV-protection creams—there are many products that have been developed for babies.

CLOTHES

Baby clothes are generally sold according to age—newborn, 3 months, 6 months, and so on. European-made clothes are usually sold in centimeter sizes starting at 50 cm. A big baby may not get any wear out of newborn size clothes, so if you're baby's weight is projected to be 10 lbs (4.5 kg) or more, you may want to start with a 3-month size. There are special ranges for very small and premature babies.

Your baby will probably dislike being dressed and undressed, so choose clothes that are easy to put on and take off. Avoid buying clothes that you need to handwash or iron—you won't have the time—and choose natural fibers as these minimize sweating and irritation. Always check that there are no raised seams or scratchy labels.

Stretch suits

The most practical stretch suits have snaps up the front and around the crotch to give easy access for diaper changing. Your baby's bones are very soft and it's essential that clothes have plenty of room in the legs and feet for proper growth.

Undershirts

These should have wide or envelope necks so that they can be slipped easily over the head. Many brands of undershirt fasten under the crotch with snaps, providing extra warmth and keeping the diaper securely in place. Once again, keep clothing loose so that your baby can grow into it.

Nightwear

Most baby nightdresses have drawstring bottoms but if not, your baby's feet may become cold so you will need socks. You may prefer to put your baby in an all-in-one sleep suit, or if it is warm, put him down to sleep in an undershirt and diaper.

Outdoor clothes

Babies lose a lot of heat from their heads, which are proportionately large for their bodies, so a hat is essential in winter and may be advisable in spring and autumn. A sun hat is essential for summer if you plan to spend a lot of time outside in the sunshine. If it's very cold and your stroller doesn't provide much protection from the elements, you will need a bunting bag. Shawls, cardigans, and mittens are all useful for the cold and should be close-knitted to prevent tiny fingers being trapped. If it gets very hot, invest in a few lightweight summer romper suits.

PREPARING FOR LABOR

As your due date approaches you'll want to prepare yourself for the birth—both physically and emotionally. Now is the time to look at things you can do that will help you be comfortable, and to address concerns you may have about giving birth.

Although you may be feeling excited about having a new baby in your life, you may not feel quite so enthusiastic about the birth itself. This is very natural, since the act of giving birth involves a highly sensitive and private part of your body, which carries with it a wealth of emotional feelings. Be prepared to react emotionally to the birthing process as well as physically, and try to work through any fears beforehand so that the birth can be a positive, unproblematic experience.

Emotional fears can affect the birth in a very direct physical way. A woman who isn't prepared for the pain of normal contractions may believe that something is wrong and become frightened. This can disrupt her breathing, increase the tension—and therefore pain—in her muscles, and may even decrease the flow of oxytocin, the hormone that causes the uterus to contract. Learning about the process of labor and good support can help a woman work with contractions rather resist them.

The best way to avoid this is to try to find and resolve any emotional problems that you might have buried deep in your subconscious mind. It's no coincidence that your fantasies and fears rise to the surface in late pregnancy to help you face problems before the birth, and you can use this opportunity to chase these out of your life for good. If you have had especially difficult and traumatic experiences, such as a history of sexual abuse or a previous negative birth experience—or if you have strong control issues—it may be beneficial to seek out some professional counseling.

5 tips to help you through late pregnancy

1   Wear light, loose clothing. You'll be feeling hotter than normal, mostly because of increased fat deposits and an increased metabolism.

2   Try to get as much sleep as possible. Supplement your nightly sleep with naps, especially if you're being woken by trips to the bathroom.

3   Keep your body hydrated by drinking plenty of fluids so that you cope better with your faster metabolism and relieve swelling feet and legs.

4   Take a break whenever you can. Sit down and put your feet up on a stool for 10 to 15 minutes, three times a day if you have swelling in your feet and legs.

5   Increase your intake of protein. Plenty of milk, eggs, meat, and fish can alleviate some of the problems with late pregnancy,

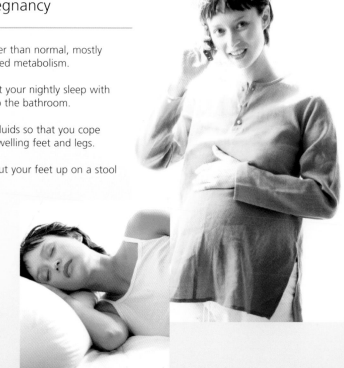

Your late pregnancy exercise program

At this point in your pregnancy, you should be keeping up your daily exercise (see page 117). From about 28 weeks onward add a few extra exercises to get you into shape for childbirth.

Tailor sitting This position helps improve pelvic flexibility in preparation for the birth. Place pillows under your thighs to support them and sit with your back straight and the soles of your feet together **1**. Draw your heels toward your perineum, using your arms to push down on your thighs. Relax your shoulders and the back of your neck and breathe deeply. Hold the stretch for a count of 12 and repeat daily.

As you get more flexible, you can remove the pillows from under your thighs **2**, and push your knees closer to the floor.

DRAWING OUT YOUR NIPPLES

If your healthcare provider hasn't already assessed your nipples, do so yourself at around 28 weeks. This is because the use of breast shells is advised for women who have flat or retracted nipples and plan to breastfeed. Grasp your breast between thumb and forefinger, about ½ to 1 inch (2 to 3 cm) outside the areola, and gently squeeze. If your nipple retracts into the areola or remains very flat, you can buy specialized shells that will help your nipples protrude. Wear them daily until you deliver.

POWER KEGELS

At around 28 weeks start building up the intensity of your pelvic-floor exercises (see page 122). Start to hold each squeeze for a count of ten, and repeat 12 times, three times a day.

By 34 weeks you're ready for more advanced exercises. Begin with six strong squeeze-and-release flexes. Next, flex the lower third of the birth canal near your vaginal opening, then the middle part, and finally the area around your cervix. Hold the flex at each level, like an elevator stopping at three floors. Release these muscles from the top down, floor by floor. Repeat six times twice a day.

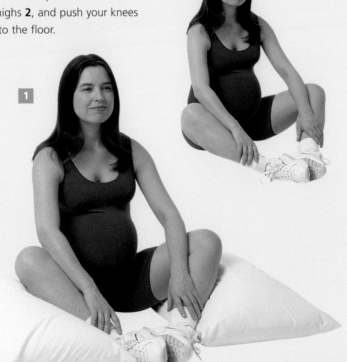

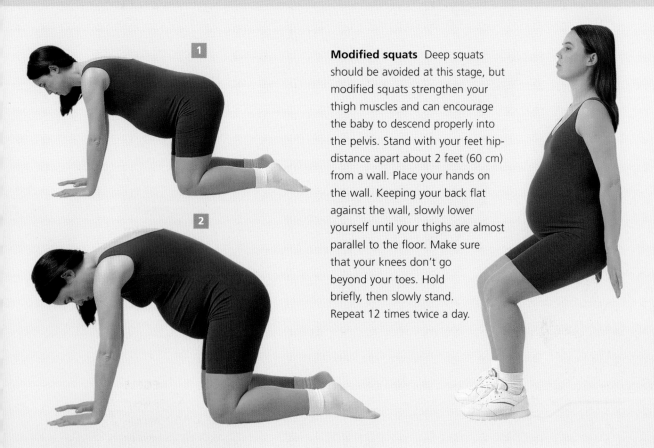

Modified squats Deep squats should be avoided at this stage, but modified squats strengthen your thigh muscles and can encourage the baby to descend properly into the pelvis. Stand with your feet hip-distance apart about 2 feet (60 cm) from a wall. Place your hands on the wall. Keeping your back flat against the wall, slowly lower yourself until your thighs are almost parallel to the floor. Make sure that your knees don't go beyond your toes. Hold briefly, then slowly stand. Repeat 12 times twice a day.

Pelvic rock This exercise can ease backache during late pregnancy and labor. Get down on your hands and knees, with your knees about hip-width apart. Begin with your neck in line with your spine and your back flat—don't let it sag **1**. Then slowly round your shoulders and back and let your head drop down **2**, tightening your abdomen and buttocks as you do so. Hold briefly, then gradually return to the start position. Repeat ten times twice a day or whenever you feel tension.

PERINEAL MASSAGE

You can use this technique daily, from around 34 weeks, to stretch the tissue around your vagina and perineum in preparation for the birth.

Always wash your hands before and after this exercise. Use a hand-held mirror to locate your vaginal opening, perineum, and urethra.

Sit or lean back comfortably, with a towel under your hips. Using a non-petroleum lubricant, such as K-Y jelly, coat your thumbs and perineal area. Place your thumbs 1 to 1½ inches (3 to 4 cm) inside your vagina. Press gently down and to the sides. Stretch until you feel a slight tingling sensation. Hold this pressure for about 2 minutes.

Maintaining the pressure, gently massage back and forth over the lower half of your vagina for 3 to 4 minutes. Take care to avoid your urethra during the massage because of the risk of urinary tract infection.

Many women find taking a tour of the birth unit beforehand very helpful. By doing this, you may be more able to picture yourself giving birth, and can emotionally prepare for the actual event.

YOUR BODY IN LATE PREGNANCY

During the last weeks of pregnancy, you'll probably find it increasingly hard to get comfortable, as your baby demands more and more space, and you're likely to experience a number of minor problems. For more information, see Chapter 2.

Indigestion is one of the most common discomforts of late pregnancy. While hormones relax the sphincter between your stomach and esophagus, your growing baby puts pressure on your abdomen, causing a reflux of gases and gastric juices into the esophagus. You can help ease this by avoiding large meals, not eating close to bedtime, and sleeping with extra pillows to prevent acid from rising up. Antacids containing calcium carbonate aren't generally effective as they cause an increase in stomach acidity.

Abdominal stretching can cause an uncomfortable burning sensation over your taut belly. Sometimes called hot spots, these are quite common and are superficial pains—if the pains are deeper within your abdomen you must inform your healthcare provider. Hot spots can be irritated by tight or heavy clothing, so avoid pantyhose and stick to loose clothing, and apply an ice pack to relieve

What position is your baby in?

Head down

This is the best position for birth, and 95 percent of babies naturally adopt it before labor. If your baby's back is facing your abdomen, this is called occiput anterior; if her back is turned toward your spine, this is called occiput posterior. This position can cause severe backache during labor.

Breech presentation

As many as 4 percent of babies settle with their bottom or feet first. This is known as a breech presentation. There are small, but significant risks to the vaginal birth of a breech baby, especially for first babies, and some practitioners will only deliver breech babies by cesarean. However, you can carry out exercises to move the baby into a head-down position (see opposite).

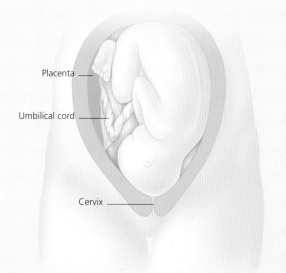

Placenta

Umbilical cord

Cervix

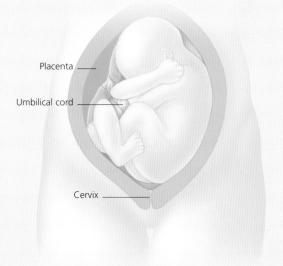

Placenta

Umbilical cord

Cervix

the burning. Worn occasionally, an abdominal support designed for pregnancy is helpful for backache, especially for women whose abdominal muscles have been stretched by frequent or closely spaced pregnancies. For exercises to strengthen abdominal muscles, see page 123.

HELPING A BREECH BABY TO TURN

When the baby is still relatively small, before about 32 weeks, she has room to change positions frequently. After this most babies settle into their preferred position (see below), and it's important to know what this is, since this can profoundly affect the birth. Your healthcare provider can tell the position of your baby by palpating (gently pressing)

Transverse lie

Another 1 percent of babies are positioned across the womb, known as a transverse or oblique lie, which make a normal vaginal birth impossible. It is sometimes possible to change these positions using the breech tilt after 32 weeks and external version after 37 weeks.

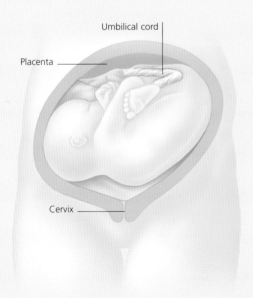

Umbilical cord

Placenta

Cervix

your abdomen. If your baby is in a breech position or a transverse lie, it may be possible to help her assume the head-down position with the following.

Breech tilt

Lie on your back with your knees flexed and place four plump pillows or cushions under your buttocks so that your pelvis is higher than your stomach. Remain in this position for a minimum of 10 minutes twice a day. Because your pelvis is higher than your stomach it will allow your baby's head to float, which will encourage her to turn so that her head moves up into the pelvis.

Visualization

On an empty stomach, concentrate on relaxing your abdomen while visualizing your baby turning. Repeat for 10 minutes twice a day. This technique was developed by Dr. Juliet DeSa Souza, who found it to be successful in turning 89 percent of breech presentations, usually within 2 to 3 weeks.

External version

If a breech baby fails to turn before you are 37 weeks into your pregnancy, many healthcare providers will perform an external version— manipulating the mother's abdomen so that the baby slowly turns. This procedure is not without risks, which your healthcare provider should discuss with you. An external version is carried out ideally at 37 to 38 weeks, when there's enough amniotic fluid to allow for a small amount of movement. Success rates vary from 50 to 70 percent.

POSITIONING THE BABY'S HEAD

Another aspect of positioning that affects the birth involves how your baby's head rotates as it descends through your pelvis. Since the top opening of a woman's pelvis is oval, with the long axis from side to side, babies enter the pelvis facing sideways. But the lower opening of the pelvis is oval with its long axis from front to back, with the largest part at the front, so the head must turn during its descent so that the baby faces the mother's tailbone; the occiput anterior (OA) position. Unfortunately, 20

PACKING YOUR BAGS

Bag for the birthing room

- Change for telephone calls, parking, and snacks.
- Cell phone.
- Phone numbers for when labor begins: coach, doula/monitrice, doctor/midwife, relatives.
- Phone numbers for after the birth: friends, relatives, insurance company, baby nurse, childbirth educator, diaper service, stationer for announcements.
- Insurance cards and pre-registration forms.
- Camera or video equipment.
- Magazines, books and other distractions.
- Snacks for you and your birth partner.
- Watch with a second hand for timing contractions.
- Lotion or powder for massage.
- Cold and warm packs for back relief.
- Slippers and heavy socks for cold feet.
- Toothbrush, toothpaste, and mouthwash.
- Hairbrush, clips, and bands.
- Pillow, if appropriate.

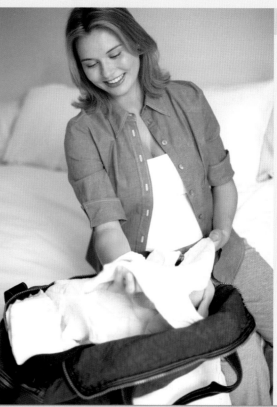

Bag for after the birth

- Robe, nightgowns, and panties.
- Maternity sanitary napkins.
- Breastfeeding supplies: nursing bra, nursing pads, nursing gown, purified lanolin for nipples.
- Changing bag and diapers for your baby.
- Baby clothes.
- Toiletries.
- Birth announcements with address list and a pen.
- Baby book for footprints and signatures.
- Extra camera film.

Bag for going home

- Loose outfit, including comfortable shoes.
- Bag for carrying home gifts and hospital supplies.
- Infant car seat.
- Going home outfit for your baby: undershirt, nightgown or stretch suit, socks, receiving blanket, and cold weather gear if needed.
- Diapers and baby wipes.

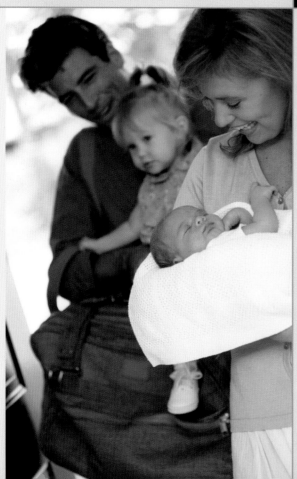

percent of babies rotate into an occiput posterior (OP) position, facing the pubic bone. This may lead to prolonged labor (see page 250).

MONITORING YOUR BABY'S WELL-BEING

Once you can feel your baby's movements—from around 18 to 20 weeks—you may want to keep a record of her levels of activity. This is particularly useful if your baby is overdue (see page 208). A kick-count sheet is a chart that you fill out daily, recording your baby's movements over a number of hours. This is a very reliable test of your baby's well-being, and you should always report a significant decrease in your baby's movement immediately, whether you are doing a kick-count sheet or not.

GETTING READY TO GO

As the excitement builds up toward the delivery date, you need to make sure that everything is at hand when you need it. At least four weeks ahead of time, you need to pack your bags, leaving room for last-minute items, and make final preparations for your trip to the hospital or birth center. If you're having a home birth, special preparations must also be made, so check with your healthcare provider.

Travel plans

Decide how you want to get to the hospital or birth center; are you confident about your transport arrangements? It's a good idea to have a back up plan. Ask a friend or keep the number of a reliable cab service handy. Map out the easiest route and try it out; you may find that you need a different one during the rush hour. It may also be necessary to find a car park with good rates. Find out which entrance of the hospital or birth center you need and who you should approach when you get there.

If you already have children, you need to prearrange a babysitter who will be able to stay at your home or collect your children straight away. Once again make sure that you have a couple of back ups ready to call on.

SAMPLE KICK-COUNT SHEET														
TIME	WEEK 39							WEEK 40						
	M	T	W	T	F	S	S	M	T	W	T	F	S	S
9 am														
9.30 am														
10 am														
10.30 am														
11 am														
11.30 am														
12 pm														
12.30 pm														
1 pm														
1.30 pm														
2 pm														
2.30 pm														
3 pm														
3.30 pm														
4 pm														
4.30 pm														
5 pm														
5.30 pm														
6 pm														
6.30 pm														
7 pm														
7.30 pm														
8 pm														
8.30 pm														
9 pm														

If less than ten movements by 9 pm, record total number here

9														
8														
7														
6														
5														
4														
3														
2														
1														

GOING OVERDUE

Extra days or weeks past your due date may provide crucial extra resting time before the birth. Only 5 percent of women deliver on their due date, with the majority giving birth a little late.

The main reason for due dates rarely being accurate is because the due date is an estimated time around 40 weeks from the start of your last period. Your baby is expected to be born within two weeks either side of the due date, and a pregnancy is only considered officially post-date after 42 weeks.

It's also common for a baby to be overdue if it's a mother's first pregnancy. A first pregnancy is prolonged, on average, eight days past the due date. The average second baby is born three days late. Poor positioning of the baby's head can also delay the baby's descent.

Many women prefer to avoid the concern of friends and family by giving a general time span for when the baby is to be born, such as the middle of June. It also helps you prepare for continuing beyond your due date. If your pregnancy approaches 42 weeks, your healthcare provider will discuss the use of induction to start labor (see page 186).

MONITORING YOUR OVERDUE BABY

Between 2 and 5 percent of pregnancies outlive the placenta's ability to nourish the baby. Since this can cause problems for the baby, it's vital that you take special precautions after 40 weeks to ensure that your baby is doing well.

- *Kick-count sheets* This is a useful test that you can do at home (see page 207).
- *Non-stress tests* These are simply the use of a fetal monitor to record your baby's heart. It's usually carried out in your healthcare provider's office.
- *Contraction stress tests (CST)* This uses a fetal monitor to record your baby's response to the stress of contractions that your doctor stimulates.
- *A biophysical profile* This is an ultrasound that measures your baby's limb and lung movement, and the amount of amniotic fluid.

5 natural ways to encourage labor

1 Exercises for positioning of the baby (see page 205) can help avoid a prolonged pregnancy.

2 Sexual intercourse can help prepare your cervix for labor. Semen is rich in prostaglandins, hormones that are known to soften the cervix. Orgasm also stimulates uterine contractions.

3 Nipple stimulation causes secretion of the hormone oxytocin, which stimulates your uterus to contract. Occasionally, nipple stimulation can cause strong, lengthy contractions and may result in decreased blood flow to the baby. This technique should be used under the supervision of a trained professional.

4 Emotional readiness is a component of labor that is rarely discussed. Women who are emotionally unprepared may subconsciously forestall birth. If you have any concerns about the effect your new baby will have on your life, discuss them with your partner or healthcare provider.

5 Certain herbs and homeopathic remedies may stimulate uterine activity. There haven't been any scientific studies to determine how safe or effective these herbs are, so don't take anything without professional advice.

6 Stripping the membranes involves introducing a gloved finger into the cervix and teasing the membranes away from the edge of the cervix. In some, but not all, studies, this procedure has been shown to reduce late births. This should only be done by your healthcare provider.

12

CHAPTER

YOUR LABOR AND BIRTH EXPERIENCE

Very soon now, you will go through the process of

labor, culminating in the birth of your baby. It's an

awesome prospect, but finding out as much as you

can about what happens during labor and birth is

invaluable. It will make you feel more in control, a

lot more confident, and more able to enjoy this

special event.

RECOGNIZING LABOR

Before real labor can begin, your body has to undergo certain changes. For most women, these pre-labor preparations take place sometime during the three weeks before or two weeks after their "due dates"—only 5 percent of women actually deliver on their due dates.

Your emotions can veer wildly before labor. You may feel thrilled by the anticipation of your baby's arrival one minute, and totally unprepared for labor, birth, and motherhood the next. All these feelings are entirely natural. It's common also to feel a little down during these last weeks of pregnancy—your baby may seem to have taken over your life and your body completely. When you feel like this, try to keep your emotions positive by treating yourself to a baby-shopping spree, or lunch with a friend.

SIGNS THAT LABOR IS APPROACHING

In the days or weeks before your baby's birth you may have a number of symptoms of your body's preparation for labor. If you are a first-time mother, these physical changes can begin weeks before true labor. With subsequent babies, these changes are more likely to happen closer to the birth.

Engagement

As the lower part of your uterus softens and expands, your baby's head descends lower into your pelvis. This is known as engagement or "dropping," and when it happens, you'll find that you have more space to breathe. Any heartburn symptoms you've had may be eased, and you won't feel uncomfortably full after a meal. Engagement usually occurs between two and four weeks before labor starts if it's your first baby; with subsequent pregnancies it often occurs as labor is about to begin.

Pelvic pressure

Once your baby's head is settled in your pelvis, you may experience some minor discomforts. You'll probably need to pass water and bowel movements more frequently because of the pressure that your baby is placing on your bladder and bowel. The

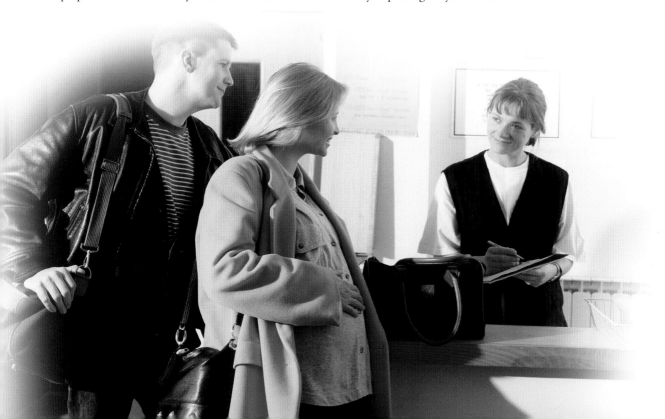

HOW THE HEAD ENGAGES

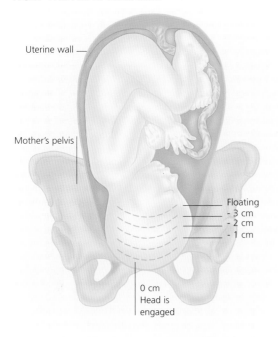

Uterine wall —

Mother's pelvis |

Floating
- 3 cm
- 2 cm
- 1 cm

0 cm
Head is
engaged

relaxation of your joints and ligaments may make
your pubic bones and back ache, and you may
experience sharp twinges as your baby presses down
on your pelvic floor. Compression of pelvic blood
vessels can cause swelling of your legs and feet.
Pelvic rocks (see page 203) and lying on your left
side can help relieve some of this pelvic pressure.

Vaginal discharge
Many women experience increased vaginal secretions
as the cervix softens. This discharge is usually egg
white, but it can be tinged pink. A yellow or frothy
discharge may signal an infection, so you should
report it to your healthcare provider.

Nesting instinct
If in the last month you find yourself seized with a
sudden desire to empty drawers, clear out closets,
and scrub the house from top to bottom, you're
simply experiencing what's known as the "nesting

instinct," an inbuilt maternal urge to prepare the
home for the imminent arrival of the baby. While
you may want to make the most of this burst of
energy, take care not to overdo it. You need to
conserve your strength for labor.

Braxton Hicks contractions
Named after the doctor who first identified them,
Braxton Hicks aren't true contractions, but
"practice" ones, designed to stretch the lower part of
your uterus—enabling your baby's head to settle
into your pelvis—and to soften and thin the cervix.
In the run-up to labor, these practice contractions
can intensify, giving you a tightening or "balling up"
sensation in your abdomen. Lying down usually
helps ease any discomfort.

Shivering or trembling
You may find yourself shivering or trembling for no
apparent reason when labor or pre-labor symptoms
arrive—often without any sensation of cold or
weakness. This can be a result of stress hormones or
an alteration in progesterone levels.

Diarrhea
Prostaglandins, which are the body chemicals
released in the process of early labor, may trigger
episodes of loose bowel movements.

SIGNS THAT LABOR IS IMMINENT
The exact cause of the onset of labor remains
unknown. The most widely held theory is that your
baby will produce substances that result in a change
in pregnancy hormones. Alternatively, you may
develop an increasing sensitivity towards the end of
pregnancy to substances in the body that produce
uterine contractions. So how do you know you're in
labor if there's no clearly defined start to it? This is
the question that every pregnant woman worries
about, but you can rest assured that when the time
comes, you will know.

HEALTH FIRST

Discoloration of fluid If, when your water breaks, it's stained yellow, green, or brown, the amniotic fluid contains meconium. This is a baby's first bowel movement and is normally passed in the hours following birth. If passed earlier, it could be a sign that your baby's in distress, so contact your healthcare provider without delay.

While the only true sign that labor has started is the onset of regular contractions, causing your cervix to dilate, there are other signs that labor's imminent.

Mucus plug and bloody show

As the cervix softens, shortens, and begins to dilate, the mucus plug that has sealed the cervix for most of your pregnancy is dislodged. This is called a bloody show—or sometimes just a "show"—and usually appears as a small amount of bright red or brownish mucus. A show may also appear as a heavier discharge or it may simply be unnoticeable. Though a show can be a sign that labor's imminent, it can occur as much as six weeks before the birth. However, if you have a show, you should contact your healthcare provider for advice.

Rupture of membranes

The amniotic sac containing the fluid around your baby usually ruptures—known as the "water breaking"—at some point during labor. Occasionally, however, it may rupture before contractions begin in earnest. Most women go into labor within 24 hours of their water breaking, as the rupture causes the release of prostaglandins, contraction-stimulating substances. Sometimes a woman may have been having contractions before her water breaks but has not been aware of them. Once the water breaks, contractions can intensify, as the baby's presenting part (the part that will be born first) now presses directly onto the dilating cervix.

If your water breaks at home, make a note of the time it broke and its consistency, and notify your healthcare provider. Amniotic fluid is usually clear and odorless, and once the bag of water has ruptured at term, it will go on leaking until delivery. If you're preterm, or if your baby was felt to be unengaged or high in the pelvis at your last exam,

TRUE OR FALSE LABOR?

Contractions are the one sure way to tell if you're in labor or not.
Use this chart to find out if your contractions are the real thing.

True labor	False labor
Contractions have a regular pattern—coming every 5 minutes.	Contractions are irregular—coming every 3 minutes, and then every 5 to 10 minutes.
Contractions become progressively stronger.	Contractions don't intensify with time.
Contractions don't abate when walking or resting.	Contractions may recede with changes in activity or position.
Contractions may be accompanied by a show.	Contractions usually not accompanied by increased mucus or bloody show.
Progressive cervical dilatation.	No significant cervical change is detectable.

your healthcare provider may recommend that you go into the hospital to be assessed before contractions start.

Once your water breaks it's important not to put anything into your vagina as there is a possible risk of infection. Showers are preferable to tub baths until active labor has begun and your baby has been assessed by your healthcare providers.

If you're aware of something pulsing in the vagina after your water breaks, this may be a prolapsed cord, so call your healthcare provider immediately and go to the hospital right away.

Regular contractions

Identifiers of true labor are that the cervix steadily dilates (opens out) and there are regular contractions. Early contractions are sometimes called "false" labor, because they occur only intermittently as they prepare the uterus for true, progressive labor. These early contractions stretch the lower uterus to accommodate the baby as she moves down the uterus. They also soften the cervix, but do not result in cervical change as regular contractions do. Labor aids or narcotic analgesia may help your body relax and allow the uterus to work more efficiently.

At some point, any brief, irregular contractions are replaced by ones that have a rhythmic pattern and longer length. These contractions are likely to be progressively contracting the upper uterus while stretching the lower part and opening the cervix. By this mechanism, the powerful upper uterus muscles push the baby through the stretchable lower uterus.

Sometimes back labor occurs (see page 251). If you experience back pain every 5 minutes, call your healthcare provider and go to the hospital.

WHEN TO GO TO THE HOSPITAL

The early part of labor can take hours. If you're not in any real discomfort, it's best to stay at home in familiar surroundings where there's plenty to do to distract yourself. If you're in a lot of discomfort, however, you may want to go to the hospital or birthing center sooner. As a rough guide, aim to go to hospital when contractions are so intense that you're unable to hold a conversation during one and

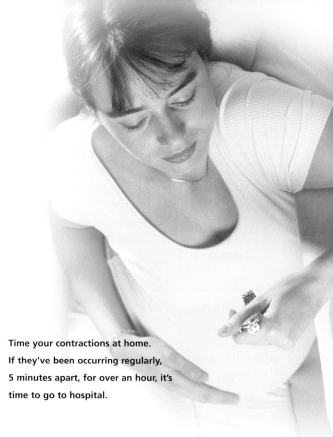

Time your contractions at home. If they've been occurring regularly, 5 minutes apart, for over an hour, it's time to go to hospital.

if you've been having regular contractions for over an hour—5 minutes apart, each lasting 45 to 60 seconds. Intense contractions that are less than 3 minutes apart are often a signal that birth is very near. If you've given birth before, keep in mind that, on average, second babies arrive in half the time that first babies take.

If your water breaks in the midst of regular contractions, this may be a signal to go to hospital. If your water breaks before regular 5-minute contractions occur, call your healthcare provider for advice. If you aren't sure whether it's false or real labor, don't feel embarrassed about going to the hospital to be assessed or asking your midwife to check you. It can be easy to misinterpret the signs of labor, especially with a first pregnancy, and it's better to err on the side of caution.

What happens when you arrive at the hospital

While admissions procedures for hospitals or birth centers vary greatly, the same things still have to happen once you're admitted. Generally, most women are asked to go to the maternity ward at once, although at some hospitals you may be asked to go to the emergency room so you can be taken to your room in a wheelchair. You may have pre-registered—some hospitals offer you the chance to do this before the birth; if not, you will do this at the check-in desk at the maternity wing. You'll then be taken to a labor and delivery suite or a birthing room, where a nurse will assess your progress by carrying out the following procedures:

◆ *Vital signs* Your pulse, blood pressure, breathing, and temperature—will be checked repeatedly throughout labor. You'll also be asked about your contractions, whether your water has broken, and whether you've recently eaten any food.

DID YOU KNOW...

A second delivery is often faster than the first
This is because the birth canal has already expanded to accommodate the first baby and there is less work for the uterus to do. On average, second labors take about eight hours and the second stage—pushing—is half the time of the first. The cervix of a second-time mother may dilate more before entering active labor.

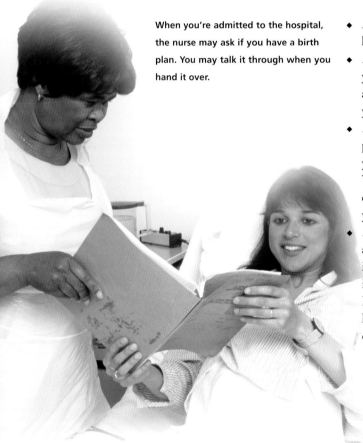

When you're admitted to the hospital, the nurse may ask if you have a birth plan. You may talk it through when you hand it over.

◆ *Monitoring* Your contractions and your baby's heart rate will be monitored in some way.
◆ *Internal exam* You'll have an exam to see whether your cervix is dilated. If you're still in early labor and everything's fine, you may be sent home until you go into active labor.
◆ *Brief history* You'll be asked what sort of pregnancy you've had and what sort of pain relief you want to have if you make that decision. You'll probably be given a hospital gown to change into, although some hospitals will allow you to wear your own clothes if you want to.
◆ *Blood sample* Your blood group will be checked and you may have an intravenous line (IV) inserted. This is routine at many hospitals in case it is needed later, for instance, for an epidural. However, you can ask to postpone the IV until later in labor, so that you are free to move about during this stage.

THE STAGES OF LABOR

Childbirth is divided into three stages. The first stage is labor, where uterine contractions work to fully dilate the cervix, so the baby can exit the uterus and pass into the birth canal. The second stage is the birth of your baby, and the third stage is the delivery of the placenta.

While every woman's experience of childbirth is unique, all birthing women will go through these three stages. The whole process averages about 14 hours for a first baby and about 8 hours for later babies. Some labors, however, progress more slowly during the first stage and then speed up at the beginning of the second stage. There are a variety of reasons why labor may slow down:

- *The baby is in the wrong position* Most babies fit best down the birth canal with their heads flexed and downward, facing the mother's side when in the pelvis, and facing her back when emerging from the pelvis. If your baby's not in this position, it can take a while for him to get into the right one. By changing position yourself and staying upright as much as possible you can help your baby adopt the best position for birth.
- *More molding and stretching is needed* Your baby's head needs to mold and your pelvic tissues need to stretch as she moves through the birth canal. This molding and stretching can take time.
- *Your contractions are weak* Rarely, uterine muscles are overstretched or infected and perhaps not contracting well. If help is needed, your healthcare provider may help strengthen your contractions with oxytocin (Pitocin).

THE FIRST STAGE

Labor, the first stage, is often divided into three phases: Early or latent labor, active labor, and transition or hard labor. For many women, these stages are distinct and noticeable. Other women may not notice such clear-cut differences.

Early or latent labor

While usually the longest part of labor, this is generally the easiest. During this time, the cervix continues to efface (thin out) and progressively dilate to 3 or 4 cm. At this stage, you may be aware of contractions, but they're usually manageable, and you may be able to sleep through them.

Contractions are usually short, lasting from 20 to 60 seconds. Initially they may be as far apart as 20 minutes, becoming increasingly stronger and closer over a six to eight hour period. This may be the point at which the mucus plug is dislodged or membranes rupture. Unless there's a medical reason for you to go early to the hospital, you'll be much more comfortable staying at home in early labor.

MORE **ABOUT** | active management of labor

Many hospitals follow a policy of active management of labor (AMOL) for first-time labors. This means that your labor is expected to proceed within a certain time-frame and your healthcare provider helps it along if it seems to be taking longer. Once labor is diagnosed—with intense contractions, 80 percent effacement (thinning of the cervix), ruptured membranes, or bloody show—women are expected to deliver within 12 hours. Frequent vaginal exams assess progress. If there's no progress one hour after labor is diagnosed, the membranes will be ruptured artificially (see page 228). If no progress is seen within two hours and the cervix is less than 1 cm dilated, a dose of oxytocin is given. In hospitals that practice AMOL, it has helped shorten the length of first labors and reduce the cesarean rate.

If you first notice the contractions at night, continue resting as much as possible. If you can't rest, find a distracting, but not taxing, activity. Don't forget to eat light snacks during this early stage. Women used to be advised not to eat at all in labor in case they needed general anesthesia, in which case it was thought that they might breathe in food. But studies have shown that this risk is very small, while eating light solids in labor can actually improve labor outcome—labor is hard work and your body needs energy in order to cope.

Your symptoms in early labor may be similar to those of pre-labor—cramps, backache, increased urination and bowel movements, increased vaginal discharge, pelvic pressure, and leg and hip cramps. Many women also experience a burst of energy, but try to conserve this energy for later on.

Active labor

This stage is reached when the cervix begins to dilate rapidly. For first-time mothers in this stage, the cervix usually dilates at a minimum of 1 cm an hour. Contractions become noticeably more intense,

DID YOU KNOW...

Grazing can help your labor
Your digestive system slows right down during labor, so it won't be able to cope with a full stomach, but "grazing" (eating small amounts frequently) will help fuel your energy levels. Choose high-energy food that's easy to digest such as toast with jelly, bananas, and broth. Avoid hard-to-digest foods such as meats, dairy products, and fats.

and if a cervical check is performed, you'll probably be 3 cm dilated. Contractions now last 45 to 60 seconds, getting progressively stronger and closer together, from occurring about every 5 to 7 minutes to every 2 to 3 minutes.

As contractions become stronger and longer, you may need to work harder to relax through and between contractions. Try moving around and changing your position to relieve muscle tension. The sheer physical effort of labor can lead to increased breathing, heart rate, perspiration, and even nausea. It's important to drink plenty of cool liquids to guard against dehydration.

Contractions will feel a lot stronger now, and you may experience increased aches and tiredness. Your membranes may rupture if they haven't already. You'll probably feel a lot less sociable now as you focus in on yourself. Women in this stage of labor sometimes feel that labor is never going to end. Try to remember that this phase is usually rapid and the cervix will be dilated soon. You also may worry about how well things are progressing, so ask your healthcare provider about anything that's bothering you. If you find this difficult for any reason, you may prefer your birth partner to ask on your behalf.

Transitional labor

Lasting between around one and two hours, transition is labor's most difficult and demanding period, during which the cervix fully dilates from 8 to 10 cm. Contractions now become very strong, lasting from 60 to 90 seconds and coming every 2 to 3 minutes. Where you might have made rapid progress though the

THE CERVIX DILATING
During labor your cervix will dilate to 10 cm, as shown in this life-size diagram.

2   4   6   8   10

active phase, everything can seem to slow down during transitional labor. Be assured, however, that the end is in sight.

Because of the intensity of this phase, dramatic physical and emotional changes can accompany it. As your baby is pushed into your pelvis, you'll experience strong pressure in your lower back and/or perineum. You may have the urge to push or move your bowels and your legs may become shaky and weak. Significant stress reactions aren't uncommon, with perspiration, hyperventilation, shivering, nausea, vomiting, and exhaustion all possible. Without meaning to, women can reject the help of their birth partners and find every touch or labor aid unacceptable during this phase.

Many women lose all inhibitions, and may verbalize their distress uncharacteristically by shouting and swearing. Keep the goal in sight. The pushing stage will be coming soon and your discomfort will be much more controllable. Keep in mind that stronger contractions bring the phase to an end faster. Don't be afraid to express yourself—make it clear what helps and what doesn't. Try also to relax; it's the key to conserving strength and the best way to help contractions accomplish their goal.

DEALING WITH PAIN DURING LABOR

Labor is just what its name suggests—hard work. It's work that's performed by a very powerful muscular organ. Because the uterine muscle is a smooth muscle like the heart or intestinal tract, most of your sensation of its activity comes from the muscles and nerves surrounding the uterus. The neighboring muscles in the abdomen and pelvis need to relax so that the uterus can accomplish its work efficiently, pushing your baby past these muscles and out of your body. The accompanying sensation can be felt as anything from serious discomfort to extreme pain.

Monitoring your baby

Being squeezed through the birth canal is a stressful, although natural, experience for your baby, so your healthcare provider may want to monitor his progress. The least invasive way of doing this is to check his heartbeat with a Doppler, a handheld ultrasound device. Tests should be carried out at regular intervals of 15 to 30 minutes during labor and then every 5 minutes during delivery.

Alternatively, an external fetal monitor that has two devices strapped to your abdomen may be used. One device detects your baby's heartbeat, the other measures your contractions. This type of monitoring can be used intermittently, so that you can move around during labor.

If your baby appears to be in distress, his progress may need to be monitored internally. After the membranes have ruptured, a small electrode is passed through your vagina and attached to your baby's head to monitor his fetal heart rate.

If your healthcare providers feel that they need more information about your baby's progress they may carry out a fetal scalp pH. A small tube is inserted through your vagina until it reaches your baby's head. A tiny prick takes a few drops of blood from his scalp which is then tested for oxygen levels. These results help your healthcare provider decide on the next course of action.

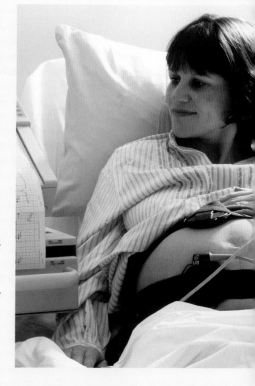

The purpose of pain

Hard work requires adequate oxygen and nutrition to keep the muscles being used pain-free. Muscles forced to work without oxygen or food will form and accumulate lactic acid, producing pain. The experience of pain may indicate that your body needs extra oxygen or nourishment. Just as you would change an activity if you suddenly developed pain while exercising, so labor pain may be a signal to change breathing patterns, to relax muscles, or increase nourishment to help the uterus work.

If you haven't prepared for childbirth, fear of the unknown can be a major problem; this is because fear leads to the stress response, which can lead to pain. Finding out what to expect in labor and birth can be very helpful to reduce this fear. If the fear is deep-seated, or, if you have seen or heard frightening experiences of childbirth, you may find it useful to discuss your concerns with your healthcare provider.

Medical pain control

There are a variety of ways to cope with uncomfortable sensations in labor. For more details, see Chapter 10. It's always best to discuss your options with your doctor before labor so you can be clear about the risks and benefits of each particular treatment. Learning about the general course of labor in advance can also help you understand the particular status of your own labor if you are considering medical therapy. Some medical treatments may be less suitable if you're close to delivery because many medications cross the placenta and can affect your baby's ability to adapt to life on his own. Also, if you know that your body may be less than an hour or two away from delivery, that knowledge might be enough to spur you on.

In labor, as in most situations, if you experience strong sensations without understanding them, they can lead to fear, stress, and pain. Understanding what your body is up to and realizing that these sensations are totally normal can help you interpret your contractions as "work" and not "pain."

Another way your mind can help the work of your body is by focusing on a goal—in this case the arrival of your baby. You also may find that distracting yourself can help you cope with a distressing body sensation. There are all sorts of mental distraction techniques you can employ, from breathing, massage, meditation, or imaging, to hypnosis.

While trying mental strategies to cope with potential body discomforts, don't ignore your body entirely. For instance, you may feel discomfort if your baby is descending in the wrong position, and if you change position you may help shift him. Or your bladder may be full, and relieving it may help your baby's descent. Nausea or weakness may be an indication of low blood sugar or dehydration. Realize that labor is an amazing time and process, but one for which your body is very well equipped. Work with your body and keep things in an appropriate, positive perspective.

Managing labor naturally

Try not to rely exclusively on medical therapy for coping with contractions. Over the centuries, women have discovered a variety of techniques and methods that can make labor more comfortable and medical intervention less likely. Some tried and tested techniques are given below. For some ways that your birth partner can help, see page 182.

- ◆ *Labor positions* Try out different positions to see which is the most comfortable. Try leaning against a wall or your birth partner; sitting on a chair the wrong way around, so you're facing the chair back; kneeling forward on a pile of cushions; or going on all-fours—good for backache. There may be times when you find it comfortable to lie down, if so, support your body with plenty of cushions, placed under your head, beneath your belly, and underneath and between your thighs (see page 71). Changing positions can also help guide the baby through the curvature of your lower abdomen and pelvis.

◆ *Breathing* A good supply of oxygen is essential in any endeavor, and childbirth is no exception. Muscles deprived of oxygen produce lactic acid, and accumulation of this acid causes pain. Not enough oxygen going to the uterus and the placenta also can lead to distress for your baby. Breathing correctly, therefore, is an important component of successful labor.

Breathing exercises—also called patterned breathing—are often taught in childbirth classes as a tool to help distract parents from other sensations of labor and to ensure that mother and baby get an adequate oxygen intake. Patterned breathing doesn't work for everyone and can be confusing if you haven't practiced it beforehand. If you'd like to find out more about it and how it works, ask at your childbirth class.

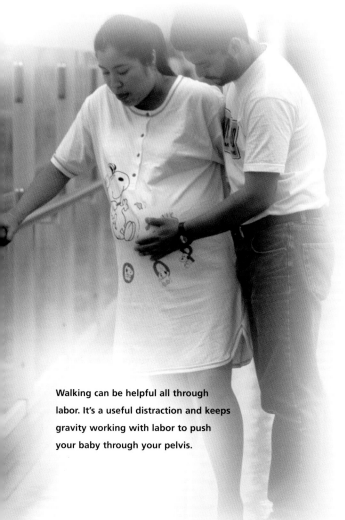

Walking can be helpful all through labor. It's a useful distraction and keeps gravity working with labor to push your baby through your pelvis.

In early labor, slow breathing helps promote and maintain relaxation. Taking deep, relaxing breaths at the beginning and end of contractions enhances the delivery of oxygen. When you breathe, try not to panic and hyperventilate (breathe too quickly), and don't hold your breath for prolonged periods.

In late labor, if the descent of your baby triggers the urge to push before your cervix is fully dilated, your healthcare provider may recommend panting or deep blowing, as if you're trying to keep a feather floating. This type of breathing also is helpful if you need to slow down pushing at the time of actual delivery of your baby's head. Breathing out stops your lungs from expanding and pushing down on your uterus at a time when pushing isn't appropriate.

◆ *Massage* Kneading or stroking muscles can help release muscle tension and promote relaxation. Relaxation, in turn, can increase blood circulation to muscles, helping ensure that they have adequate oxygen. Between contractions, massage can provide a pleasant tactile sensation to help lift your spirits, while during contractions massage can help take your mind off the pain.

If you're suffering from lower back pain, you may like to ask your birth partner to gently rub the area, particularly around the sacrum (where your spine joins your pelvis). He or she should make a series of large circles using the heel of his or her hands followed by smaller circles made with the thumbs.

◆ *Relaxation techniques* Relaxation counters your body's automatic reaction to the stress response. This is an innate "fight or flight" response, which has protected human life since time began. However, the stress response is not at all helpful in labor, because it causes the muscles to tense in preparation for action, expending energy at a high rate; and it diverts the body's blood supply to vital body organs—the heart and brain—and away from the uterus.

The mental effort required to slow down breathing and relax muscles can also serve as a distraction from painful contractions. Relaxed

Birth positions

When it comes to giving birth, an upright position is best, as it enlists the aid of gravity to help push your baby out. You may want to stick to one position or try a few out; do whatever makes you feel most comfortable. There's a variety of positions in which you can give birth, and you may want to assume one or more of these during labor to ease pain or help the baby's progress.

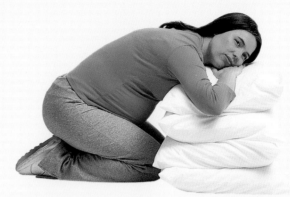

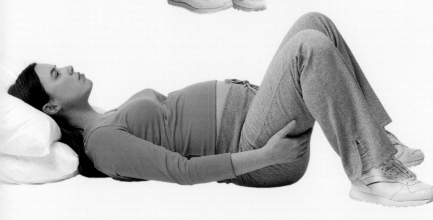

Knee-chest position If you have a large baby, this can help relieve backache and rotate a backward-facing baby. It may be useful to slow down the baby's descent if he is coming too fast. Go down on your knees and rest your arms on a pile of pillows or beanbag. If you have backache, try rocking your hips from side to side.

Squatting The most commonly adopted position, squatting encourages your baby to descend rapidly and may widen your pelvis by as much as 2 cm. You don't have to put as much effort into bearing down, but it can be a tiring position to hold for any length of time. Having your birth partner support you from behind or using a birthing stool can help.

Lying on your back Lying on your back is the position traditionally preferred by obstetricians, as it permits ease of intervention. It may also be the safest position for a highly anesthetized mother. However, it doesn't make use of gravity, and pressure from the baby on your back may increase the risk of backache and perineal injury.

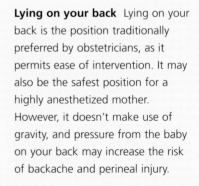

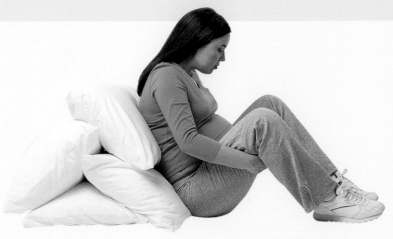

Sitting This is a good position if you're tiring, and one that can be used with continuous electronic monitoring, if your baby requires it. Sit as upright as possible with pillows supporting your back and keep your legs apart.

This position is frequently used in settings with birthing beds. It can also work well if an epidural has been used.

Lying on your side If you have had an epidural, or if you're tiring, this is a good position because it can make contractions more effective and slow down the baby's descent if he's coming too quickly.

Lie on your side on the floor, resting on a beanbag or some pillows. If your upper leg gets tired, you can ask your birth partner to help support it.

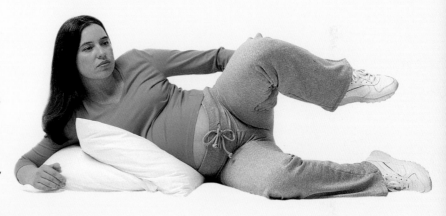

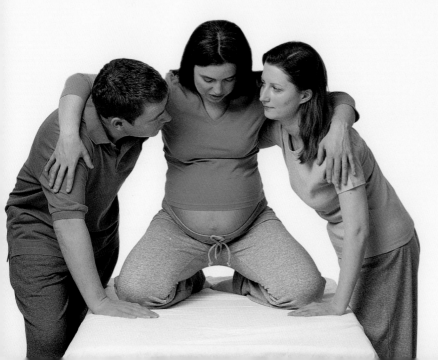

Kneeling with support If your baby's in an occiput posterior position (facing backward) this can help him rotate. Kneel on the bed between your birth partner and healthcare provider. Put your arms round their shoulders for support as you bear down.

muscles make it much easier for your uterus to do its work so that they are also more likely to stretch as your baby passes through your pelvis.

It's important to learn relaxation techniques before the birth. Understanding what happens during labor can help you relax, too. If you know that the powerful sensations you're experiencing are normal, this can help your mind relax and this can, in turn, help your body release tension.

- *Water* Immersion in water can provide substantial pain relief during labor and even help progress it (see page 181). Most hospitals or birth centers that use water for pain relief during labor keep it at body temperature or less—higher temperatures have been associated with fetal distress. Sometimes even a brief spell in water can

advance labor so rapidly that you give birth while you're in the water. Delivery under water doesn't appear to be a problem. Most doctors recommend bringing your baby above water immediately after birth for his first breath, as the placenta may begin to separate within seconds of delivery, and your baby will need oxygen quickly. Infants are born with an intact "diving reflex," which allows them to hold their breaths while submerged—they won't take their first breaths until they hit the colder air above the surface.

THE SECOND STAGE

Once you are through the transition period of labor, the time has come to push your baby out. The second stage usually takes an hour, but can take as

The moment of birth

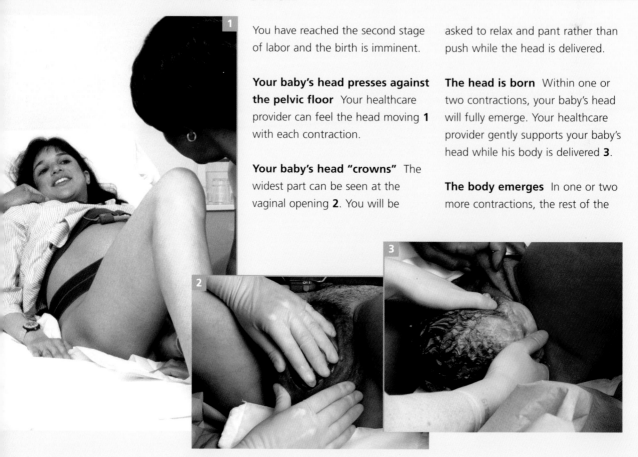

You have reached the second stage of labor and the birth is imminent.

Your baby's head presses against the pelvic floor Your healthcare provider can feel the head moving **1** with each contraction.

Your baby's head "crowns" The widest part can be seen at the vaginal opening **2**. You will be

asked to relax and pant rather than push while the head is delivered.

The head is born Within one or two contractions, your baby's head will fully emerge. Your healthcare provider gently supports your baby's head while his body is delivered **3**.

The body emerges In one or two more contractions, the rest of the

little as ten minutes or as much as three hours. As with early labor, the second stage may be significantly lengthened if anesthesia has been given.

Even after a long, exhausting labor, many women find a renewed burst of energy in the second stage, as they've achieved full dilation of the cervix and know that birth is imminent. Now you can take a much more active and mentally distracting role, which can make you feel a lot more positive.

The second stage can have another significant plus: Bearing down with contractions can make discomfort seem to disappear. As long as the second stage isn't too fast and allows the perineum to stretch gradually, it can be a time of pressure, not pain. Often the extreme pressure of the baby's tight fit and the subsequent compression of nerves leads to a form of anesthesia itself. For many women, this nerve compression blocks the sensation of perineal tears, surgical incisions, and repairs.

Contractions in the second stage still last for 60 to 90 seconds but may come every 2 to 4 minutes, so you have more time to rest in between. Your position can influence their pattern—staying upright can intensify contractions; reclining and knee-chest positions may slow them down.

You'll have an overwhelming urge to push, but wait until your healthcare provider says that it's okay. You'll feel huge pressure on your rectum, and a tingling, burning feeling as your baby's head appears at the entrance to your vagina. Your emotions may veer now from exhaustion and tearfulness to excitement at the thought of meeting your baby.

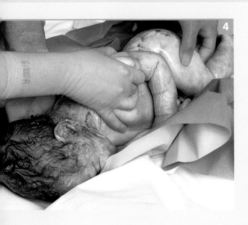

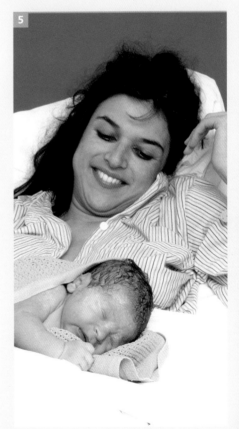

body appears. He may be covered with vernix and have streaks of blood on his skin **4**.

Your baby is handed to you
Once your baby has been checked, the cord is cut and he will be wrapped and given to you **5**. Lay him on your stomach so that he can be comforted by your familiar heartbeat and breathing rhythms.

CUTTING THE CORD
Your healthcare provider may clamp and cut the cord immediately, or he or she may wait until the cord stops pulsating. Sometimes your healthcare provider may then pull gently on the cord to help you deliver the placenta by pushing during a contraction.

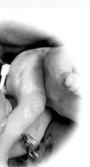
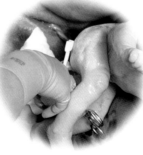

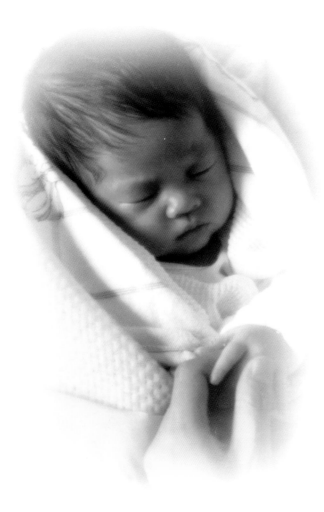

After the birth, your baby may appear to have a bluish tinge, but his color will soon be normal.

important as timing with the contraction. Shorter pushes—for about 5 to 6 seconds—are usually fine and allow more oxygen to enter your bloodstream.

Sometimes the front lip of the cervix may not have fully dilated when the urge to push first appears. This may occur because the baby has descended too rapidly or is positioned awkwardly. Pushing against an undilated cervix can cause swelling and hinder progress. To reduce a cervical or anterior lip, as it's called, try lying on your left side, or going on all fours for a few contractions. Sometimes "blowing" breathing can help you avoid pushing against the lip: This is breathing as if you're blowing out a candle, and it prevents you from holding your breath, which would result in downward cervical pressure. Moving to a knee-chest position can reduce the pressure on the cervix and pelvic muscles, decreasing the urge to push.

The baby's coming

The first sign that your baby's about to be born is the distension (stretching) of your anus and perineum. With each contraction, your baby's head becomes increasingly visible at the vaginal opening. Once it has stopped slipping back, it remains at the opening, and this is called crowning.

In just a brief period of time, the perineum thins from approximately 5 cm thick to less than 1 cm. This is totally natural, and the distension reverses within minutes after the birth. You may feel this distension as strong pressure, possibly with some mild stinging as your baby's head—or buttocks if he's breech—stretches the vaginal opening. This is the point when you may be offered an episiotomy if it looks like you're going to tear badly.

As your baby is born, slow, controlled pushing is best, as it allows the perineum to stretch gradually, helping prevent tears. Your healthcare provider may even tell you not to push so your uterus can achieve the final expulsion with less force.

Time to push

If you've been given the go-ahead to push, bearing down when the urge occurs will bring satisfying relief from pent-up sensations. Many women's bodies tell them before their healthcare providers do that their cervix has fully dilated and it's time to push. As your baby presses on your pelvic-floor muscles, receptors trigger an urge to bear down. The urge to push is often mistaken for the need to have a bowel movement, because the pressure of the baby on your rectum stimulates the same receptors as a bowel movement.

Usually the urge to push occurs two to four times within the course of a contraction, or you may feel one long, continuous urge. Take a deep breath, relax your pelvic muscles, and bear down with your abdominal muscles. The length of the push isn't as

Cutting the cord

After your baby is born, his umbilical cord usually will be clamped in two places and cut in between. It's not vital to clamp and cut the cord immediately, but it enables your healthcare provider to check your baby, if necessary. It also gives you more freedom of movement with your baby. Many healthcare providers prefer to wait until the pulse has stopped beating before cutting the cord. If baby and mother are doing well, this is a reasonable alternative.

THE THIRD STAGE

The third stage of labor sees the complete removal of the pregnancy with the delivery of the placenta. For most deliveries, this is relatively automatic and requires little effort or concern.

Delivering the placenta

While you get to know your baby, the uterus still has work to do. As soon as your baby leaves your uterus, the uterus continues to contract, causing a massive decrease in volume, which usually shears the less flexible placenta from its walls. Further contractions push the placenta out. Here again, gravity can assist in this process, and women who remain upright tend to need less intervention. If you're lying down, your healthcare provider may massage your uterus to help expel the placenta, or he or she may ask you to bear down and push.

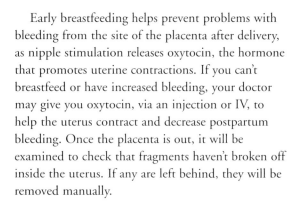

At birth, the placenta weighs about 1 lb (0.5 kg). The fetal side is smooth and covered with blood vessels. The side that was attached to your uterus is dark red and looks like raw liver.

Early breastfeeding helps prevent problems with bleeding from the site of the placenta after delivery, as nipple stimulation releases oxytocin, the hormone that promotes uterine contractions. If you can't breastfeed or have increased bleeding, your doctor may give you oxytocin, via an injection or IV, to help the uterus contract and decrease postpartum bleeding. Once the placenta is out, it will be examined to check that fragments haven't broken off inside the uterus. If any are left behind, they will be removed manually.

IMMEDIATELY AFTER BIRTH

Your baby is finally born and you'll feel a range of strong emotions—relief, elation, excitement, even disbelief that you're now a mother. You may feel cold and shivery and you'll certainly be very hungry and thirsty after all that hard work.

Before you leave the birthing room, you'll be stitched if you had an episiotomy or tear. Most women hardly notice this is happening, they're so preoccupied with their babies, but you'll be given a local anesthetic, if necessary. You'll be freshened up, and offered a fresh gown. Don't be alarmed to find you start bleeding heavily. This is perfectly normal and the discharge, called lochia, will subside over the next few weeks (see page 321). In the meantime, you may need to wear maternity pads.

After spending time with you, your baby will be taken away briefly for a bath, a pediatric exam, and needed procedures. You'll then be transferred to a postpartum room unless you gave birth in a labor, delivery, recovery, postpartum (LDRP) room, in which case you will remain where you are. Your baby will be brought back to you and a bassinet will be made available next to your bed.

Special deliveries

Breech

Breech babies are positioned so that their legs or bottoms are closest to the cervix. This position can make delivery difficult because the baby's head is the largest part of his body and it could get trapped if the body slips through a partly dilated cervix. Vaginal delivery is possible with breech presentation but sometimes breech babies need to be delivered by cesarean section to avoid trauma to baby or mother.

Twins and more

The prospect of giving birth to two or more babies can be daunting to say the least. However, many women give birth to twins vaginally without any problems and the birth tends to be faster than with single babies. However, extra care has to be taken with a multiple birth, so an anesthesiologist will be standing by in case you need a cesarean. The first baby may deliver vaginally without any problem, but the second baby may be positioned awkwardly and need assistance. The second baby should arrive 10 to 20 minutes after the first. If progress is slow, you may be given oxytocin (Pitocin) to speed up delivery, or your baby may be helped out with forceps. The placenta or placentas may follow soon after, or you may be given an injection to speed up their delivery. If you're expecting triplets or more, you'll most likely have them delivered by cesarean.

Posterior

A baby who descends into the birth canal with his head downward and his back toward his mother's spine—referred to as occiput posterior (OP)—may be harder to deliver. Posterior babies present a slightly larger head diameter for passing through the narrow birth canal and posterior labors may take longer or involve greater back pain. Not infrequently, however, the baby turns in mid-labor or during the stage of pushing. If your baby doesn't turn spontaneously, your healthcare provider may be able to encourage the baby to rotate once the cervix is completely dilated.

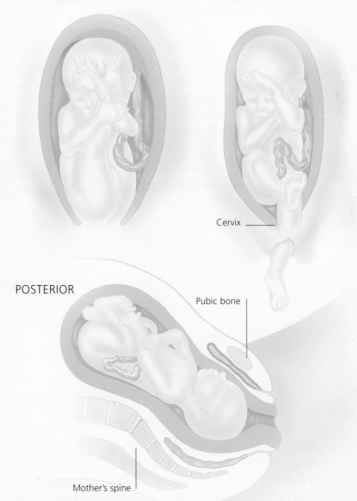

FRANK BREECH

FOOTLING BREECH

Cervix _____

POSTERIOR

Pubic bone |

Mother's spine |

SPECIAL MEDICAL INTERVENTIONS

Not every labor starts or progresses as it should. In these instances, medical intervention may be necessary to assist your baby's birth.

Although your healthcare provider will try to respect your wishes if you have planned for as natural a birth as possible, there may be instances when intervention is medically necessary. It may involve induction, an episiotomy, the use of forceps or vacuum extraction, or a cesarean section.

INDUCTION OF LABOR

Occasionally your healthcare provider may recommend inducing your labor, usually because of some medical risk to you or your baby. The most common reason why your healthcare provider may want to perform an induction is if you're overdue. It's felt that beyond one to two weeks past your due-date the placenta may cease to function well, and the baby may be at risk of decreased oxygen and malnutrition. Alternatively, induction may be suggested if you have a medical problem such as pre-eclampsia, or if your baby seems to be having difficulties such as an abnormal heart rate. In addition, if your membranes have ruptured but labor doesn't ensue within 24 hours, your healthcare provider may fear a risk of infection.

If your healthcare provider wants to get your labor started, there are three ways he or she will probably go about it. You may be given prostaglandins, you may have your membranes ruptured, or you may be given an IV of oxytocin. Many women need all three methods. Some healthcare providers use more natural alternatives.

Prostaglandin

Your body naturally produces many different types of prostaglandin, some of which are important in stimulating changes in the cervix and uterine contractions. Prior to labor, the cervix becomes softer, more compliant, and begins to shorten and open. These changes can be caused either by your body producing prostaglandin, or can be stimulated by synthetic prostaglandin.

The most common way of giving prostaglandin is into your vagina. Your healthcare provider will first ensure your baby is well by monitoring his heart rate for about 30 minutes. He or she will then perform a vaginal exam to establish exactly how "ripe" your cervix is (how soft and short it is and how far open).

Synthetic prostaglandin can be administered as pills, vaginal or rectal suppositories or gels, or within mechanical dilators, such as balloon catheters and

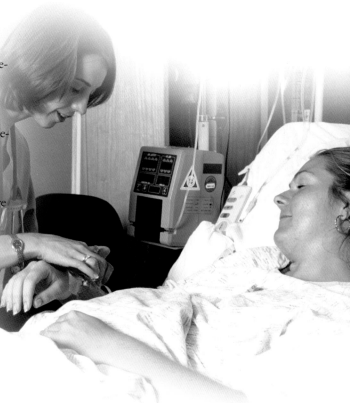

In some hospitals an intravenous (IV) line may be fitted routinely in case you need medication during labor.

osmotic dilators (like sterile tampons). Some women start to have contractions soon after the first dose of prostaglandin, whereas other women appear to have no response for some hours. You'll be examined again either the following morning—some inductions, especially if it's your first baby, start in the evening—or three to six hours after your first dose of prostaglandin. If your cervix has changed sufficiently for your healthcare provider to rupture your membranes, that will be done at this stage. If it's not possible to rupture your membranes, you may be given a further dose of prostaglandin.

Artificial rupture of membranes

One of the most common methods of either inducing labor or speeding it along is to artificially break the bag of membranes surrounding your baby. This is called artificial rupture of membranes (AROM) or amniotomy, and is often carried out during a vaginal exam. It should be no more painful than a routine exam, and is done using a 10-inch (25-cm) long, plastic instrument with an end like a crotchet hook. This is inserted through your cervix, gently catches the thin bag of membranes, and bursts it to let the amniotic fluid out. This action increases the amount of prostaglandin produced locally, which will speed up labor.

Pitocin (oxytocin)

This is the hormone that's most widely used to induce labor once the cervix has softened. A synthetic version of the same hormone produced by your body to initiate contractions, Pitocin is usually administered via an intravenous line (IV). If your labor is induced by this method, the dose will be progressively increased until your contractions show a regular pattern and cervical change is underway. Pitocin may be continued throughout labor or discontinued when labor is established. It may also be used to get labor started again if it seems to have stalled. Pitocin usually requires continuous monitoring, as it may be associated with fetal distress. If you do have an IV and are attached to a fetal monitor, you won't be able to move around and change position as easily.

Coping with induction

Induced labors are almost guaranteed to last longer—at least in the latent phase. Consequently, if you are induced, you should adjust your mental expectations and expect a longer labor. Some inductions take days and can still result in a normal vaginal delivery. Don't get discouraged. Prepare to distract yourself for a longer period of time while waiting for active labor.

Many women also feel that Pitocin-induced contractions are stronger—this can be the case if the contractions induced are too close together. When the uterine muscle contracts, its blood supply is temporarily squeezed and less oxygen gets to the muscle. For some women, Pitocin can be discontinued once active labor is in progress.

Natural alternatives to induction

There are a number of alternatives to medical therapy for induction, including nipple stimulation, membrane stripping, and mechanical dilators. However, health professionals sometimes disagree about the effectiveness of these techniques.

Nipple stimulation causes the release of oxytocin in the body. It can be carried out manually or with the aid of a breast pump. But you should speak to your healthcare provider before you try this yourself.

Membrane stripping involves introducing a gloved finger into the cervix and teasing the membranes away from the edge of the cervix. This should only be carried out by a health professional.

Mechanical dilators are usually used in conjunction with prostaglandins, but you may find that your healthcare provider uses the dilator on its own or in combination with saline. Mechanical dilators ripen the cervix directly, or indirectly, by increasing the body's own secretion of prostaglandins or oxytocin. In a typical dilation device a balloon catheter is inserted through the vagina and the cervix into the space between the amniotic sac and the uterine wall. The balloon is then inflated to keep the catheter in place.

Other natural induction techniques include sexual activity, herbal remedies, and positioning exercises. For further information, see page 208.

EPISIOTOMY

There are several reasons why an episiotomy (a cut to enlarge the vaginal opening) might be necessary during labor: if the perineum hasn't stretched sufficiently during the pushing stage; the baby's head is too large; it's a breech birth; the baby is in distress; or forceps need to be used. If your healthcare provider feels that an episiotomy is necessary, you'll be given a local anesthetic in the perineal area.

ALTERNATIVE EPISIOTOMY CUTS

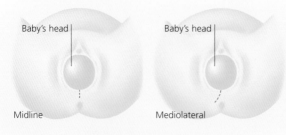

Baby's head

Baby's head

Midline

Mediolateral

When the area is numb, the cut will be made with scissors when the head is crowning and the perineum is stretched taut. There are two types of incision that might be used: The midline cut is straight down toward the rectum, while the mediolateral cut is angled a little to the side, away from the rectum. Although the midline cut is easier to repair and causes less blood loss, there is a slight risk that too much pressure may cause it to tear through to the rectum. For this reason, the mediolateral may be used.

FORCEPS AND VACUUM EXTRACTION

If your baby has entered the birth canal at an awkward angle or is in distress, or if you have a medical condition such as heart disease or are too exhausted or over-medicated to push effectively, your healthcare provider may decide that forceps or a vacuum extractor should be used to help the baby out and shorten the second stage.

If your healthcare provider is using forceps, and you haven't already had an epidural, you will be given local anesthetic or pain medication to numb the area. Then an episiotomy may be performed.

Your healthcare provider will then gently slide one side of the forceps at a time into your vagina. These fit around the sides of a baby's head, in much the same way your hands would if you were to place them along your baby's cheeks. While you push your healthcare provider will help pull the baby out.

If a vacuum extractor is to be used, your healthcare provider will attach the rubber or plastic cup to the top of the baby's head. Suction is created by a pump, and the healthcare provider gently pulls on the instrument to help the baby along while you push. Although the vacuum extractor involves less risk of trauma to the mother, forceps might be preferred if speed is an issue.

HAVING YOUR BABY BY CESAREAN

Sometimes circumstances exist where labor itself may be considered a danger to mother or baby; in these instances, cesarean delivery will be pre-planned. Other times, emergencies develop during labor or unexpectedly before labor, and the baby will need to be delivered by emergency cesarean.

With a planned cesarean section, a date is set, your family can gather, regional anesthesia can be used, and risks are generally decreased. In the case of

ASSISTED DELIVERY

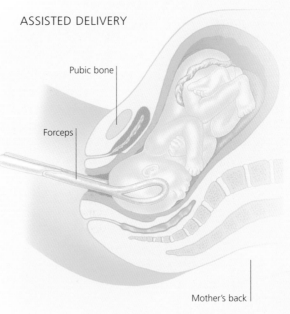

Pubic bone

Forceps

Mother's back

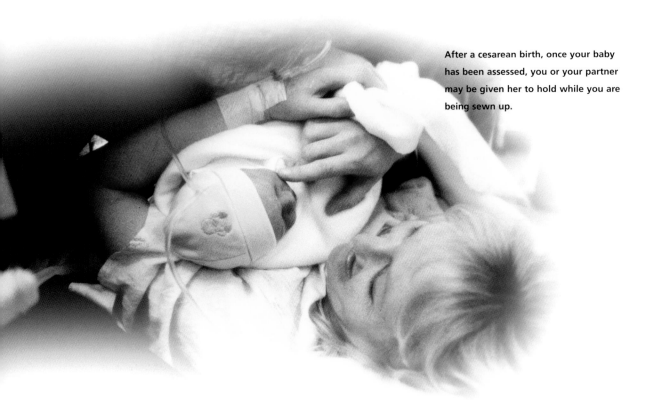

After a cesarean birth, once your baby has been assessed, you or your partner may be given her to hold while you are being sewn up.

an emergency cesarean, there's often little time for mental preparation, you may need to be put to sleep with general anesthesia, and your family may or may not be able to attend.

Why you may have a planned cesarean

The most common cause for planned cesarean is repeat cesarean section. Many physicians worry that unscheduled vaginal births after cesareans may be too risky in a small hospital setting due to lack of emergency surgery facilities. Many mothers worry that a prolonged and possibly painful first labor, which led to their original cesarean section, may be repeated if they reattempt labor.

A cesarean may also be planned if your baby is lying in a position other than head down, or when he is expected to be too large to pass through your pelvis—a situation technically known as macrosomia. Sometimes a baby or his mother may have an anomaly or injury that might be re-injured or damaged as a result of a vaginal delivery—for example, the mother may have a prior pelvic-floor muscle injury, or the baby may have a bleeding disorder, hydrocephaly, or an abdominal wall defect.

What happens during a planned cesarean

The night before your cesarean, you should not eat or drink anything, not even water, for at least eight hours. This helps avoid anesthesia complications. You may be admitted to the hospital at least two hours before the surgery, and this often takes place early in the morning.

In the hospital before the procedure, a nurse will take a health and pregnancy history. An intravenous (IV) will be started in your arm; to keep you hydrated and able to receive necessary medications.

Depending on your medical condition and the reason for the cesarean, you'll be given either a general or a regional anesthetic. A general anesthetic is an anesthetic gas mixed with oxygen that is given through a tube in your throat via your mouth. It puts you to sleep and you won't remember anything. Regional anesthetics include epidural and spinal anesthesia that blocks pain from the waist down (see page 179). If you have a regional anesthetic, you'll be awake and alert and able to see and, perhaps, hold or touch your baby. It's preferable for you to meet the anesthesiologist before your surgery so that you can discuss all the options.

Before surgery, a catheter (a small tube) will be placed in your bladder to drain urine during your cesarean and for several hours following surgery. Before the operation begins, the nurse will shave a small area of your lower abdomen, where the incision will be made. Your healthcare provider should talk to you about the type of incision before the surgery (see page 232).

Depending on the hospital's policy, one or two support people may accompany you into the operating room. If they do join you, they should: sit or stand by your head to communicate with you; follow the staff's instructions; remain in one spot; and refrain from touching anything.

Your abdomen will be prepared with an antiseptic wash and sterile drapes. An incision will be made with a scalpel through the skin in the lower abdomen. The muscles of the abdomen aren't usually cut but are separated in the midline and pushed aside. The bladder may be pushed down to protect it from instruments. Another incision will be made in the uterus. You may hear a whooshing noise as the amniotic fluid is sucked out.

Once your uterus is open, your baby will be lifted out through the incision. Frequently at this time, the top of the uterus is squeezed—just as you would do when pushing—and you'll feel pressure and a tugging sensation. The baby will be handed to another member of the team, who will give him a full physical and some basic tests, including the Apgar score (see page 287). You may be able to see your baby right away or after he has been assessed.

After the doctor has removed the placenta, your uterus and the layers of the abdominal wall will then be sewn closed. These sutures are absorbable and won't need to be removed. Your skin will then be closed with either sutures or staples. Once this is done, you will probably be united with your baby before you leave the surgical suite.

Once surgery is completed, and you and your baby are ready to be moved, you will be taken to a recovery area called a post anesthesia care unit (PACU) where you will be able to hold, bond with, and breastfeed your baby. For information about recovery from a cesarean, see page 324.

DID YOU KNOW...

You can help avoid an unnecessary cesarean
Research has shown that nearly 1 million cesareans carried out in the United Stated each year are medically unnecessary. Once you've gone into labor you can help avoid a cesarean in several ways: don't arrive at the hospital too early; walk and change position frequently; labor in an upright position; practice relaxation techniques and natural pain relief; try to rest between contractions.

Why you may have an emergency cesarean

This may be necessary for babies at risk of birth trauma such as extremely premature babies or those in distress, or when a serious medical condition, such as pre-eclampsia (see page 254) makes rapid delivery necessary.

What happens during an emergency cesarean

Although the surgical process involved in an emergency cesarean is much the same as a planned one, the circumstances can make a cesarean birth more stressful for the mother. The staff may seem more rushed, your birth partner may be asked to leave the room, and you may be given general anesthesia. If the baby is in an awkward position or if it's necessary to work fast, a larger incision may be necessary. However, try to trust in the skill of your healthcare providers and believe that the outcome—the safe delivery of your healthy baby—is more important than the birth process.

Pain relief options for cesareans

Cesarean deliveries are safest for the mother and baby if they can be performed with regional—epidural or spinal—anesthesia (see page 179). Less medicine goes to the baby, the mother can be awake to greet her newborn, and family members can be present. There's also no need for a respirator (a tube inserted into the mouth to aid breathing).

Sometimes, however, general anesthesia is necessary for the mother's or baby's safety. Usually, general anesthesia is a combination of IV medication and anesthetic gas administration. During the surgical procedure, general anesthesia usually requires the use of a respirator to protect the mother from aspiration (inhaling food particles and stomach acid into her lungs) and serious pneumonia. General anesthesia is faster and may be a necessity if it's an emergency, for instance, if the baby's in distress. Some mothers may require general anesthesia for certain medical conditions such as back problems that may rule out regional anesthesia.

Alternative incisions

During a cesarean birth, the doctor will make two separate incisions: one through the skin and abdominal wall and the other, beneath this, through the uterine wall. The scar that you see on the outside doesn't necessarily mirror the incision that has been made on the uterus beneath it.

The skin incision that is most often used is the "bikini" incision, made across the lower abdomen, just above the pubic hairline. This is preferable because it leaves a small, unnoticeable scar. Rare circumstances may require a vertical skin incision from the pubic area to the umbilicus (belly button). This might be used if the doctor needs a large area in which to work or when the baby must be removed quickly.

Similarly, the most common uterine incision is the low transverse (side-to-side) incision, which is made across the lower part of the uterus (see top right). As this is the segment of the uterus that stretches rather than contracts, incisions made here have less risk of re-opening or rupturing in future labors. Many women who have this incision have a vaginal birth the next time. A disadvantage of this incision is that it takes longer to perform, so it may not be used in the case of emergency cesareans, where time is critical.

UTERINE CESAREAN INCISIONS

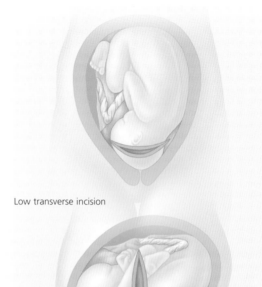

Low transverse incision

Vertical incision

A vertical uterine incision allows more room to avoid birth trauma to mother and baby if the baby's in an awkward position, if it's a multiple pregnancy, or if the lower uterine segment isn't stretched enough to allow delivery through the transverse incision. If you require a vertical incision and it extends into the upper portion of the uterus, you will need to have a cesarean for future deliveries as there's a higher risk—greater than 2 percent—of scar separation in future labors.

YOUR BABY'S EXPERIENCE OF BIRTH

Birth is not only a lengthy and physically demanding process for you, but it involves considerable changes for your baby as she adapts to life outside the uterus.

Your baby is well prepared for her journey to the outside world. For instance, because the plates of her skull aren't fixed, her skull is able to "mold" to the shape of the birth canal as she travels through it. Your baby's skull will then recover its normal shape within 24 to 48 hours of delivery. It also appears that the neural connections that would lead a baby to interpret birth sensations as "pain," may not have developed at the time of labor.

ADAPTING TO LIFE

The pressure on your baby's body as she squeezes through the narrow birth canal is actually helpful in preparing her to live outside the uterus. Pressure on her head causes the release of thyroid and adrenal hormones that help her regulate her temperature after birth. The compression of a baby's chest while in the birth canal helps expel fluid and mucus from her lungs. This pressure also prevents her from breathing and inhaling fluid and blood as she passes through the birth canal. This helps prepare her to take her first breath upon emerging.

As your baby passes through the birth canal, there is short-lived hypoxemia (lack of oxygen) as her umbilical cord is compressed. Once outside your body, your baby's chest is able to expand and the pressure on her head is released, both of which promote the instinctive response to hypoxemia which is inhalation. This is the impetus to breathe.

Your baby's first breath

To provide her own oxygen supply after the cord is clamped and cut, major changes have to take place in your baby's heart and lungs. While she was in your uterus, her oxygen was supplied from your blood vessels in the placenta and not by her breathing. As her heart had to pump blood along the umbilical cord as well as around her body, the blood was largely diverted from her lungs.

The first time that your baby breathes, it initiates major changes in her body. As her lungs fill with air, the tiny air sacs in the lungs begin to expand. The oxygen causes the blood vessels in the lungs to relax, and this initiates an increase in the flow of blood. The openings in her heart that permitted diversion of blood from her fetal lungs, close shortly after birth. Your baby's umbilical cord stretches and, as this occurs, arteries close down, otherwise your baby would lose blood when the placenta separates.

Your baby's first cry

Although not all babies cry when they are born, the shock of birth usually produces some reaction from a newborn. Your baby may cry for several minutes after delivery, or may give a startled shriek and then settle down. If, however, she is sedated by pain-relief medication you were given, she may not cry until some time after the birth.

DID YOU KNOW...

Your baby instinctively looks for your nipple

Your baby's ability find your nipple immediately after birth is remarkable. Research has shown that a baby connects the smell of the fluid on his hands with the smell of his mother's nipples. If placed on the mother's belly, he makes crawling movements to try to reach the breast. He also may use his touch and sight to try and find the breast. This is why the first hour can be crucial for successful breastfeeding.

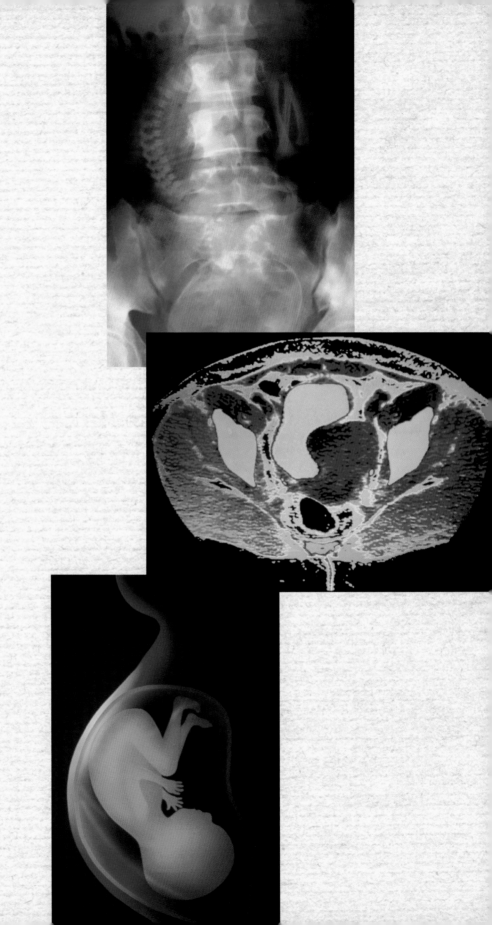

PART III

PRENATAL REFERENCE

PRENATAL TESTS

During your pregnancy, your healthcare provider may recommend a variety of tests that are intended to confirm that your baby is developing normally. The decision whether to have these tests or not is yours—you do not have to agree to any procedure you are not comfortable with. Understanding the procedures, why the tests are offered, and what they will tell you, will enable you to make an informed decision.

SCREENING TESTS

These procedures consist of ultrasound or blood samples to check for abnormalities in the baby and/or disease in the mother. Their attraction for many women is that unlike diagnostic tests they're non-invasive and therefore pose no threat to the baby. However, screening tests won't give you a definite "yes" or "no" if, for instance, you want to know if your baby has Down syndrome. They can also give "false positives," indicating there's a problem with the baby when everything's in fact fine, or "false negatives," indicating that everything's fine with the baby when it isn't.

Ultrasound

This technology makes use of sound waves and their echoes to create a picture of the uterus and the baby inside it. Ultrasound examinations are painless, and the sound waves used are safe for both you and your baby.

An ultrasound exam can be performed either transvaginally, using a special ultrasound probe inserted into the vagina, or trans-abdominally, using a transducer that is moved across the mother's abdomen. The choice of which approach to use will depend on the reason your doctor has requested the ultrasound. An ultrasound carried out in the first trimester of pregnancy will frequently be done transvaginally. The advantage to this approach is that the probe is closer to the baby at this early point in pregnancy so that a much clearer view is obtained. Some women worry that a transvaginal probe inserted into the vagina could harm the baby. While understandable, there's no basis for this concern

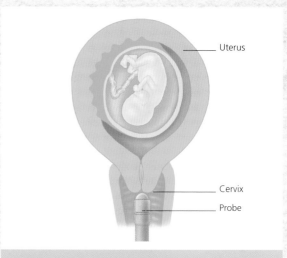

Uterus

Cervix

Probe

During a transvaginal ultrasound exam a special probe is inserted into the vagina to give a clear picture of the baby in the first trimester.

and it's completely safe. Occasionally, your doctor will request a transvaginal ultrasound exam in the second trimester specifically to look at the cervix.

Ultrasound exams carried out after the first trimester are usually done transabdominally since the baby can be seen clearly in the abdomen by this time. Gel is spread over the abdomen, and the transducer is moved around through the gel. The amniotic fluid surrounding the baby provides the liquid needed to transmit the sound waves to create a clear, detailed picture. Picture quality varies, depending on maternal fat, scar tissue, and the position of the baby.

Basic ultrasound

This is usually carried out before 12 weeks, for the following purposes:

- *Locate the pregnancy* The overwhelming majority of pregnancies are located inside the uterus. Occasionally, however, the pregnancy may be located outside of the uterus. This is called an ectopic pregnancy (see page 274) and can be dangerous if undetected.

- *Establish an accurate due date* An ultrasound can show whether the baby is any larger or smaller than the date your last menstrual period would suggest. If the crown to rump measurement, which measures the baby from his head to his rear, is more than three to four days from what your last menstrual period would suggest, your healthcare provider may change your due date. An ultrasound in the first trimester is more accurate than one later on in confirming or establishing your due date.

- *Check on the baby's condition* By five to six weeks into your pregnancy, you can actually see your baby's heart beating by ultrasound. Once

a fetal heartbeat has been seen, the risk of miscarriage drops significantly—to about 3 percent. Prior to five weeks, the actual baby may not be visible—instead, the ultrasound may show only the gestational sac.

- *Detect some abnormalities* Typically, a complete ultrasound examination to detect birth defects in the baby is usually not performed until between 16 to 20 weeks. Occasionally, however, some problems may already be visible by 11 to 12 weeks. Much of the brain, spine, limbs, abdomen, and urinary tract structures may be seen with transvaginal ultrasound. In addition, the presence of a thickening behind the neck of the baby—known as an increased nuchal translucency—may help indicate an added risk for certain genetic or chromosomal conditions (see page 238).

- *Check the number of babies* An ultrasound shows whether you're carrying one, two, or more babies. If you have twins, the appearance of the membrane separating the babies, as well as where their placentas are located, helps to

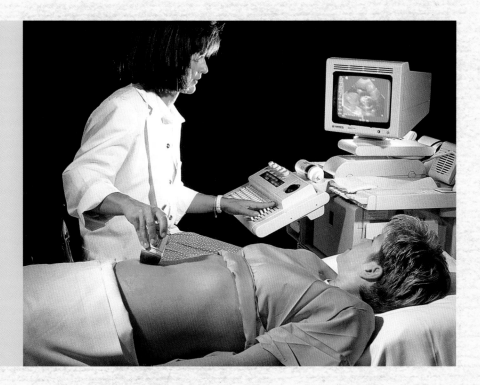

Transabdominal ultrasound is a painless procedure which is most commonly used after the first trimester to check on the well-being of your baby.

indicate whether the babies share one placenta—called a monochorionic placentation—or each have separate placentas—called dichorionic placentation.

◆ *Check the ovaries* An ultrasound can reveal whether or not your ovaries appear normal. Sometimes, a small cyst is seen, called a corpus luteal cyst. This is a cyst that forms at the site on the ovary where the egg was released. Over the course of the first trimester, it gradually disappears. Other types of cysts, unrelated to the pregnancy, also may be found during an ultrasound exam. Whether these cysts need to be removed during pregnancy or afterward depends on their size and appearance.

◆ *Check the uterus* An ultrasound exam can evaluate the shape of the uterus and appearance of the cervix. It can also determine if you have fibroids. These are commonly seen benign overgrowths of the muscle of the uterus and they won't usually cause any problems with your pregnancy.

Targeted ultrasound
This fetal anatomy scan may be performed at around 16 to 20 weeks and is much more detailed than the first trimester ultrasound. It is used to check the following:

◆ Number of babies.
◆ Gestational age.
◆ Growth rate.
◆ Fetal heart rate.
◆ Amount of amniotic fluid.
◆ Location of placenta.
◆ Fetal anatomy including brain and skull, heart, chest cavity, and diaphragm, stomach, abdominal cavity, and abdominal wall, face, kidneys, and bladder, arms and legs, and spine.
◆ The baby's gender—after 15 to 16 weeks—although this isn't always possible to see.

Some doctors feel that ultrasound is the single most important advance in modern obstetrics. Although it has truly revolutionized prenatal care, it isn't perfect. For example, even in the most experienced hands, it can't detect all birth defects.

Fortunately, though, many of the ones it can't detect are minor. Women often ask if an ultrasound can diagnose chromosomal abnormalities, such as Down syndrome. The answer is that sometimes ultrasound can increase the index of suspicion that there may be a chromosomal abnormality, but the only way to definitively diagnose whether or not one exists is to perform an invasive test such as amniocentesis or chorionic villus sampling (see page 242).

A doctor (an obstetrician, a perinatologist, or a radiologist) or an ultrasound technologist may perform the ultrasound. Sometimes a technologist does a preliminary exam, and the doctor comes in later to check on images or review the printed pictures. Typically, the examiner measures the baby first and then studies his anatomy. Whether and how often you need an ultrasound depends on your particular risk factors and your healthcare providers' preferences. Some recommend that all women have an ultrasound exam at around 20 weeks, while others feel that it's unnecessary if your risks for having problems are low.

Further ultrasounds
A number of ultrasound examinations may be needed if any of the following arise:

◆ If you're carrying twins or more.
◆ If your doctor suspects the baby is too small or too large for its age.
◆ If your doctor suspects that you have too little or too much amniotic fluid.
◆ If you're at risk for preterm labor.
◆ If you have diabetes, hypertension, or other underlying medical conditions.
◆ If you're bleeding.

Nuchal translucency screen
This test involves the use of ultrasound to measure a special fluid-filled area behind the baby's neck. Experiments with this procedure in the United Kingdom have suggested that Down syndrome can be identified this way in up to 80 percent of cases. A nuchal translucency scan can only be performed by doctors specially trained in

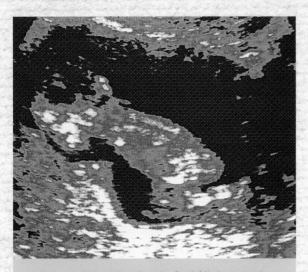

Ultrasound is used so that the fluid-filled area at the back of the neck can be measured during a nuchal translucency screen, offered at around 12 weeks.

◆ Underestimation of the age of the baby (how pregnant you are).

◆ The presence of twins or more.

◆ The cause of bleeding that may have occurred earlier in the pregnancy.

◆ Neural tube defects (spina bifida, anencephaly, and others).

◆ Abdominal wall defects (protruding of the baby's abdominal contents through a defect in the abdominal wall).

◆ Rh disease or other conditions associated with fetal edema (abnormal fluid collection in the baby).

◆ A rare fetal kidney condition known as congenital nephrosis.

◆ Fetal death.

◆ Other fetal abnormalities.

Remember that the MSAFP test is only a screening test. Most women with an elevated MSAFP have a normal baby and continue to have a completely normal pregnancy. Only about 5 percent of women with a positive maternal serum screen are actually found to have some abnormality, and only 5 percent of these have a baby with a neural tube defect. On the other hand, the test isn't perfect, and therefore it can't identify 100 percent of abnormal fetuses. To reduce the risk of getting a false positive result, a positive test should be repeated—especially if it's only mildly elevated or under 3.0 MOMs—and an ultrasound should be performed to confirm the age of the baby. If a test comes back elevated a second time, a detailed ultrasound exam should be done to look for any detectable abnormalities. In fact, many doctors believe that a detailed scan at 20 weeks is better than MSAFP as it stops the mother being worried by false positive results.

If you have two elevated MSAFP tests or a very high single test, you may want to have an amniocentesis (see page 243) to check the level of AFP in the amniotic fluid. The amniotic fluid can also be checked for a substance called acetylcholinesterase, which is present if the baby has an open neural tube defect. In most cases, the amniotic fluid MSAFP is negative and the

the procedure. When measurements of nuchal translucency are combined with blood screening tests (see below) the accuracy of these tests are increased. While in certain parts of the world, specifically the United Kingdom, this test is routine, in other parts it's considered fairly experimental. In the United States, for example, there is currently a large study being carried out, called the "FASTER TRAIL," which is evaluating the test's accuracy.

MATERNAL BLOOD TESTS
Maternal serum alpha-fetoprotein screen
Alpha-fetoprotein (AFP) is a protein made by the baby, which also circulates in the mother's bloodstream. Doctors use a simple blood test to check the level of maternal serum alpha-fetoprotein (MSAFP) between 16 and 20 weeks. The test result is affected by race, and preexisting diabetes, so it has to be adjusted for those factors. MSAFP can usually indicate whether a pregnancy is at risk for certain complications. An elevated MSAFP—expressed as more than 2.0 or 2.5 multiples of the median (MOMs)—may indicate:

pregnancy continues normally. Some studies suggest that women who have an abnormal MSAFP and then a normal amniotic fluid MSAFP may be at risk for preterm delivery, low birth weight babies, or hypertension. So if you fit the pattern, your doctor may suggest that you and your baby be closely observed, either with ultrasound or with other tests. This area is fairly controversial in the field of obstetrics, and not all practitioners follow the same routine.

Note: In mothers of twins, MSAFP greater than 4.0 or 4.5 MOMs is considered elevated. In triplets and quadruplets, the measurement hasn't been well-studied.

Serum screening

Another test that can be performed with the same sample of blood that's used for the MSAFP is a screening test for Down syndrome. This can also help identify women at risk of having babies with other chromosomal abnormalities, such as trisomy 18 or trisomy 13 (an extra copy of either the number 18 or 13 chromosome).

This test is performed by measuring two, three, or even four substances in the blood: MSAFP, human chorionic gonadotropin (HCG), estriol (a form of estrogen), and Inhibin A. The results of these various tests are used to calculate a risk for Down syndrome. In women under the age of 35, the test detects Down syndrome about 60 percent of the time when it's present—but it will miss 40 percent. In mothers over the age of 35, the accuracy goes up from 60 to 80 percent. This test is only a screening, and cannot diagnose a birth defect, so even if the result is abnormal, the baby is unaffected in the majority of cases. If you have an abnormal test result, you are only carrying one baby, and your dates are correct, your doctor may suggest an amniocentesis.

First trimester serum screening

This test checks the levels of PAPP-A, a substance produced by the placenta, and HCG, a hormone in the mother's blood. It may help screen for Down syndrome in the first trimester. But studies are still underway to determine the rate at which such a test can identify Down syndrome.

Hepatitis B

Your blood will be routinely checked for this at your first prenatal visit. Caused by a virus, this liver infection is usually caught from blood—as

BLOOD TESTS FOR INHERITED CONDITIONS

If you or your partner have a family history of an inherited disease you may be offered a blood test to help diagnose whether your unborn baby is at risk (see page 246).

A blood test may also be recommended if there is a higher-than-average chance that you and your partner could be carrying a defective gene for a particular disorder, even though there is no known history of the condition in your family. In the United States, it is recommended that all Caucasians

are tested for cystic fibrosis—a defective CF gene is carried by 1 in 25 Caucasians of European descent. Jewish couples whose families originate from Eastern Europe may be offered testing for Tay-Sachs and possibly Canavan's disease. Tay-Sachs is also associated with other ethnic groups including Cajun Indians and French-Canadians. African-American couples may be tested for sickle-cell anemia, and those whose families originate from the Mediterranean may be offered a

test for thalassemia—a hereditary form of anemia.

Blood tests are also used to identify diseases that can be passed on from only one carrier parent, such as hemophilia, or from an affected parent, as in the case of Huntington's disease.

Your healthcare provider will be able to advise you about genetic testing, and may refer you to a genetic counselor.

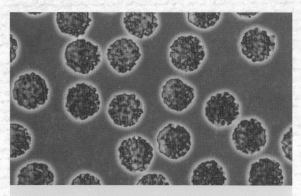

The hepatitis B virus (show above) is the cause of serum hepatitis, or hepatitits B, which is usually transmitted through blood or unprotected sex.

little as a few drops—or unprotected sex with an infected person. About 1 percent of pregnant women in the United States, 0.3 percent in Canada, and 2.2 percent in Australia are carriers of the hepatitis B virus. If you carry this virus, it could infect your baby at delivery. To reduce your baby's risk of infection, she will be given a vaccine immediately after delivery.

Syphilis

Although syphilis is very uncommon these days, there is still a chance that you may have been unknowingly infected in the past and have never shown any symptoms, which is why a routine blood test to check for syphilis is given during pregnancy. The organism that causes syphilis can be transmitted to your baby from early in pregnancy and can result in facial abnormalities and mental retardation. Fortunately, once identified, syphilis can be treated early in pregnancy with antibiotics —usually penicillin— which will not only prevent your baby from being affected but will also cure you of this disease.

Glucose tolerance test

A form of diabetes—known as gestational diabetes—is a complication of pregnancy. Gestational diabetes is detected in different ways. In some practices you may be given a sugary drink at your first visit and have a blood sample taken one hour later, which is sent for laboratory testing. In other clinics, you may have a blood sugar test every three months or you may be tested only if you fall into one of the risk groups or are found to have sugar in your urine.

INVASIVE DIAGNOSTIC TESTS

Depending on your age, your medical and obstetrical history, your family history, and other factors, you may want to undergo one or more invasive tests designed to detect certain genetic diseases or conditions. A number of such tests are available, including chorionic villus sampling (CVS), amniocentesis, and fetal blood sampling —also known as percutaneous umbilical blood sampling (PUBS). These tests can evaluate the chromosomes of your developing baby.

Abnormalities in the number or structure of chromosomes can lead to problems in the baby. The most common chromosomal abnormality in liveborn babies is Down syndrome, which is associated with severe mental retardation. The invasive tests mentioned above can detect such abnormalities by yielding a karyotype, an enlarged picture of the individual chromosomes.

In addition, the DNA obtained from these procedures can be used to test for certain genetic diseases you may be at risk from, based on your family history or your ethnic background; for example, Tay-Sachs, cystic fibrosis, or sickle-cell disease. However, unless a couple is specifically at risk for one of these rare genetic disorders, this specialized testing won't be routinely done.

Traditionally, in the United States, and Canada, women who are aged 35 or older—or who will be at their due date—are offered the chance to undergo one of these invasive prenatal tests to check for abnormalities. Thirty-five is the target age, because a woman's risk of having a baby with a chromosomal abnormality increases significantly after she reaches that age. It's also the age at which the risk of miscarriage from the procedure itself is roughly equal to the chance that the baby has a chromosomal abnormality. However, while the risk of a chromosomal abnormality is much less for women under the age of 35, most babies with Down syndrome are born to women under this age, because far more women under 35 are having babies than women over the age of 35.

What if you are advised that you have an increased risk of a chromosomal problem but you find the risk of miscarriage associated with the test unacceptable or you have decided that you

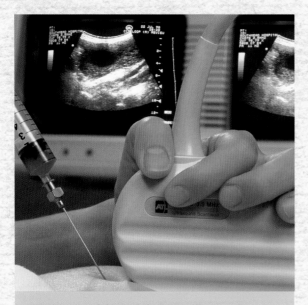

During transabdominal chorionic villus sampling (CVS), ultrasound is used to determine the position of the placenta, and to guide the needle through the abdomen and the uterine wall to the edge of the placenta, without harming the baby.

wouldn't wish to terminate a pregnancy even in the case of an abnormality—can you refuse? You can—you have the right to decide whether or not to agree to any procedures that are offered—but you need to bear in mind that even if pregnancy termination isn't something you would consider, prior knowledge of an abnormality can give you more time to make preparations for a child that may have special needs.

If you are under the age of 35 and want to have your baby tested for chromosomal abnormalities, this is completely reasonable, as long as you understand the risks and benefits of the testing. However, be aware that some insurance carriers may not cover the cost, which can amount to several hundred dollars or more, depending on where you live.

Chorionic villus sampling (CVS)
Tiny, finger-like pieces of tissue known as chorionic villi make up the placenta. They develop from cells arising out of the fertilized egg, so they have the same chromosomes and genetic makeup as the developing baby. A sample of chorionic villi will enable your healthcare provider to see whether or not the chromosomes are normal in number and structure. DNA from the chorionic villi can also be used to test for some genetic diseases, if the baby is thought to be at risk.

The main advantage CVS has over amniocentesis is that the results are available earlier in the pregnancy. This means that if the test reveals an abnormality in the baby, and if pregnancy termination is an option, it can be done earlier, which is easier for the mother, both physically and emotionally.

How it's performed
CVS is typically done between 10 and 12 weeks of pregnancy and can be performed in one of two ways—either by withdrawing placental tissue, which contains chorionic villi, through a hollow needle inserted through the abdomen—transabdominal CVS—or through a flexible catheter inserted through the cervix—transcervical CVS. Ultrasound is used to guide the doctor to the right location and to avoid injury to the baby as the procedure is performed. The tissue is then processed in a laboratory and a karyotype (a picture of the chromosomes) is prepared. The decision on whether to perform CVS through the abdomen or the cervix depends on where the placenta is located within the uterus and the general shape and position of the uterus itself.

Risks and side effects

Regardless of whether the CVS is performed through the cervix or the abdomen, neither method is riskier than the other, although having an invasive test always slightly raises the risk of miscarriage. Studies show that the experience of the person performing the procedure is important in reducing this risk.

In the early 1990s, some people were concerned that babies tested with CVS could be at a greater risk of limb defects. Since that time, an international registry has collected data on more than 200,000 mothers who have undergone CVS and found no evidence of an increase in limb defects among their babies when the test was done after 9 weeks. That is why CVS is not performed before week 10 of pregnancy.

Some vaginal bleeding may occur after CVS and should not be a cause for concern, although you should report it to your healthcare provider if it lasts for three or more days. There is also a very slight risk of infection, so you should tell your healthcare provider if you have a fever in the days following the procedure.

Results

CVS results may be available in seven days, although it can take 2 to 3 weeks for a full report. These will provide a complete picture of the genetic makeup of your baby.

Amniocentesis

This test involves withdrawing amniotic fluid from the uterus, which contains cells from the baby that can be used to obtain information about the baby's chromosomes.

Amniocentesis to test for genetic abnormalities is usually done at 15 to 20 weeks. It primarily tests to see that 23 chromosome pairs are present and that their structures are normal. It doesn't routinely test for all possible genetic diseases or structural abnormalities. It may also be used to test for specific genetic disorders for which the baby is known to be at high risk—for example, if both parents are known to be carriers of cystic

fibrosis, or Tay-Sachs disease, or if one parent is a carrier for a genetic disease that can be passed by just one parent, such as Huntington's disease.

Amniocentesis will be offered if you had an elevated MSAFP—if you had abnormal results from the Down syndrome screening, or if your ultrasound exam was abnormal, indicating, for example, poor fetal growth or some form of suspected structural abnormalities.

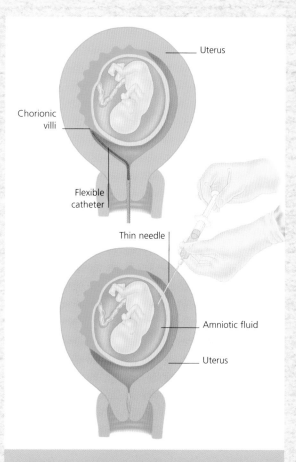

Uterus

Chorionic villi

Flexible catheter

Thin needle

Amniotic fluid

Uterus

CVS (top) and Amniocentesis (bottom) are both screening tests that can be carried out if an abnormality is suspected. Amniocentis is more commonly used than CVS as there is less risk to the baby. With both tests ultrasound is used to guide the doctor to the right location in the uterus and to avoid injury to the baby.

Further amniocentesis

You may be offered amniocentesis later in pregnancy to test for:

- *Preterm labor* An infection within the amniotic fluid may be a cause of preterm labor. If this is suspected the amniotic fluid can be sent to a lab for tests to look for any such infection. If an infection is present, your doctor may suggest the immediate delivery of your baby to minimize any harm to either you or the baby.
- *Other infections* Some pregnant women may be at risk of developing such infections as toxoplasmosis, cytomegalovirus (CMV), or parvovirus. The amniotic fluid can be tested for evidence of such problems in women who are considered to be at risk.
- *Rh sensitization* Rh-negative women who have become Rh-sensitized are sometimes given a test known as delta OD-450, in which the amniotic fluid is examined for evidence of broken-down fetal red blood cells.
- *Lung maturity studies* Sometimes your doctor needs to find out whether the baby's lungs are mature enough for the baby to be delivered. Certain tests of the amniotic fluid can determine the maturity of the lungs. An amniocentesis that is done later on in the pregnancy—for example, in the third trimester for lung maturity—doesn't carry the same risk of miscarriage. It carries only a very tiny risk of infection, rupture of membranes (breaking the water), or onset of labor.

How it's performed

The procedure may be performed in your doctor's office, or you may be referred to a center that specializes in ultrasounds and procedures such as amniocentesis. The ultrasound scan is used to identify a "pocket" of amniotic fluid away from the baby. A thin needle is inserted down through your abdomen and the wall of the uterus, into the amniotic sac. About 15 to 20 cc (1 to 2 tablespoons) of amniotic fluid is withdrawn, after which the needle is removed.

Some women think that the needle is inserted through the navel, but it isn't. The exact point of insertion depends on where the baby, the placenta, and the amniotic sac are located within the uterus.

Many women have heard that an amniocentesis needle is exceptionally long, and they fear that such a long needle causes pain. But the needle's length, which enables it to reach the amniotic sac, doesn't make it painful. It's the thickness of a needle that determines how uncomfortable it is. An amniocentesis needle is very thin, so any discomfort should be minimal.

The procedure only lasts about 1 to 2 minutes, although it may feel longer. It's mildly uncomfortable but not terribly painful. Most women report that it isn't as bad as they expected it to be. Generally a slight, brief cramping sensation is felt as the needle goes into the uterus, followed by a strange pulling sensation as the fluid is withdrawn through the needle. While some doctors choose to give local anesthesia, others feel that the discomfort caused by the injection of the anesthetic agent isn't worth the benefit. After all, the anesthesia only numbs the skin, and doesn't numb the uterus where any discomfort will be felt. Afterward, your doctor may advise that you rest for one to two days and avoid strenuous activity and sex during this period.

Risks and side effects

There is a small risk of miscarriage with this test. After the procedure some women experience cramping for several hours. The best treatment for cramping is rest. You may experience a little leakage of amniotic fluid through the vagina—no more than a teaspoonful. A small leakage of fluid that then stops is usually all right, but if you experience a big gush of fluid, you should call your healthcare provider immediately. You may also experience spotting which lasts a few days.

Many parents worry that having an amniocentesis will harm the baby, but the chance of this happening is extremely rare, given the use of ultrasound guidance.

Results

The amniotic fluid cells taken during the amniocentesis must be incubated and cultured, which takes some time. Results are usually available in 1 to 2 weeks. Under certain circumstances, some laboratories will perform a preliminary, rapid test called a Fluorescent in Situ Hybridization (FISH) which takes 24 to 48 hours for a result. A FISH isn't a final result, and only tests for certain common chromosomal abnormalities. When a FISH is carried out there is usually an additional cost involved for the result. FISH is most commonly used if there is a high suspicion of a chromosomal abnormality like Down syndrome, trisomy 18 or trisomy 13.

Fetal blood sampling

This procedure, which is also known as percutaneous umbilical blood sampling (PUBS) or cordocentesis, involves the withdrawal of fetal blood from the umbilical cord. Usually performed after week 18 of pregnancy, the test lets your healthcare provider obtain blood for rapid chromosomal diagnosis when a fast result is critical. It is also sometimes carried out in order to diagnose some fetal infections, to detect evidence of fetal anemia, or to diagnose and treat a condition called hydrops, in which fluid accumulates abnormally in the baby.

Some babies develop anemia, which can be treated within the uterus with a blood transfusion. The transfusion is done during a fetal blood sampling and blood is actually transfused into the umbilical cord. Conditions that may lead to anemia include certain infections, such as parvovirus, genetic diseases (see page 246), or some blood group incompatibilities (see page 90).

How it's performed

The procedure, which is carried out by an experienced maternal-fetal medicine specialist, is performed under ultrasound guidance. It's similar to an amniocentesis, except that the needle is directed into the umbilical cord rather than into the amniotic fluid.

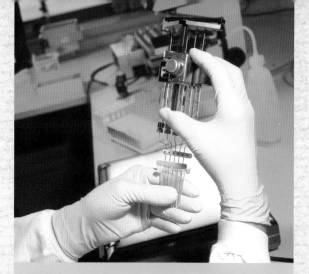

Fetal blood is taken from the unborn baby's cord during percutaneous umbilical blood sampling (PUBS) for testing in the laboratory (see above). The blood can be used to diagnose a number of different conditions.

Risks and side effects

The risk of loss of the baby is higher than for amniocentesis. Other risk factors include infection and rupture of the membranes.

Results

It usually takes three days for the results to come through. Although there is no definitive research at present on the test's reliability, the results are thought to be highly accurate.

GENETIC COUNSELING

You could be referred for genetic counseling before, during, or following a pregnancy if you think you may be at increased risk of having a baby with an abnormality. It's this sort of referral that is covered here. Ideally, genetic counseling should take place before conception. Decision making is better if it's not rushed, and it takes time to gather together all the relevant information and get any test results.

WHY YOU MAY WANT COUNSELING
The purpose of genetic counseling is to:
♦ Determine the probability of your baby having a congenital (present at birth) abnormality or genetic disorder.
♦ Explain the effects of the disorder and the amount of risk to the baby.
♦ Outline any treatments available.
♦ Highlight what prenatal tests are available to detect the problem.
♦ Explain possible courses of action.
♦ Help you reach a decision appropriate for you.
Many fetal abnormalities can be diagnosed prenatally. However, prenatal tests are entirely optional and can be declined. If a mother chooses to have a prenatal test and is told there's a possible problem, or if the baby is found to have a serious abnormality—either during pregnancy or after delivery—the implications can be discussed at a genetic counseling session with a doctor, midwife, or genetic counselor.

Many people mistakenly believe that all types of congenital abnormalities (those present at birth) happen more often to babies born to older mothers. In fact, most abnormalities aren't related to the mother's age, and, as most babies are born to women under 40, these babies represent the largest population with congenital abnormalities. However, older mothers do have a greater risk of having babies with Down syndrome and other chromosomal problems.

Why you might be referred
Couples who are at a higher-than-average risk of having a baby with an inherited disease or congenital abnormality should be referred for genetic counseling before pregnancy or in the early stages of pregnancy. Such people would include those who:

♦ *Have had children with abnormalities* If the mother or someone else in the family has had—or lost—a baby with an abnormality, this should be reported to the doctor. Counseling may be offered to discuss if and how this affects the chances of having another baby with the same problem.

♦ *Are from particular ethnic groups* Some genetic disorders are more common in certain racial or cultural groups. For example, people of Ashkenazi Jewish origins are at above average risk of carrying a gene for a degenerating neurological disorder called Tay-Sachs disease. Afro-Caribbeans, on the other hand, are at higher-than-average risk of carrying the gene for sickle-cell disease, and people of Asian or Mediterranean descent are at increased risk of carrying the gene for thalassemia.

♦ *Are known carriers* If either of the parents carry an abnormal gene or an unusual chromosome is found—via testing because of ethnic origin, family history, repeated miscarriage, or a general screening program—then the healthcare provider should recommend genetic counseling to determine what significance this has for children and other family members.

♦ *Are married cousins* If the expectant parents are first cousins, they will share one in eight of their genes—second cousins share 1 in 32. Therefore there's an above average risk of both having the same abnormal gene, so the chances of the baby having a recessively inherited genetic condition are also higher than average.

It is important to remember, however, that most marriages between cousins produce normal, healthy children.

- *Have had repeated miscarriages* A mother can be referred for chromosome testing if she's had repeated miscarriages, as an unusual chromosome pattern in one parent can be the cause. Testing isn't usually offered until there have been two or three losses, because miscarriage is common and doesn't usually indicate a problem in either parent.
- *Have had harmful exposure* If the mother suspects that shortly before or during her pregnancy she could have been exposed to something hazardous, such as X-rays, chemicals, or certain medications, which could have harmed the unborn baby, her healthcare provider should be told immediately, as genetic counseling may be necessary.
- *Have had a potential problem found on a prenatal test* If an ultrasound scan or other prenatal test detects an abnormality, a referral will be made to a genetic counselor.

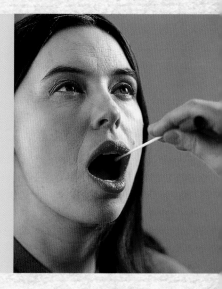

A saliva sample may be used for gene or chromosome testing when assessing the risks of an inherited disease. The inside of the cheek is rubbed with a cotton swab which is then sent to a laboratory for analysis.

What happens during a counseling session

You will be asked questions by a geneticist, specialist nurse, or genetic counselor about your relatives, in order to construct a family tree to find out if any disorders seem to "run in the family" and to assess the chances of your baby inheriting such a condition. To get more detailed information, both partners and other family members may be asked to give a blood sample or a saliva sample for gene or chromosome testing.

If your baby is thought to be at high risk of having a genetic or chromosomal abnormality, amniocentesis (see page 243) or chorionic villus sampling (see page 242) will be offered, or if the mother is over 20 weeks pregnant, fetal blood sampling may be offered.

If, once all the information and test results are available, the unborn baby is found to have a disorder, you will be told how the disorder will affect him, what treatments are available, and whether a termination of pregnancy is an option.

You won't be told what to do. All the tests are voluntary, and whatever course of action you decide upon is acceptable. The counselor or healthcare provider will put forward the pros and cons of different options, and will be able to give you any further information you may require, but won't make the decisions.

How diseases are inherited

A baby has two genes for each characteristic: one from the mother and one from the father (see page 17). It's likely that the parents and the child will carry some abnormal genes—most people do—but the abnormal genes probably won't cause problems. An abnormal gene is only likely to cause problems if it's dominant, if it's recessive and the baby has inherited two copies of the affected gene, or if it's X-linked and the baby is a boy (see page 248). The figures given are average risks for the different types of inheritance. Keep in mind, that just as one couple can have six boys or six girls in a row, so a couple could have many children with a problem, for which the risk is one in two or one in four, or they could have many normal, problem-free children.

New mutations

Sometimes a baby is born with a dominant or X-linked problem, which neither parent has—a

DOMINANT GENES

Examples of diseases: Huntington's disease, achondroplasia, and myotonic dystrophy.

If a person carries an abnormal dominant gene, he or she will probably know already because the person will have the problem—unless the effects aren't apparent until later in life. If such a gene is carried, every egg or sperm produced has a 50:50 chance of containing this abnormal gene.

Chances of baby inheriting problem: Each child has a one in two chance of being affected.

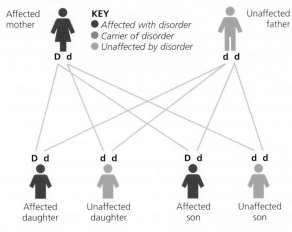

D = Abnormal, dominant gene d = Normal gene

RECESSIVE GENES

Examples of diseases: cystic fibrosis, thalassemia, and sickle-cell disease.

An abnormal recessive gene won't affect the mother's or father's health provided that the matching gene is normal. However, if a baby inherits two copies of the abnormal gene, one from each parent, he'll be affected. If he inherits one copy, he'll be a healthy carrier of the problem—like his parent.

Chances of baby inheriting problem: Each child has a one in four chance of being affected. Each unaffected child has a two in three chance of being a carrier.

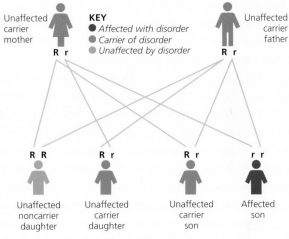

R = Normal gene r = Abnormal, recessive gene

X-LINKED GENES

Examples of diseases: hemophilia, Duchenne muscular dystrophy, and color blindness.

If a woman carries an abnormal gene on an X chromosome, she probably won't have a problem, as her other X is likely to carry a normal version of the gene. A man carrying an abnormal gene on his X chromosome will suffer from the disorder, as he won't have another X chromosome with a normal version of the gene.

Chances of baby inheriting problem: If the mother is a carrier, a daughter has a one in two chance of being a carrier. Her sons have a one in two chance of being affected. If the father is affected, all daughters will be carriers, sons will not be affected.

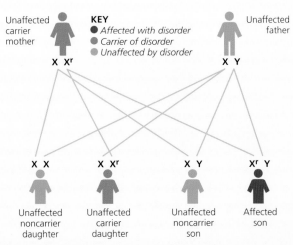

X = Chromosome with normal gene Y = Chromosome without gene
X^r = Chromosome with abnormal gene

new mutation. Mutations arise from a mistake in the copying of a gene during the egg or sperm production process. If you have a baby with a new mutation, although your future children won't be at high risk of having the problem, the affected child could pass on the gene to his children.

CHROMOSOMAL PROBLEMS

It's extremely important for a baby to inherit the correct number (46) of chromosomes—an additional chromosome means thousands of extra genes; an absent one, thousands of missing genes.

Trisomies (including Down syndrome)

If a baby inherits an extra copy of a chromosome, he'll have three copies instead of the normal two. This condition is called trisomy. Most trisomies cause a pregnancy to miscarry, but some allow a baby to develop. The most common of these is Down syndrome, also called trisomy 21 because the baby has three copies of chromosome 21. Edwards syndrome (trisomy 18) and Patau syndrome (trisomy 13) are rarer and more serious disorders. The risk of having a baby with Down syndrome increases with a woman's age: at 20 it's about 1 in 1500, at 30 it's 1 in 900, and at 40 it's increased to about 1 in 100.

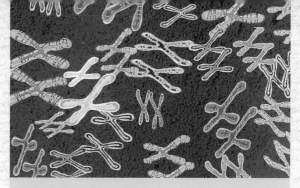

The male sex chromosomes are seen here as bright yellow (centre left) with the larger X chromosome below the small Y chromosome. The Y chromosome is responsible for masculine characteristics.

Extra sex chromosomes

Studies show that at least 1 baby in 1000 has an extra sex chromosome. Such babies are usually normal in appearance and behavior, and many progress through life without being diagnosed as having an extra chromosome. However, some of these children may have problems—for example, males with an extra X chromosome are infertile. If prenatal tests show that your baby has extra X or Y chromosomes, you will be offered genetic counseling to discuss the implications.

Translocations

About 1 person in 500 has one or more chromosomes on which pieces have been swapped with another or have broken off. Such rearrangements are called translocations. A balanced translocation will cause no problems, since all the genes are present, but in a different location. If there is an unbalanced translocation (with extra or missing genetic information) a miscarriage will usually occur—if the baby is born he could suffer major physical and intellectual problems. People with balanced translocations are at increased risk of producing eggs or sperm with unbalanced translocations.

MULTIFACTORIAL OR POLYGENIC DISORDERS

Many abnormalities, such as spina bifida (see page 375) or heart defects (see page 374), aren't usually caused by an abnormal gene or chromosome but arise from a combined effect of many different genes and the environment. These are called multifactorial or polygenic disorders. When a baby is born with one of these disorders, the risk of recurrence that the parents are given is based on observations of what has happened to other couples in the past who have had similarly affected children.

COMPLICATED LABORS

Every woman's experience of labor is different, and every baby's experience of birth is unique. Some babies take their time to be born; others pop out without any fuss. Then there are the babies who arrive late, and those who arrive early. Occasionally, problems occur which affect the progress of labor.

PRETERM LABOR

Not all labors occur at term (between 37 and 41 weeks after your last menstrual period). If regular contractions start before 37 weeks and occur at a rate of six or more in an hour and don't abate with rest, you may be having preterm labor. Because the baby may not be mature enough to cope on her own if she's delivered too early, you should be examined as soon as possible.

Just as with term labor, no one knows exactly what causes preterm labor but there appear to be many possible causes or contributing factors. Among these are:

- Uterine infection, which can trigger the release of prostaglandins, that may induce labor.
- Problems with or inadequacy of the placenta which may cause the baby to release substances that bring on early labor.
- Uterine anomalies such as large fibroids, which decrease the ability of the uterus to stretch and accommodate the growing baby.
- Expecting more than one baby.
- Polyhydramnios (excessive amniotic fluid) (see page 262).

Preterm contractions may feel as strong as labor at term, possibly because they're unexpected. Some women experience them as persistent or rhythmic low back pain or pelvic pressure; others as menstrual-like cramps, or groin pulling. Increasing vaginal discharge may be a sign that the cervix is dilating, especially if it's blood-tinged.

Management

If you suspect you may be having preterm contractions, plenty of fluids and bed rest can sometimes relieve the symptoms. Resting also allows you to attend to your body. In particular, keep a hand on your lower abdomen, over your uterus. If you feel repeated episodes of tightening or balling up and they persist when you're resting, call your healthcare provider.

SLOW LABOR

There are several types of labor in which progress is slow or non-existent. These include:

Prolonged latent (early) phase

This occurs when the cervix has failed to dilate, or has only dilated by a small amount, after 20 hours of labor with a first pregnancy, or 14 hours with a second one. This may be because the cervix is unprepared, the baby isn't properly positioned, or the mother is excessively sedated. Alternatively, contractions may be false labor.

Healthcare providers often treat a prolonged latent phase with sedation or rest in order to help distinguish false from true labor. Walking may also achieve this distinction and may help position

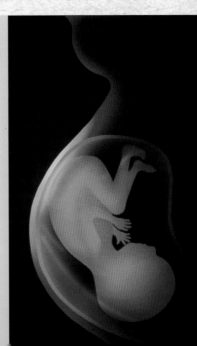

The baby can be seen in this artwork in the head-down position in the uterus, ready for birth.

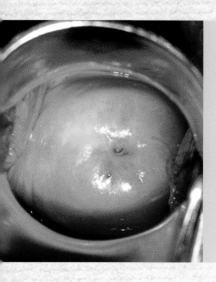

During pregnancy the opening of the cervix (centre left) remains tightly closed. Hormones and an increased blood supply gives the cervix a deep pink color.

the baby properly. Don't tire yourself out, however; you will need to save some energy for active phase labor and pushing.

Protracted active phase

The active phase of labor begins when the progressive dilation in the cervix proceeds at one or more centimeters per hour. This usually occurs when you've dilated to between 3 and 5 cm. Once active phase labor occurs, complete dilation is usually reached within four to eight hours. Contractions are much more intense during this phase as they work to fully dilate the cervix and guide the baby farther into the pelvis—usually 1 cm deeper per hour.

Protracted active phase occurs when progress stalls and it takes over an hour to dilate 1 cm. This can happen if the baby is in the wrong position, or with overmedication or epidural analgesia. You may be given Pitocin, a synthetic form of oxytocin, to help stimulate contractions. If labor is still not progressing, the baby's head may be too large to fit through the pelvis—known as cephalopelvic disproportion (CPD)—and a cesarean section will be necessary.

BACK LABOR

Many women feel their contractions most strongly in their backs. This is usually because the baby isn't in the most common position for labor but in the occiput posterior position, in which he faces away from his mother's spine and the occiput (back of head) presses against the spine. Back labor can be relieved by getting into the knee-chest position, pelvic rocks, walking, or keeping upright to encourage the baby to descend—babies often turn when they descend. Back massage and occasionally acupressure, and water therapy can also help. For information on all these, see Chapter 12.

FAST LABOR

Occasionally, the cervix dilates very rapidly, so that it becomes fully dilated within a very short time. This abrupt labor—taking three hours or less from start to finish—doesn't usually cause any problems to the baby. Very occasionally, however, a rapid labor can deprive the baby of oxygen, or result in tearing or other damage to the cervix, vagina, or perineum. Medication may be given to slow labor down so that the baby can be delivered safely without any damage to the mother.

VAGINAL BREECH LABOR

A vaginal breech labor is always considered a trial labor, and is allowed to proceed only as long as it progresses normally. Up to the second stage the labor is treated the same as a head-down labor. Depending on the baby's exact breech position (see page 226) your healthcare provider will decide on the safest way to proceed once the second stage is reached—usually a cesarean is required. If a vaginal breech birth does go ahead, the legs and lower half of the body are usually delivered naturally, then forceps are often used to deliver the shoulders and head, and a large episiotomy may be needed.

PREGNANCY COMPLICATIONS

Many women suffer minor health problems during pregnancy, but more serious complications occasionally arise. When these occur, treatment is usually required, so it is important to report any unusual symptoms to your healthcare provider immediately.

BLOOD DISORDERS

Anemia

A common condition in pregnancy, anemia occurs when there aren't enough blood cells circulating in the mother's blood. Many pregnant women will develop some degree of anemia at some point, but in mild cases, it doesn't cause any problems. And, because your body diverts all its resources in favor of your baby, she is unlikely to be lacking in iron. However, if anemia occurs as a result of hereditary abnormalities in hemoglobin, this can threaten the health of both you and your baby.

The most common anemia of pregnancy is dilutional anemia. The amount of blood circulating around the body increases by as much as 40 to 50 percent to sustain the growing baby. This dramatic rise is mainly achieved by an increase in the serum or liquid component of blood. Unless red cells increase at the same rate, they will be diluted in the blood, leading to dilutional anemia.

Iron deficiency is the other major cause of anemia in pregnancy. Because you need to produce enough red blood cells for both you and your baby, you need more iron during pregnancy—30 mg a day, which is twice the pre-pregnancy requirements—to maintain blood volume. Most women don't have enough stored iron in their bodies and it's very difficult to ingest sufficient amounts. Consequently, a large percentage of women will eventually become anemic in pregnancy.

Iron deficiency anemia also can be caused by folic acid deficiency, blood loss, and chronic illness. Unless nutritional intake of iron is supplemented during pregnancy, a woman will be deficient in iron stores at the time of birth, placing her at risk if postpartum bleeding occurs. Anemia during pregnancy also can result from a diet deficient in folic acid, the B vitamin needed to produce red blood cells.

Symptoms
- Fatigue, loss of energy
- Pallor
- Decreased ability to fight illness
- Dizziness, fainting, shortness of breath

Treatment
During pregnancy, iron deficiency anemia is treated with an iron supplement. In addition, iron-rich foods—molasses, baked potatoes, red meat, kidney beans, spinach, fish, chicken, and pork—should form a major part of your diet. To increase iron absorption, vitamin C is needed, so take your iron pill with orange, tomato, or vegetable juice.

Rarely, a woman unable to absorb adequate iron may require intravenous or injectable iron preparations. Folic acid or vitamin B12 may also be taken in the form of pills or by injection. In severe cases, blood transfusions may be needed, especially if labor and delivery are near.

Deep vein thrombosis

Commonly called DVT, this is a condition which occurs when a blood clot blocks a vein in one of the legs—usually the calf vein or a vein in the upper leg or groin area.

Symptoms
- Pain, tenderness, and swelling of the calf, upper leg or groin
- Swollen area feels warm

Treatment

If you suspect you may have DVT, you need to go straight to the hospital. This condition shouldn't be ignored, because if left untreated the clot can travel to the lungs causing a pulmonary embolus, which can be life-threatening. A special ultrasound scan called a Doppler is available that will quickly tell doctors if a DVT is present. Treatment usually consists of blood-thinning injections or medication.

It's easy to confuse DVT with the common and harmless condition of superficial thrombophlebitis. Sometimes the small surface veins in the lower legs become rather red and sore in pregnancy especially if you're overweight. Soothing cream and support tights are all that is needed in these cases.

Gestational diabetes

This is a type of diabetes unique to pregnancy in which the body fails to make enough insulin to cope with the increased blood sugar. In pregnancy the placenta produces a hormone, human placental lactogen, which acts against insulin and can therefore expose a tendency to diabetes. For women with gestational diabetes, the main complication is that the baby can become very large. Delivery is often recommended by no later than 40 weeks gestation.

You're at risk of gestational diabetes if you've had it before, if you're over 35, overweight, or Asian, if your previous baby was over 8 1bs 13 oz (4 kg), if you have a parent or sibling with diabetes, a previous baby with an abnormality, or a previous stillbirth. The actual diagnosis for gestational diabetes is based on testing the sugar levels in your blood when fasting and after eating a fixed amount of sugar.

Symptoms
- Sugar in urine
- Excessive thirst
- Excessive urination
- Fatigue

Treatment

Most women with gestational diabetes can control their sugar levels by following a sensible, relatively sugar-free diet. For some women this is insufficient, not because they don't stick to the diet but because of the pregnancy itself. These women will need to start having at least twice daily insulin injections or oral medication to control their blood sugar. This is managed with the hospital diabetic team who will teach you how to check your own sugar levels and how to give yourself injections.

High blood pressure (hypertension)

If a woman's blood pressure is elevated before pregnancy, this is known as chronic hypertension. If a woman's blood pressure is elevated only during pregnancy, this is referred to as pregnancy-induced hypertension (PIH). PIH affects about 8 percent of pregnancies and can develop any time after 20 weeks, but it generally does close to the due date. It will only resolve itself after delivery.

Many doctors tend to refer to PIH and pre-eclampsia as one and the same thing. While PIH is less of a risk to mother and baby than pre-eclampsia, PIH often progresses to pre-eclampsia, therefore the distinction between them often doesn't matter.

A deep vein thrombosis (DVT), caused by a clot in a vein in the upper leg, appears as an inflamed area that is warm to the touch.

Symptoms

There are usually no symptoms of high blood pressure until some organs, such as the kidney and eyes, are affected by the decreased blood supply that can accompany hypertension. Because untreated hypertension can eventually lead to serious complications (see below), blood pressure checks are routine at prenatal visits.

Pre-eclampsia

A syndrome that occurs only in pregnancy, pre-eclampsia is characterized by high blood pressure, protein in the urine, and increased swelling of the legs and feet. Six to eight percent of pregnancies are affected, and 85 percent of these are first-time pregnancies. Mothers who are over 40, teenage mothers, and mothers with diabetes, or kidney, or rheumatologic disease such as lupus, or a history of blood pressure problems also are at higher risk.

Many women with pre-eclampsia feel perfectly well and only realize they have this condition because they are told their blood pressure is high. If the following symptoms develop the condition becomes more serious.

Symptoms

- Sudden excessive lower leg edema (swelling) or excessive weight gain
- Persistent headaches
- Flashing lights, blurred vision, or spots before your eyes
- Upper abdominal pain on right side of the body, just below ribcage

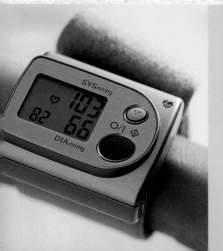

A simple home blood pressure monitor can be used to keep a check on your blood pressure, if you are thought to be at risk for pre-eclampsia.

Treatment

The cause of pre-eclampsia remains unknown and consequently no treatment has been consistently shown to prevent or treat it. Birth is the only cure, with induced delivery for women who are close to their due dates or who are severely affected by the disease. Low dose aspirin (75mg daily) may reduce your risk of developing pre-eclampsia. Make sure you attend all your prenatal appointments, so any problems can be detected early. Relax and try not to get stressed as this can raise your blood pressure. Eat well and healthily—cut back on sodium and fat, take in more fruit, vegetables, and calcium, and drink plenty of water. You may be asked to monitor your own blood pressure so you can instantly spot any dramatic change.

Eclampsia

Pre-eclampsia can develop into eclampsia, a rare but very serious condition.

Symptoms

- Seizures
- Possible coma

Treatment

Eclampsia is a medical emergency, and oxygen and drugs will be given to the mother to prevent any further seizures occurring. Urgent delivery of the baby is usually required to enable proper treatment of the mother.

HELLP syndrome

A life-threatening condition, HELLP syndrome is a unique variant of pre-eclampsia. It stands for its characteristics: H is for hemolysis (the breaking down of red blood cells); EL for elevated liver enzymes; and LP for low platelet count. HELLP syndrome occurs in tandem with pre-eclampsia, but because some of its symptoms can occur before those of pre-eclampsia—namely high blood pressure, protein in the urine, and swelling—they can be mistaken for other conditions. As a result, the right treatment may not be given, leaving both mother and baby in a very vulnerable state.

Six to eight percent of all pregnant women in the United States develop pre-eclampsia. Between two and 12 percent of these go on to suffer from HELLP syndrome. Older white women with more than one child are most at risk of getting HELLP, but it can affect any pregnant woman. If for some reason the diagnosis of pre-eclampsia is delayed the likelihood of developing HELLP syndrome will be even higher.

Symptoms
- Headache
- Nausea, vomiting
- Abdominal soreness and pain in the right upper section—from liver distention

These symptoms may or may not be present:
- Severe headache
- Visual disturbances
- Bleeding
- Swelling
- High blood pressure
- Protein in the urine

Treatment
The only effective treatment for women with HELLP syndrome is delivery. The quicker pre-eclampsia is detected and managed, the better the outcome for mother and baby.

UTERINE PROBLEMS
Fibroids
Benign growths on the wall of the uterus, fibroids are more common in older women than younger women, and don't usually affect pregnancy. Pregnancy hormones can make fibroids grow bigger, and occasionally they may cause problems, such as preventing the baby from growing properly. The position of the fibroid may make a vaginal delivery impossible.

Symptoms
- Pain
- Abdominal tenderness
- Slight fever

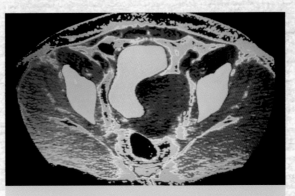

A large fibroid, a benign tumor, can been seen (round black area) in the uterus (yellow), on this color-enhanced CT scan. Fibroids may occasionally cause problems during pregnancy.

Treatment
If fibroids are causing discomfort, pain-relieving medications are usually the only treatment during pregnancy. The size of fibroids usually shrinks in the weeks after delivery. If they continue to be a problem, they may be surgically removed some months after delivery.

It's considered unsafe to remove fibroids at the time of a cesarean section, because of the risk of severe blood loss and the possible need for hysterectomy to control bleeding.

BOWEL PROBLEM
Anal fissure
Occasionally pregnancy or a difficult delivery can lead to a tear in the anal mucosa (lining of the anus). Bowel movements can reopen this tear, resulting in bleeding and intense pain; continual opening prevents healing and can result in scar tissue. Anal fissures are usually linked to bowel problems; constipation or frequent stools can cause straining and exacerbate the problem. Anal fissures also can be caused by syphilis, tuberculosis, Crohn's disease, and tumors.

Fissures can be confused with hemorrhoids, painful swellings at the anus caused by enlarged veins and venereal warts, which have similar symptoms. Anal fissures are generally diagnosed with an anoscopy, which allows examination of the anal canal. They can usually be prevented by keeping bowel movements regular and soft. Eating plenty of fiber and taking stool softeners, such as docusate, can help achieve this.

Symptoms
- Pain during and after a bowel movement
- Bright red bleeding
- Constipation

Treatment
Anal fissures can be acute or chronic, and it's important to get them treated as early as possible or complications can set in. Treatment depends on the severity of the condition. Acute or recent fissures are usually treated with a bulk-forming laxative, and a local anesthetic cream. In severe cases, a surgical procedure may be necessary. After treatment, it's important to follow a high fiber diet, eat regularly, and drink plenty of fluids.

DIGESTIVE PROBLEMS
Hyperemesis gravidarum
Rarely, morning sickness can develop into this more extreme condition. Approximately 1 in 200 women in early pregnancy need to be admitted to hospital because they're vomiting excessively and need to be rehydrated by intravenous drip. If left untreated, hyperemesis gravidarum can result in low levels of potassium in the bloodstream and prevent the liver from functioning properly.

Symptoms
- Excessive nausea and vomiting
- Weight loss
- Dehydration
- Dark yellow urine
- Passing small quantities of urine

Treatment
Fortunately, treatment by admission to the hospital, stopping all oral intake, and giving rehydrating fluids via a venous line (a drip) is

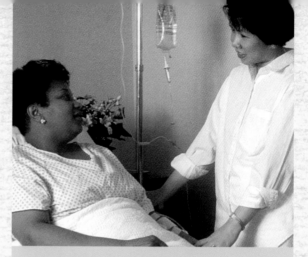

Dehydration, caused by hyperemesis gravidarum, may require a stay in hospital so that rehydrating fluids can be given through a venous line.

usually very successful. Food is then slowly reintroduced and you will be discharged home after a matter of a few days.

INFECTIONS
It is worth remembering that most women go through pregnancy with no infections, that most maternal infections have no effect on the baby, and that significant infections are very rare.

At your first prenatal visit you may be offered screening for certain infections—rubella (German measles), syphilis, and hepatitis B. Some women will also be offered screening for human immunodeficiency virus (HIV) and toxoplasmosis (see page 257). You don't have to be screened for any of these infections, but the more you know, the more you can protect your health and that of your unborn baby. If you aren't immune to rubella, for example, you should be vaccinated after pregnancy, and during pregnancy you should avoid potential infections.

Cytomegalovirus
A member of the herpes virus family, cytomegalovirus (CMV) is the most common congenital (present at birth) infection in the United States. Between 25 and 60 percent of

preschool children carry the virus, which is spread by contact with saliva, urine, and feces. About 1 percent of newborns are infected every year. The vast majority aren't affected by the virus but about 8000 babies a year develop lasting disabilities such as mental retardation, deafness, and blindness.

A woman who contracts CMV for the first time during pregnancy—in the United States about 1 to 3 percent of pregnant women do—has a 30 to 40 percent risk of passing it to her baby. Women who contracted CMV at least 6 months before getting pregnant appear to have little risk of developing complications. A lab test can determine whether a woman has had the infection before, while a culture can be grown from a urine specimen to detect active infection. If CMV is diagnosed, the baby can be tested for the infection by amniocentesis. In newborns, the virus can be identified in body fluids within 3 weeks of birth.

Symptoms
- Sore throat
- Fever
- Body aches
- Fatigue

Treatment
At present, there's no preventive treatment for congenital CMV, but a new antiviral drug called ganciclovir may help babies with the infection. In the meantime, the risk of contracting CMV can be reduced by observing careful hygiene, such as thorough hand-washing after contact with the saliva and urine of young children.

Toxoplasmosis
Although quite rare in the United States and Canada, toxoplasmosis is an infection that can seriously affect the fetus. It can be caught through contact with outdoor cats, and by eating under-cooked meat and unwashed vegetables. If a pregnant woman becomes infected, the chance that she will transmit the infection to her baby, and the possible effects it may have depend largely on when she contracts it. If it's during the first

trimester, the chance that the baby will become infected is less than 2 percent, although the effect it has on the baby's development is greater. If the infection isn't contracted until later in pregnancy, the chance that the baby will become infected is higher, but the effects of the infection are much less severe. There may be some general symptoms (see below), but it is possible to have the infection without knowing it.

While some doctors routinely screen for toxoplasmosis in early pregnancy, others don't. It often depends on your own particular risk factors such as whether you own an outdoor cat.

Symptoms
- Feeling generally unwell
- Slight fever
- Swollen glands
- Rash

Treatment
If blood tests show that you have developed toxoplasmosis either immediately prior to conception or during pregnancy, you should meet with a maternal-fetal medicine specialist or your own doctor to discuss the possible implications. You may need to be given certain antibiotics to decrease the chances of transmitting the infection

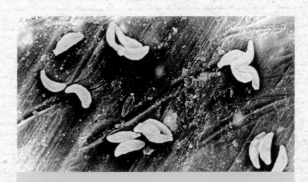

Toxoplasmosis bacteria can be seen here as yellow crescent-shaped parasite cells. If a pregnant woman becomes infected, it can affect her unborn baby.

to the baby, and possibly have an amniocentesis (see page 243) in the second trimester to determine if in fact the baby has contracted the infection. The good news is that recent studies from France have shown that even if the unborn baby is infected, treatment with the appropriate antibiotics gives an excellent chance that the baby will still be fine.

Listeriosis
Caused by listeria, a bacteria found in unpasteurized milk and cheese, raw and under-cooked meat, poultry, fish and shellfish, and unwashed raw vegetables, listeriosis can cause serious illness in pregnancy, which can lead to preterm birth, miscarriage, stillbirth, or infection of the baby. Listeriosis is hard to detect, as symptoms can appear any time between 12 hours and 30 days after contaminated food is eaten, and may be ignored, as they are similar to those of flu, or mistaken for normal pregnancy side effects.

Symptoms
- Headache
- Fever
- Muscle aches
- Nausea and diarrhea

Treatment
Infection can be prevented by avoiding eating any food that could be contaminated (see page 111). If the infection is present, antibiotics will be needed to treat and cure listeriosis.

Rubella (German measles)
Also known as rubella, German measles is a relatively mild infection normally, but in pregnancy it can have very serious implications, as it can cause birth defects ranging from deafness to encephalitis (inflammation of the brain) and heart defects. Fortunately, most women are immune to the disease, either from a vaccination or from having had it as a child.

Ideally, if you are not immune, you should be vaccinated against rubella before getting pregnant and then wait three months before trying to conceive. If you received the vaccine before being aware you were pregnant, the chances that it will harm the baby are very low. A detailed ultrasound may be carried out at 18 weeks to check your baby's progress.

Symptoms
- Rash first appearing on the face and spreading to other parts of body
- Fever
- Swollen glands

Treatment
If you contract rubella during pregnancy, the risk to your baby depends on when you caught it. If it was in the first month, there's a one in two chance the baby will be affected. By the third month, the risk drops to one in ten. Unfortunately, nothing can be done during the pregnancy to protect your baby. Your healthcare provider will explain your options and what tests are available.

Chickenpox
As most adults in the United States and Canada have had chickenpox as a child, there's a very good chance you're immune to it. If you have had chickenpox you will not get it again even if you are in contact with someone with chickenpox or shingles. The infection is caused by the varicella virus, which can appear as chickenpox or as shingles—chickenpox is the illness you get the first time you catch the virus, while shingles is a reactivation of this virus. There's a very small risk to a baby if the mother becomes infected. However, occasionally, a rare but devastating condition known as congenital varicella syndrome can cause severe birth defects, which can be fatal.

Symptoms
- Itchy blister-type rash
- Fever
- Malaise
- Fatigue

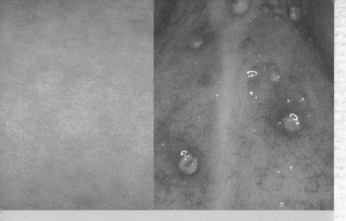

A rash is a symptom of both rubella (left) and chickenpox (right). Although most adults are immune to these diseases, they can cause serious complications if a woman becomes infected with them during pregnancy.

Treatment

If you aren't immune to chickenpox and catch it in pregnancy, you'll be offered an injection of VZIG (antivaricella antibodies), as the disease can lead to pneumonia in adults. You may be admitted to hospital for observation and treatment. You also can be given antiviral drugs to treat the infection. If you catch chickenpox just before delivery, the virus can be passed to the baby and make him very ill. In this case your baby can be given VZIG at birth.

Yeast infections

An increase in vaginal discharge is usual in pregnancy as mucus production increases. As long as the discharge is thin and white—although it may be yellow when dry—it's probably normal. However, hormonal changes in pregnancy can encourage germs in the vagina to overgrow, resulting in yeast infections caused by a microscopic fungus called Candida albicans. Candida is very common—25 percent of women have candida in their vagina.

Symptoms

- Thick, curd-like, white discharge
- Burning, and redness and itching of the vulva

Treatment

While candida won't affect your pregnancy, if the infection isn't treated, your baby can contract oral yeast (thrush) while passing through your vagina at birth. Candida can be treated by vaginal creams, ointments, suppositories, and oral medication. Many of these are available over-the-counter, but before using any medication check with your healthcare provider. To alleviate symptoms and prevent candida from occurring, avoid feminine hygiene sprays, and bath preparations. Cut down on carbohydrates and sugar, as they encourage yeast growth. Wear cotton underwear and cotton crotch pantyhose, and avoid synthetic fabrics and tight pants. Always wipe from front to back after going to the toilet. Eating live yogurt (containing lactobacillus acidophilus) each day can help reduce the risk.

Urinary tract infections (UTIs)

UTIs include infections of the bladder and the kidneys, such as cystitis, the ureters (the tubes that lead from the kidneys to the bladder), and the urethra (the tube that carries urine from the bladder to outside of the body). UTIs are very common in pregnancy. Infection can be mild to severe, ranging from bacteria in the urine to kidney infection. As UTIs can be present and not have any symptoms, urine specimens are routinely tested throughout pregnancy to detect bacteria in the urine. If bacteria are found—referred to as asymptomatic bacteriuria (ASB)—taking antibiotics can prevent a mild infection from affecting the kidneys.

Symptoms

- An urgent need to urinate
- A sharp pain or burning sensation on urination
- Very little urine is eliminated, and it may be tinged with blood, be cloudy or smell bad
- The need to urinate returns minutes later
- Soreness may occur in the lower abdomen, in the back, or in the sides
- Back pain, chills, fever, nausea, and vomiting if infection spreads to kidneys

Treatment

Untreated UTIs can trigger contractions, and possibly preterm birth. You should contact your healthcare provider, as antibiotic therapy is usually necessary for treatment of UTIs. To help prevent a recurrence, drink plenty of water to help flush germs from the system. Empty your bladder frequently and, as you do so, lean forward on the toilet to make sure that the bladder is completely emptied—stagnant urine is the perfect breeding ground for bacteria. Fresh cranberry juice can help prevent urinary tract infections, as it makes urine more acidic, and so less agreeable to germs.

JOINT PROBLEMS
Carpal tunnel syndrome

The carpal tunnel is in front of the wrist and houses the tendons and nerves that run to the fingers. When the hand and fingers swell in pregnancy, in common with other tissues, the carpal tunnel swells, too, putting pressure on a nerve. This pressure results in the sensation of pins and needles spreading down into all the fingers except the little finger. Symptoms tend to be worse at night, but usually ease during the day as the joints are used and become more supple. It should disappear in the days following delivery.

Symptoms
- Pain in the wrist
- Pins and needles extending from wrist down into hand
- Stiffness of fingers and joints of hand

Treatment

Sleeping with your hands raised on a pillow can prevent fluid building up. On waking, dropping your hand over the side of the bed and giving it a vigorous shake can help disperse fluid and ease stiffness. Wearing a splint on the wrists can help.

Symphysis pubis dysfunction

The pelvic girdle is made up of three bones—one at the back and two at the front—joined by ligaments. The bones meet to form three "fixed"

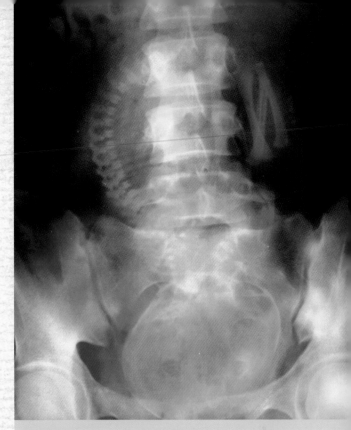

Pressure from the baby, seen here in the head-down position in the pelvis, sometimes causes the symphysis pubis joint (below the baby's head) to separate.

joints, one at the front, called the symphysis pubis, and one at each side of the base of the spine. In pregnancy, the pregnancy hormone relaxin loosens all the pelvic ligaments to allow the baby easier passage at birth. However, these ligaments can loosen too much, making the pelvis move, especially when weight is put on it. The weight of the baby makes this worse and sometimes the symphysis pubis joint actually separates slightly. The result is mild to severe pain in the pubic area, and is called symphysis pubis dysfunction (SPD). This condition can develop at any time from the first trimester onward.

SPD sometimes occurs if you've been immobile for a long time, or extremely overactive. It also may occur after an activity such as swimming breaststroke or lifting something incorrectly.

Symptoms
◆ Pain, usually in the pubis and/or the lower back, but can be in the groin, inner thighs, hips, and buttocks
◆ Pain is made worse when weight is on one leg
◆ A sensation of the pelvis separating
◆ Difficulty when walking

Treatment
Unfortunately, SPD is untreatable during pregnancy as it's due to the effect of hormones. The condition should improve, however, as your body returns to its pre-pregnancy state. In the meantime great care should be taken not to make SPD worse. Avoid putting weight on one leg as much as possible—sit down to get dressed, get into the car by putting your buttocks on the seat first, and then lifting your legs into the car. Avoid breaststroke when swimming, and keep your knees together when turning over in bed. If the pain is severe, ask your healthcare provider about painkillers, and arrange to see a physical therapist, who may advise a pelvic support belt.

Special care needs to be taken during labor and birth. Your legs need to be kept as close together as possible. Good birth positions are on all fours, kneeling up against the back of the bed, or side-lying with the top leg supported.

PROBLEMS WITH BABY
Growth problems
Sometimes a baby seems to be growing too slowly or too rapidly. Both can cause problems. How well a baby grows can be affected by a number of factors. For example, if you smoke, your baby will generally be smaller than average, while if you have diabetes you are likely to have a larger baby. If abnormal growth is suspected, a common way of confirming that there is a problem is to measure from the pelvic bone to the top of the uterus. However, the accuracy of this method is now known to be relatively poor. If a growth problem is suspected, ultrasound is likely to be used to more accurately measure your baby's size and growth for your dates.

Baby too small
Apart from the actual measurement of size, the ultrasound scan will be used to look for other important features. The amount of fluid around the baby will decrease if the placenta is functioning poorly. A very small baby may move less often, will practice its breathing less, and may be less active. In conjunction with a heart rate trace from the baby, these features comprise the biophysical profile (BPP). A normal BPP suggests that the baby is currently healthy.

Another very useful test when trying to decide whether a poorly growing or small baby is healthy is the umbilical artery Doppler estimation. This is also an ultrasound scan and can tell how fast the blood moves along the umbilical cord. When the speed is reduced it suggests that the placenta isn't functioning well.

When a decision about delivery is made, lots of factors will be taken into account. These will include how mature your baby is, how ill the baby is suspected to be, and your health. Some very ill babies will need to be delivered by cesarean. When a baby is ill and needs to be delivered prematurely you may be given steroid injections to help the baby's lungs mature.

Baby too big
Taller or heavier mothers tend to have larger babies than shorter or lighter mothers. But there are some serious conditions that cause a baby to become overlarge. The most common is if the mother has diabetes.

Many mothers worry about whether they'll be capable of delivering a large baby. Ultrasound isn't always very accurate in the measurement of large babies, and, in assessment of a baby's weight, there's about a 10 percent error. If your baby is big and you are near the end of your pregnancy you may be offered an induction of labor, to try to deliver your baby before he becomes even bigger. If your baby is large for your dates but you still have some time to go before the birth, it's best to discuss with your doctor a plan, taking into account your views, and his or her advice.

Polyhydramnios (hydramnios)

About 2 percent of pregnant women have too much amniotic fluid, a condition known as polyhydramnios. Most cases are mild and are a result of a gradual buildup of fluid during the second half of pregnancy. About half the time, polyhydramnios goes away and women will deliver healthy babies with no problems. Rarely, polyhydramnios can be a warning sign that there's a birth defect or that a medical problem such as gestational diabetes has developed.

Polyhydramnios may also occur in conditions that cause fetal anemia or certain viral infections. If polyhydramnios is severe, it may make the uterus contract and trigger preterm labor.

Symptoms

- Larger than normal uterus
- Abdominal discomfort
- Indigestion
- Swelling in the legs
- Breathlessness
- Hemorrhoids

Treatment

Polyhydramnios is normally diagnosed with ultrasound. If the condition is advanced, amniocentesis may be performed to remove excess fluid. If membranes rupture, there's a risk of cord prolapse where the cord is delivered before the baby, so you should contact your healthcare provider immediately.

Oligohydramnios

This is a condition in which there's too little amniotic fluid in the uterus. Most women with this condition will have a normal pregnancy, but occasionally it can signal or result in problems. In early pregnancy there is a slight risk of umbilical cord restriction, or the development of a club foot in the baby because there isn't enough room for normal growth. Later in pregnancy it can be a sign of fetal distress. Rarely it accompanies some form of fetal defect, such as problems with the digestive or urinary systems.

Symptoms

- The uterus may be smaller than average
- Less frequent fetal movement
- Slowed growth

Treatment

Maternal oral and IV hydration and bed rest may help the condition. Sometimes the fluid may be replaced through amnioinfusion—a process in which the amniotic fluid is "topped up" with warm saline solution, pumped directly into the amniotic sac through a catheter into the uterus. This treatment is considered experimental and doesn't help in all cases. If detected at a time when it is safe to deliver the baby, labor will be induced. Women with this condition should take extra care of themselves, and be sure to rest, eat properly, and drink lots of water.

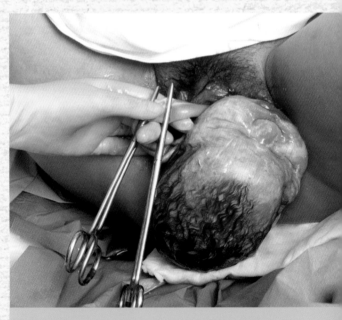

Sometimes the umbilical cord becomes wrapped around the baby's neck and immediate delivery is necessary. When this occurs, the cord is clamped and then cut as soon as the head is born.

Knotted cord

Sometimes the umbilical cord becomes knotted or tangled in the uterus, even wrapping around the baby's neck. This can reduce the baby's blood supply, so it's vital that any cord problems are resolved quickly.

Symptoms
◆ Decrease in fetal activity

Treatment
If the blood supply to the baby has been stopped for some reason, immediate delivery, usually by cesarean, is necessary.

Cord prolapse

Rarely, the baby's umbilical cord can fall into the birth canal ahead of the baby's head or other parts of the baby's body. A prolapsed cord can be very harmful to the baby. When the cord is squeezed, the baby's supply of blood and oxygen is cut off, which can have very serious consequences.

Prolapse is more likely to happen: if polyhydramnios is present; during delivery of the second baby of twins; if the baby is breech or in a transverse lie; or if the membranes rupture, either naturally or during a vaginal exam before the baby descends into the pelvis.

Symptoms
◆ Decreased heart rate, usually detected by a fetal heart monitor

Treatment
If the cord is still pulsating and can be seen or felt in the vagina, the doctor will support the part of the baby delivering first to take pressure off the cord. To assist with this you may be asked to get on your knees and bend forward. The doctor will keep a hand in the vagina until the baby is delivered the fastest way possible, usually by emergency cesarean section or possibly with forceps or vacuum extractor if the baby is in the right position for these to be used.

Fetal distress

This is a term used to describe any situation in which the unborn baby is thought to be in jeopardy—usually through decreased oxygen flow. The distress can be caused by a variety of problems including: maternal illness such as anemia, hypertension, heart disease, low blood pressure; a placenta that is no longer functioning well or has separated prematurely from the uterus; umbilical cord compression or entanglement; fetal infection or malformation, and prolonged or excessive contractions during labor.

Symptoms
◆ A change in fetal movements
◆ Absence of fetal movement
◆ Fetal heartbeat changes

Treatment
Immediate delivery is usually recommended. If vaginal delivery is not imminent, then an emergency cesarean is likely to be performed. The mother may first be given medication to slow contractions, which will increase oxygen to the baby, and to dilate her blood vessels, which will improve blood flow to the baby.

PRE-EXISTING MEDICAL CONDITIONS

If you had a medical condition before you became pregnant, it may affect the way your pregnancy is managed. Your healthcare provider will want to ensure that your treatment is safe for you and your baby. Sometimes special precautions are necessary, and you may require more frequent prenatal checks.

RESPIRATORY DISEASES
Asthma
This is the most common respiratory disease encountered in pregnant women, occurring in between 1 and 4 percent of all pregnancies. The effect of pregnancy on asthma is highly variable, causing symptoms to worsen in 22 percent, improve in 29 percent, and remain unchanged in the remainder of cases. In general, asthma tends to improve from 36 weeks, and it is highly unusual to suffer a severe asthma attack during labor. In well-controlled asthma, there is little or no effect on the pregnancy.

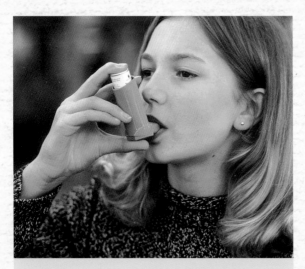

There is no evidence to suggest that the use of asthma inhaler pumps can cause any harm to your baby during pregnancy.

Management
If you have asthma, it can worsen in pregnancy if you don't continue to use your usual medication. You can continue to use an asthma inhaler pump, and even if steroid tablets are needed to control asthma, they won't do any harm. Long-term use of steroids can very occasionally cause high blood pressure or raised blood-sugar levels, but both of these can be treated.

IMMUNE DISORDERS
Anti-phospholipid syndrome (APS)
Also known as lupus, APS is an autoimmune disorder in which antibodies that harm the body are made. The antibodies make the blood sticky and can cause small or large blood clots. This syndrome may also accompany another disorder called systemic lupus erythematosus (SLE) and it's then called secondary anti-phospholipid syndrome. APS is a serious condition as it can cause miscarriage, pre-eclampsia, blood clots as well as stillbirth.

Management
APS can be treated with low-dose aspirin—75 mg daily—and, for some women, daily injections of heparin. If you have this condition, you will need to be treated by an obstetrician who will closely monitor your pregnancy and the growth of your baby. It is important to discuss your condition with your healthcare provider as soon as pregnancy is confirmed as with the correct treatment the chance of a successful pregnancy is over 70 percent, whereas without treatment up to 70 percent of pregnancies will miscarry.

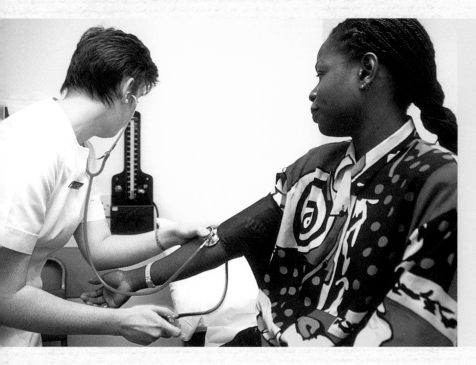

Women who suffer from chronic hypertension require frequent blood pressure checks during pregnancy because of the risk of pre-eclampsia.

CIRCULATION/BLOOD DISORDERS
Chronic hypertension
If you already had high blood pressure before you got pregnant, the condition is described as chronic hypertension. This is more common in women over the age of 40, African-American women, and those with mothers or sisters with high blood pressure. Certain medical conditions can make hypertension more likely, such as diabetes, renal disease, and being overweight.

The main risk of hypertension during pregnancy is the increased risk of developing pre-eclampsia (see page 254). The risk of pre-eclampsia in women with preexisting hypertension is around 20 percent. In general, unless pre-eclampsia develops, the risks of hypertension to the mother and baby are small.

Management
As your pregnancy will be considered high-risk, your doctor will want to keep a close eye on you, which will probably entail more checks and tests than usual. It's important to discuss your medication with your doctor as early on as possible, as certain blood-pressure drugs aren't safe

in pregnancy. Your blood pressure is likely to decrease in the first three months. As the pregnancy progresses it's not unusual to need to increase the medication or even add in a second or even third type of drug.

With hypertension, it's important to have expert medical supervision and to take good care of yourself, which means following a low-fat diet, getting plenty of rest, and doing relaxation exercises such as yoga. This way you're increasing your chances of a healthy pregnancy.

Heart disease
Most women planning to have a family have a healthy heart. In the past, the most common form of heart disease was due to an infection called rheumatic fever which can damage the heart valves. This is no longer a common illness in the United States or Canada, although some women may have experienced it as children if they were brought up in a developing country. If you were born with a heart abnormality, it's important that you discuss this with your doctor. It may be that the only precaution that is required is to give you antibiotics during childbirth to prevent you

getting an infection on your heart. On the other hand, if you have a complex abnormality, it may be that pregnancy will have some dangers and these can be discussed prior to conception.

If you or your partner were born with a heart defect you should mention this to your healthcare provider at your first prenatal visit. Later, a detailed scan of your baby's heart can usually show if he has inherited a similar problem.

Management
If you've had rheumatic heart disease, you'll probably have a replacement heart valve. If so, the main problem with pregnancy is the management of your anticoagulation. You will likely be on warfarin to stop a clot forming in your heart around the new valve. Warfarin is a very useful drug but shouldn't be used between weeks 6 and 14 of pregnancy, so your cardiologists will change to a form of heparin. This is another anticoagulant that can only be given by daily injection but doesn't cross the placenta. Some doctors continue the heparin until delivery; others prefer to put women back onto warfarin from 14 to 36 weeks and then change back to heparin again until delivery.

Sickle-cell disease
An inherited abnormality of the red blood cells, sickle-cell disease occurs predominantly in African-American people and developed as a natural protection against malaria. If you inherit sickle-cell from just one parent, it has little effect upon your health but protects you to a certain extent from malaria. If you inherit sickle-cell from both parents, you can become unwell with sickle-cell disease.

Sickle-cell disease causes problems with joint pains and anemia, which start from childhood. Pregnancy can be a special problem as it puts extra stress on the body and can precipitate sickle crisis. Common complications include joint pains, breathlessness, chest pain, and chest infection for the mother, and growth restriction and premature delivery for your baby.

Management
Your healthcare providers will work together with you to monitor your pregnancy closely and decide when blood transfusions are useful. You may be treated with folic acid and penicillin throughout the pregnancy, and you're likely to be induced at 38 weeks' gestation.

SEXUALLY TRANSMITTED DISEASES
Bacterial vaginosis (BV)
While BV is classified as a sexually transmitted disease (STD), you don't have to be sexually active to get this vaginal infection. You may be tested for BV at your first prenatal visit. If BV is left untreated there may be an increased risk of preterm delivery. The main symptoms are a watery white or gray discharge, which has a highly unpleasant or fishy smell. However, it's possible to have BV and not experience any symptoms.

Management
BV is usually treated with antibiotics, but it can also be treated with prescription pills or with the use of vaginal creams.

Chlamydia
This is a bacterium that is generally transmitted by sexual intercourse. The symptoms in men can be minimal which means that they may not be aware that they're infected—although infected men may suffer pain when passing urine. In women, the symptoms can be nonexistent, although some women have a vaginal discharge and may experience pain on passing urine. Sometimes women experience severe pelvic pain and become unwell with acute pelvic inflammatory disease. The severity of the symptoms doesn't appear to be related to the risk of the long-term effect of infertility.

Management
If you have had chlamydia in the past, and both you and your partner have been treated so that there's no risk of reinfection, the only concern in pregnancy is how the infection may affect your

fallopian tubes. If your fallopian tubes have been damaged you may suffer an increased risk of an ectopic pregnancy. If you have progressed beyond 12 weeks of pregnancy, or you have had a scan showing the pregnancy is situated in your uterus and is not ectopic, the previous infection will have no detrimental effect on the pregnancy.

If you have untreated chlamydia in pregnancy there's a slightly increased chance of preterm birth and a small risk that your baby may become infected during delivery. If he's infected he may develop a sticky, infected eye, and then, between one and three weeks after delivery, he may develop a chest infection. Chlamydia in pregnancy should be treated with erythromycin, not tetracycline, as the latter can affect your baby's bone growth.

Gonorrhea
You'll be routinely tested for this serious STD at your first prenatal visit. Gonorrhea can cause blindness and serious infection in an unborn baby. Symptoms include abnormal bleeding, a burning sensation during urination, vaginal discharge, and severe itchiness in the vaginal area.

Management
Gonorrhea is usually treated with antibiotics, and you'll be tested again later in pregnancy to make sure you no longer have the infection.

Hepatitis B
This viral liver infection is carried in blood and body secretions and is most commonly transmitted by having sex with an infected person, infection during childbirth, or using dirty needles. If you've been infected you're likely to carry the virus forever and remain infectious to others. In the long-term hepatitis B can cause liver damage. In some parts of the world, such as West Africa and Southeast Asia, hepatitis B is widespread.

Management
Treatment consists of plenty of rest, a healthy diet, and regular blood tests. Your partner should be tested as well, as he can be immunized against this

virus if he hasn't already caught it. Hepatitis B can be transmitted to your baby at the time of birth, but this can be prevented from developing by giving your baby a course of vaccinations, starting immediately after the birth.

Herpes simplex virus (HSV)
There are two types of herpes simplex virus: type 1 typically affects the lips and causes cold sores, and type 2 affects the genitalia. Both types can be transmitted by close contact such as kissing or sexual intercourse. In both types you will suffer from small painful ulcers on the skin, which can occur at any time but typically are preceded by a tingling feeling. If your partner has HSV, he should wear a condom during intercourse so you don't become infected. This is especially important during pregnancy.

Management
If you have genital herpes (HSV type 2) it can be transmitted to your baby during childbirth. This is usually only a problem if you have your first ever attack during childbirth. If you already have HSV, your body will have developed antibodies, which will be transmitted to your baby before he's born and therefore give her protection until he's three months old. If your baby is affected by HSV

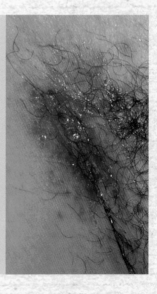

Type 2 herpes simplex virus affects the genitalia and the area around the groin. It can be seen here as an inflamed area with crusting yellow scabs.

during childbirth she could develop a brain infection known as encephalitis. This presents as lethargy and poor feeding but can develop into a life-threatening illness.

To protect your baby, most healthcare providers recommend a cesarean section if you have your first ever attack of HSV in labor, and your membranes haven't ruptured. If you have a recurrent attack, which is much more common, the advice is less certain. Some doctors will recommend a cesarean section, but the risk of your baby becoming unwell is less than 1 in 100, so many doctors are now suggesting that a normal delivery will be safe as long as the baby is treated with Acyclovir—an antiviral medicine— immediately after delivery.

Human immunodeficiency virus (HIV)/AIDS

Unprotected intercourse is the most common form of transmission of HIV/AIDS, but it can also be transmitted by the use of dirty needles, through a blood transfusion with infected blood, and during childbirth.

Management

If you have HIV—commonly known as being HIV positive—there's a 15 to 25 percent risk that your baby will become infected. This risk can be reduced to 1 to 2 percent with appropriate treatment, and HIV testing is now recommended in many hospitals. The treatment consists of anti-viral medication—either one medicine or three depending on the amount of virus in the woman's blood—cesarean section, and refraining from breastfeeding. In some circumstances, for example, if you're on triple therapy and your viral load is undetectable, vaginal delivery may be just as safe for your baby. If you're on treatment before you get pregnant, your doctor may suggest changing your regime. If you're put on just one drug during pregnancy—usually zidovudine—you can usually stop treatment after delivery.

Understandably, confidentiality may be an important issue for you, so you will need to decide who you want involved in discussions

RISK FACTORS

Around 15 to 25 percent of HIV-positive pregnant mothers will pass HIV to their babies, with 70 percent of infections occurring at the time of delivery, and the other 30 percent prenatally. Risk factors include:

- Clinical stage of HIV
- Substance abuse
- Vitamin A deficiency
- STDs and other co-infections
- Preterm delivery
- Placental disruption
- Invasive fetal monitoring
- Duration of membrane rupture
- Vaginal delivery

about your care. Your usual healthcare provider will need to know about your treatment as he or she will be concerned with your and your baby's long-term care.

Syphilis

You'll be offered testing for this disease at your first prenatal visit; however, the good news is that the instances of syphilis in pregnancy are currently lower than ever.

Treatment

A course of antibiotic treatment given in the first trimester is usually successful in preventing any harm to the baby.

Trichomoniasis

While this STD isn't too serious, it can increase the risk of preterm delivery so it is very important to have treatment. The main symptoms are a greenish, frothy vaginal discharge with a fishy smell, and itching.

Management

An oral medication is usually given, which is safe for use in pregnancy.

NEUROLOGICAL DISORDERS
Epilepsy
If you have epilepsy, the chances are that you'll enjoy an uncomplicated pregnancy. You may have severe morning sickness, but as long as your medication is carefully supervised, you have every reason to expect a positive outcome.

Management
It's important to see your doctor prior to conception so that your medication can be reduced, if possible, and altered to the best combination for pregnancy. There's an increased risk of having a baby with an abnormality and this can be reduced by taking an increased dose of folic acid (5 mg daily) for three months before you get pregnant and continuing until the baby is born. If you're already pregnant, it's important to see your doctor as early as possible. Some anticonvulsant medications can affect your ability to absorb vitamin K, which is necessary to help the baby's liver work well after delivery, so you should take vitamin K tablets or have shots from 36 weeks, and your baby should have a vitamin K injection after delivery. Seizures can increase in pregnancy and your medication may need to be changed to take account of this.

Multiple sclerosis
A degenerative neurological condition of unknown origin, multiple sclerosis (MS) consists of relapses and periods of remission. There is no evidence that pregnancy affects the long-term prognosis of MS, although relapse after delivery isn't uncommon.

Management
While MS doesn't appear to affect pregnancy, regular prenatal care is important. You can be more prone to anemia and infections such as UTIs (see page 259). Keep yourself as healthy as possible by getting plenty of rest, and avoid stress and overheating. If you're on medication, check with your healthcare provider that this is safe to take in pregnancy, as some MS medications aren't.

INFECTIONS
Chronic fatigue syndrome
Also known as myalgic encephalopathy (ME), this is a chronic debilitating illness that appears to start after a viral infection, although the nature of the infection and the cause of the chronic fatigue are unknown. If you have ME, you will need to discuss the use of any medication you are taking—including herbal and homeopathic—with your healthcare provider in case it has a detrimental effect on your pregnancy.

Management
Some women with ME find that their symptoms improve during the pregnancy, possibly as a result of the hormonal changes; but they tend to suffer a relapse after delivery. The delivery itself can be daunting. You need to plan well and consider an epidural to reduce the stress and tiredness that a long painful labor can bring. There's no reason why you shouldn't try for a normal delivery, but you may need help in the second stage if you're too exhausted to push.

The important thing to consider with ME is ensuring that you have sufficient support during the pregnancy, which you are likely to find very tiring, especially after delivery. Don't hesitate to accept offers of help from your partner, mother, sisters, and friends.

OTHER CHRONIC CONDITIONS
Diabetes
This is a tendency to have high blood-sugar levels. This condition can also develop during pregnancy (gestational diabetes, see page 253). Whether your diabetes is controlled with tablets or with insulin injections, the risks for your baby are similar. The main risks for the baby—apart from the increased risk of abnormalities—are macrosomia (growing too large) and stillbirth. The main risks for you are hyperglycemia (sugar going too high) and hypoglycemia (sugar going too low), which is common if you're suffering morning sickness. You're also at increased risk of pre-eclampsia. Because of the risk of stillbirth, many obstetricians

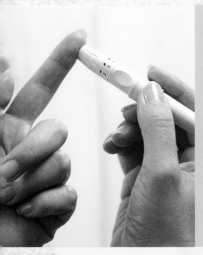

A home testing kit can be used to measure your glucose levels. A drop of blood is drawn from your finger, using a small lancing device (left). The blood drop is applied to the target area of the electrode and the monitor displays your glucose result (bottom).

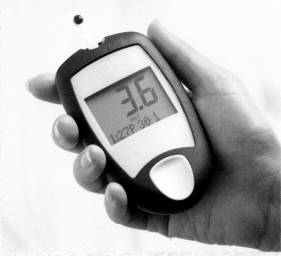

insulin you need increases every week as the placenta grows, up until about 34 weeks.

It's important to follow a healthy, balanced, stable diet to help you predict how much insulin you will need. Don't worry if you need to increase your dose of insulin, it doesn't mean that you're eating too much.

Kidney failure

Many women have problems with their kidneys. Most are relatively minor problems such as urinary infections and cystitis (see page 259), but more serious problems such as kidney failure can occur. If you have kidney failure, the way it affects your pregnancy will largely depend on the severity of your condition.

Management

Women with kidney failure should discuss the implications of pregnancy with their renal physician and a maternal-fetal medicine specialist. The chance of a successful pregnancy depends on how well your kidneys are working. If you have had a transplant and your new kidney is working well then you have an excellent chance of having a healthy baby. Most drugs used to prevent rejection are safe for use in pregnancy; your healthcare provider should be able to advise you about any medication you are taking.

If you're awaiting transplant and you're on dialysis the results aren't as good. Many women on dialysis don't even manage to get pregnant, and those who do have difficult pregnancies, with most babies born very premature. Women with moderate kidney damage are at risk of pre-eclampsia and should discuss these risks with their healthcare provider to try to minimize the risks associated with this condition.

Thyroid disease

The thyroid gland can be overactive or underactive—both extremes are bad for your health and may affect your pregnancy. If your thyroid isn't working properly you are likely to be on medication to regain the balance. Although

will recommend delivery by 38 weeks and will suggest that if you haven't delivered by then you should be induced.

Management

It's vital that you control your sugar levels prior to and in the first few months after conception, as this will decrease the chance of your baby developing an abnormality. Once you're pregnant your tablets will be switched to insulin injections. The aim during pregnancy is to control your sugar levels as tightly as possible, achieving a 3 hour post-meal sugar level of less than 120mg/dL. Increasing the number of daily injections from two to four often achieves this. The amount of

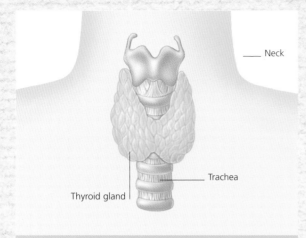

Neck

Trachea

Thyroid gland

The thyroid gland is situated in the neck, and is responsible for the production of a hormone called thyroxin, which regulates your metabolism.

this shouldn't affect your pregnancy, your healthcare provider will monitor you closely until after your postpartum check.

Management
Hypothyroidism (an underactive thyroid) can be easily treated with replacement thyroxine. You should have your levels checked every three months during the pregnancy, but you're unlikely to need to have your dose changed.

If you have hyperthyroidism (an overactive thyroid) you may need treatment with carbimazole or propylthiouracil. Both these drugs control the activity of the thyroid. If you're first diagnosed in pregnancy you may need a large dose to start with, but this is usually reduced after a few months. Both drugs cross the placenta, and in rare cases cause the baby to have a swollen thyroid gland and to become hypothyroid. Using the lowest effective dose reduces this risk.

If you have thyroid disease it's important to have your levels checked six weeks after delivery as your thyroid can become inflamed at this stage—a condition known as postpartum thyroiditis—and your medication may need altering.

Cancer
There is no indication that pregnancy directly affects the course of cancer, but it does add a complication, as the treatment you need may not be good for your baby. If the cancer is discovered after you are already pregnant you may have to consider whether to continue with the pregnancy. This will depend on the type of cancer, how advanced it is, and the effects the best treatment will have on you and your baby.

Management
During pregnancy your healthcare providers will need to find a balance between the treatment that's best for you and the safety of your baby. Chemotherapy during the first trimester increases the risk of birth defects. During the second and third trimesters, chemotherapy may lower your baby's birth weight, but the degree of risk for other complications varies depending on the medication used. Radiation therapy may or may not affect your baby, depending on the location of the cancer, the strength of the exposure and how advanced your pregnancy is. The most vulnerable period for your baby is between 8 and 15 weeks. Surgery is usually possible during pregnancy and does not often cause a risk to your baby. However, if inflammation or infection occur in the abdomen, this increases the risk of preterm labor.

MEDICAL EMERGENCIES

Most pregnancies are straightforward and proceed without any problems. Just occasionally, complications do occur that could put the mother and baby at risk. Fortunately most of these, if detected early enough, can be successfully treated. If you don't feel well or something doesn't seem quite right, don't hesitate to call your healthcare provider for advice.

SYMPTOMS YOU SHOULDN'T IGNORE
Abdominal pain

The odd ache and mild transient discomfort is to be expected during pregnancy, but any persistent abdominal pain that causes discomfort or seems in any way out of the ordinary needs to be urgently evaluated by medical staff.

Sharp lower abdominal pains just to one side or both sides of the uterus, may just be stretching of the ligaments (round ligament pain) but could signal ectopic pregnancy, miscarriage, placental abruption, or preterm labor. Constant abdominal pain associated with hardening or tense feelings in the uterus is of particular concern and needs urgent treatment.

The first sign of an ectopic pregnancy is often lower abdominal pain, cramping or a dull ache, which may just be one-sided or all around the abdomen. Shoulder pain and pain around the rectum, particularly on opening the bowels, often feature as well. Vaginal bleeding is common but normally it's not very heavy. Urgent hospital treatment is needed, because the internal bleeding can be very dangerous.

Upper abdominal pain in the area of the liver (on the right side, just below the rib cage) could be a sign of serious pre-eclampsia and needs immediate medical assessment. It can also be a sign of gallstones or indigestion, which are obviously much less serious. However, this type of pain should never be ignored.

Groin pain or lower backache can be the sign of a kidney infection and needs to be treated urgently with strong antibiotics. A high fever or chill may accompany the pain, which indicates that treatment in hospital with intravenous antibiotics is needed.

A pulmonary embolus—blood clot on the lung—(shown in an X-ray above) is a serious condition that needs urgent medical treatment.

Chest pain

A pain in the chest should never be ignored. It could indicate a pulmonary embolus (a blood clot in the lung) or pleurisy. Both conditions need urgent treatment.

Chills and fever

If you have a fever over 100°F (37.8°C) without other symptoms you should call the doctor the same day. If your fever is over 102°F (38.9°C), you need immediate treatment, as you may have an infection that requires antibiotics and rest. If the fever remains high for a prolonged length of time, the baby's development could be hindered.

Excessive lower leg puffiness (edema) or excessive weight gain
These symptoms shouldn't be overlooked as they can be associated with pre-eclampsia.

Excessive vomiting and/or diarrhea
Contact your doctor if you keep being sick or have diarrhea. There's a risk of dehydration if you can't keep anything down, while excessive diarrhea depletes you of body fluids, which is dangerous. You may need to go to the hospital and have an IV to replace lost fluids. If the vomiting is accompanied by fever, or the diarrhea contains blood or mucus, call your doctor immediately.

Fall or car accident
As a rule, falls aren't always harmful, as the baby is well protected inside the uterus, surrounded by amniotic fluid, but if you do fall over, call your healthcare provider as soon as you can and explain what happened. If you experience contractions, leaking fluid, or any bleeding, call your healthcare provider right away.

Headaches, flashing lights in front of the eyes, or double vision
These are all indications of pre-eclampsia and dangerously high blood pressure and require urgent hospital treatment.

Itching all over
This may be a sign of obstetric cholestasis especially if there is jaundice (yellow skin and dark urine). There's no danger to the mother, but there is an increased risk to the baby. For this reason, doctors advise close monitoring of the baby if cholestasis is diagnosed, and normally an early delivery is recommended.

Leaking of fluid from the vagina
This should be reported immediately, because this could be a leakage of amniotic fluid and indicate that the membranes have ruptured. This could be a sign of premature labor and leaves the baby exposed to infection.

Painful or burning urination, accompanied by fever, chills, and backache
You may have a urinary tract infection, a condition that should be treated with antibiotics.

Seizures
A seizure as a result of high blood pressure is a medical emergency and requires oxygen and drugs to prevent any further seizures occurring. Call the emergency services without delay as urgent delivery of the baby is usually required to enable proper treatment of the mother.

Swollen or painful leg
A painfully swollen leg that's warm to the touch may be a deep vein thrombosis (DVT). Call your healthcare provider immediately if you suspect you may have this condition (see page 252). It can be confused with the common and harmless condition of superficial thrombophlebitis—that affects the small surface veins in the lower legs which become rather red and sore in pregnancy, especially if you are overweight. Ultrasound will distinguish between the two conditions.

Slowing or absence of fetal movements
Feeling the baby move usually occurs at around 16 to 20 weeks of pregnancy. After 28 weeks you should be aware of at least ten movements every day. If your baby seems to have been less active over the last 24 hours, or there have been fewer than ten movements over a period of 12 hours during the day, call your doctor and go straight to the hospital for evaluation. Your baby's heartbeat will be recorded for 20 to 30 minutes on a fetal monitor to ensure that all is well. Reduced fetal movements can be a sign that the baby is under stress, so should never be ignored. On the other

hand, the vast majority of babies start to move vigorously as soon as fetal monitoring begins, and there is nothing wrong.

Thirst and infrequent urination

If you experience a sudden increase in thirst accompanied by little or no urination, this could be a sign of dehydration or gestational diabetes, a potentially dangerous condition for both mother and baby. Contact your doctor, who will then arrange for you to be evaluated.

Vaginal bleeding

A small amount of painless vaginal bleeding in the early weeks of pregnancy is common (see page 20). However, if the bleeding is heavy, it's best to call your doctor so it can be evaluated. Any bleeding associated with pain could indicate a miscarriage or ectopic pregnancy so you should contact your doctor urgently. Very heavy vaginal bleeding or bleeding associated with severe pain needs immediate attention, and you should go straight to the ER.

ECTOPIC PREGNANCY

This is a serious condition that occurs when a pregnancy develops outside the uterus, normally in a fallopian tube. It can mimic a miscarriage, because the symptoms and signs can be very similar, in that abdominal pain and vaginal bleeding occur. Normally any vaginal bleeding is light, but the abdominal pain is often more severe and may also involve shoulder pain or rectal pain.

Pain in early pregnancy should always be investigated by ultrasound to exclude an ectopic pregnancy. Blood tests are often required to monitor the levels of human chorionic gonadotropin (HCG) in the blood before this type of pregnancy can be diagnosed. Treatment is usually by laparoscopy (key-hole surgery), although a drug called Methotrexate is now being used to treat some ectopic pregnancies in a number of hospitals.

MOLAR PREGNANCY

Also called a hydatidiform mole, this is a rare type of pregnancy complication affecting around 1 in 2000 pregnancies. The cells in pregnancy called trophoblasts, which normally form the placenta, grow out of control and stop the fertilized egg from developing normally. The uterus becomes full of very abnormal tissue, which produces high levels of HCG hormone. The diagnosis can be confirmed by an ultrasound examination. Symptoms include a brownish discharge, severe morning sickness, an unusually large uterus, and absence of a fetal heartbeat.

Once the diagnosis is made, a dilation and curettage (D & C) will be carried out to remove abnormal tissue from the uterus, as in rare cases it can spread to other parts of the body. Close monitoring of HCG hormone levels will be necessary for several months to ensure that all the tissue has gone away. Attempts to conceive again should be delayed for a year until all traces of the pregnancy hormone have disappeared.

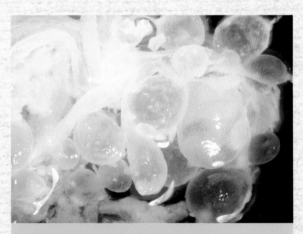

A hydatidiform mole is formed when the tissue surrounding the embryo degenerates, forming a collection of fluid-filled sacs (above).

BLEEDING IN PREGNANCY

Approximately one in four women will experience vaginal bleeding during their pregnancies. The bleeding can vary from spotting or staining to a substantial blood loss that requires urgent hospital treatment. While it's important to treat any bleeding in pregnancy seriously, remember that in at least 50 percent of cases no harm is going to come to the pregnancy.

EARLY BLEEDING (BEFORE 12 WEEKS)

Bleeding or spotting in the first few weeks of pregnancy is particularly common but doesn't necessarily mean that there's a problem. A good indicator is the amount of pain associated with the bleeding. Painless vaginal bleeding is much less of a concern than bleeding that is associated with cramping lower abdominal pain and/or backache over several hours. If you have vaginal bleeding, your healthcare provider will carry out various investigations. You may have a pelvic exam, an ultrasound, or a blood test in order to measure levels of the pregnancy hormone human chorionic gonadotropin (HCG). As the pregnancy progresses, HCG levels increase, so you may have to have more than one test. Often no cause for the bleeding can be found and the pregnancy continues without any problems. A small number of women go on to experience slight bleeding on and off throughout their pregnancies for no obvious reason.

Any woman who has a rhesus negative blood group should receive anti-D immunoglobulin in the event of bleeding, to protect against forming antibodies against the fetal blood.

Implantation bleed

Occasionally a small amount of vaginal bleeding occurs for 24 to 48 hours as the fertilized egg implants itself into the wall of the uterus around ten days after conception. This is a natural process and is of no concern.

Hormonal bleeding

Some women experience a light period-like bleed, at around 4 and 8 weeks of pregnancy, thought to

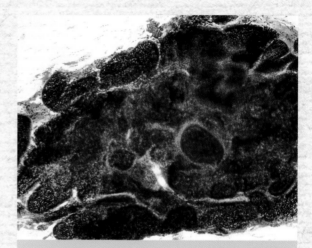

Cervical erosion occurs when a layer of cells normally found on the inner lining of the cervix appear on the outside. Above can be seen an abnormal growth of cells caused by cervical erosion.

be related to implantation. Occurring just at the times that their periods are expected, this is why some women don't realize that they are pregnant.

Cervical erosion

Spotting during early pregnancy may be caused by a cervical erosion, which occurs when the cells on the inner lining of the cervix extend onto its surface and become inflamed. Bleeding can occur after sexual intercourse because the cervix is softer and more delicate during pregnancy. Unless an infection is suspected, a cervical erosion won't affect your pregnancy.

LATER BLEEDING

Vaginal bleeding in pregnancy between 12 to 24 weeks is much less common than in the first three months. Miscarriage at this stage in pregnancy is considerably less likely. Later miscarriages—after 20 weeks—may be a result of an infection or an abnormality in the uterus, such as an incompetent cervix (see page 279), or in the placenta.

Bleeding after 24 weeks of pregnancy should always be reported to your healthcare provider. Often there's no cause for concern if the bleeding is light, particularly if it has occurred after sexual intercourse or an internal examination. However, admission to the hospital for observation for 24 hours is normal if a woman reports vaginal bleeding, especially if any pain is associated with the bleeding. The following conditions should be investigated if bleeding occurs later in pregnancy:

Marginal placental bleed

Painless bleeding can occur as a result of a rupture in one of the small blood vessels at the edge of the placenta. Usually the bleeding settles quickly, although a small blood clot can form near the cervix and lead to a brownish vaginal loss for a few days afterward. Sometimes it can be painful, as the blood irritates the uterus and causes mild contractions. There is no undue cause for concern, and rest and observation are usually prescribed.

Placenta previa

When the placenta lies low in the uterus, it can partly or completely cover the cervix. Many women are told that they have placenta previa (a low-lying placenta) when they attend for a routine 20-week scan, but during the last few weeks of pregnancy the placenta tends to move up so that it no longer blocks the cervix. However, in one percent of pregnancies, the placenta remains covering the cervix. In this position the placenta is less well attached to the uterine wall and is more likely to bleed from one or more of the huge number of blood vessels that cross the placental surface. Fortunately, although it can be heavy, the bleeding often stops of its own accord. If this

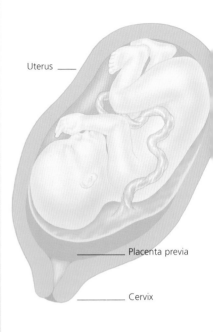

In placenta previa, the placenta lies low in the uterus and may partially, or completely, cover the cervix (see above). There is a risk to both the mother and baby from excessive bleeding.

Uterus

Placenta previa

Cervix

happens to you, you'll be advised to rest in bed until the baby is born so that you can be treated quickly should you bleed heavily again.

Placenta previa happens more to women who have had more than one child, who have had a cesarean, or who are carrying twins or triplets. Bleeding is usually painless but can be extremely heavy. It may start lightly enough as an early warning but suddenly become very heavy, requiring emergency treatment for the mother, including a blood transfusion.

Placental accreta

A very rare complication of pregnancy, where the placenta grows into the deeper layers of the uterine wall and becomes firmly attached. There are three variants of this condition—the most common is accreta, where the placenta becomes directly attached to the uterine wall. Occasionally the placenta extends deeper into the uterine muscle—this is known as placental increta. In the third, very rare variant, the placenta extends through the entire wall of the uterus—this is known as percreta.

Placental accreta most commonly occurs in women who have had a cesarean or have scarring from uterine surgery or placenta previa.

Often there are no symptoms until the third stage of labor, when the placenta doesn't separate from the uterine wall. Rarely, the condition causes rupture or partial rupture of the uterus. Treatment involves surgical removal of the placenta. Very rarely, if the bleeding cannot be controlled, a hysterectomy is required.

Placental abruption

This is when the placenta separates or shears away from the wall of the uterus. Usually the bleeding is associated with severe abdominal cramps but not always if the placenta only separates a small amount. The amount of bleeding experienced is variable but can be heavy with clots.

A particularly dangerous form of abruption is called a concealed abruption. This rare condition occurs when the placenta separates in the middle portion, causing a large blood clot to build up between the placental surface and the wall of the uterus. Usually the mother experiences severe pain and feels very faint. No bleeding is seen because all the blood loss is captured behind the back of the placenta. Urgent medical treatment is essential and immediate delivery of the baby is necessary.

Uterine rupture

Very occasionally a rupture or tear occurs in the uterus during pregnancy. Sometimes, the uterus may rupture during labor. Usually the cause of the rupture is a weakness in the uterine wall caused by a scar from a previous cesarean or a repaired uterine rupture. Abnormalities of the placenta, such as placenta previa, or placental accreta, can also increase the risk of uterine rupture. Being induced during a VBAC labor also greatly increases the risk of rupture.

The first sign of a rupture is usually a searing pain in the abdomen, accompanied by a feeling of something "tearing" inside, and some vaginal bleeding. If the rupture occurs during labor, contractions will probably slow down or cease.

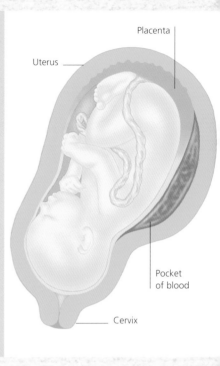

Separation of the placenta from the uterus, known as placental abruption, can lead to a pocket of blood forming between the placenta and uterus, which requires urgent medical treatment.

Placenta

Uterus

Pocket of blood

Cervix

When a rupture occurs, an immediate cesarean delivery is required, followed by surgical repair of the uterus. Rarely a hysterectomy is necessary.

After a rupture you will be closely monitored and antibiotics will be given to prevent infection.

MISCARRIAGE

Sometimes a pregnancy ends in miscarriage. There are a lot of reasons why this may happen—in the early weeks it is often the body's way of rejecting a fetus that could never develop healthily. Occasionally it is caused by a problem that occurs during pregnancy, or because of a preexisting medical condition. Recurrent miscarriages need to be investigated, as treatment may be required.

Loss of a baby before the baby is able to survive outside the uterus is known as a miscarriage. The most likely time for a miscarriage to occur is before 12 weeks, when doctors tend to refer to the miscarriage as being an "early or first trimester" miscarriage. Early miscarriage is very common, affecting about one in five pregnancies. The figure is probably even higher than this because a woman may not even be aware that she's pregnant before she miscarries with what seems like an extra-heavy period. If you smoke, are an older mother, have had previous miscarriages, or have fibroids, lupus, or diabetes, you face an increased risk of miscarriage.

At least half of all miscarriages in the first trimester are caused by chromosomal abnormalities that prevent the fetus from developing into a healthy baby. Infections, uncontrolled diabetes, thyroid problems, uterine abnormalities, or a woman's production of certain antibodies also can cause an early miscarriage.

Vaginal bleeding, accompanied by lower backache or cramping abdominal pains, similar to period cramps, which may be constant or occur intermittently, may be a sign of a threatened miscarriage. Despite these symptoms it's still possible that the pregnancy isn't going to miscarry.

But, once the uterus starts to expel the pregnancy then it's inevitable that a miscarriage will follow. The cervix opens and pieces of liver-like tissue are passed. In this case, vaginal bleeding and pain may be quite severe.

Ultrasound is the most common way to establish whether a pregnancy is continuing normally. A pelvic exam is helpful because a closed cervix indicates the pregnancy may be all right.

A complete miscarriage

When the uterus has expelled the pregnancy entirely, a miscarriage is complete. The bleeding and pain subside and an ultrasound scan will show that the uterus is completely empty.

Incomplete miscarriage

When the uterus doesn't completely expel all of the pregnancy and pieces of tissue are retained a miscarriage is described as incomplete. It's usually obvious on ultrasound, but doctors may make the diagnosis if bleeding is very heavy or if tissue can be seen in the cervix on examination.

At this stage you'll probably be offered a minor procedure under anethetic to clean out the uterus known as a dilation and curettage (D & C). This may involve dilating (widening) the cervix and scraping tissue away from the endometrium (the lining of the uterus).

Alternatively, the tissue may be left to expel itself naturally over the next few days as long as you're not bleeding too heavily and you're well enough to cope with this.

Missed miscarriage or blighted ovum

Occasionally a miscarriage occurs without any symptoms, or with very minor signs such as a small amount of brownish vaginal discharge. This type of miscarriage is usually detected by ultrasound, because an empty sac can be seen inside the uterus, meaning that the fetus has never formed—this is called a blighted ovum. To be absolutely sure, your doctor may wish to re-scan you in seven to ten days to check that a baby is not going to develop in the sac. Occasionally a fetus can be seen inside the sac but the heart has

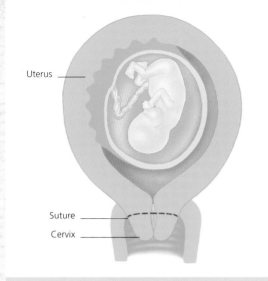

Uterus

Suture

Cervix

If cervical incompetence has been diagnosed a cerclage, (see above) may be inserted to reinforce the cervical muscle. Cerclage is most successful if it is performed early in pregnancy.

stopped beating, indicating that the fetus has clearly died at a very early stage. You will then be offered a D & C to remove the remains of the pregnancy, or you may be given the option of waiting to see if your body will naturally expel the pregnancy over the next few days.

INCOMPETENT CERVIX

Believed to be responsible for 20 to 25 percent of all second trimester miscarriages, an incompetent cervix is one that opens under pressure of the growing uterus and baby. It can be caused by a genetic weakness of the cervix; extreme stretching of or severe lacerations to the cervix during one or more previous deliveries; a cone biopsy for cervical cancer; or cervical surgery or laser therapy. It is usually diagnosed when a woman has previously miscarried in the second trimester or when ultrasound or a vaginal exam shows the cervix shortening and opening during pregnancy.

If the condition is known, or is identified during pregnancy, a procedure known as cerclage will be carried out—the opening of the cervix is stitched or sutured to keep it closed. The procedure is performed through the vagina under local anesthetic or epidural at around 12 to 16 weeks of pregnancy. The stitches or sutures are usually removed a few weeks before the estimated date of delivery; in some cases they remain in place until labor has begun. With cerclage the chances of carrying a baby to term are excellent.

COPING WITH MISCARRIAGE

It can feel devastating to lose a much-longed-for pregnancy. To grieve is natural, as is feeling sad and depressed. Often hospitals treat the situation as routine, which can be very distressing.

It can be hard to accept that miscarriage is very common and that it is usually nature's way of dealing with pregnancies where defects have arisen in the very early stages of the baby's development. Never feel guilty that somehow you were to blame; this is a natural

process and not a situation that you have caused. The happy fact is that next time you have an excellent chance of a successful pregnancy.

Remember to continue taking folic acid and keep up a well-balanced nutritious diet. There is no reason to wait before conceiving again, although many couples do take a rest before trying for their next pregnancy.

A small number of women experience repeated miscarriages. If you've had three or more

miscarriages in a row, ask your healthcare provider to arrange for you to be referred for some extra tests. Some women carry antibodies in their blood that prevent a pregnancy from implanting properly, and treatment can be given in early pregnancy to help.

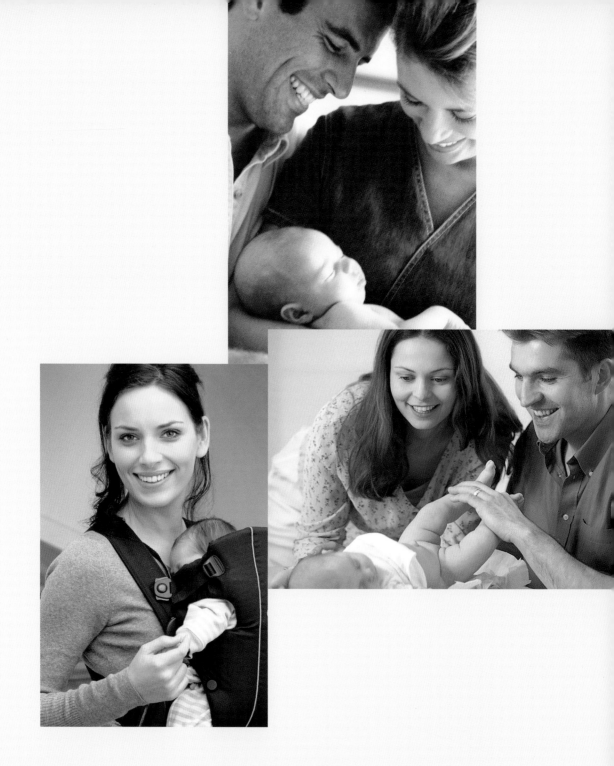

PART IV   NOW YOU'RE A FAMILY

YOUR MARVELOUS NEWBORN

After all the months of waiting, your baby is finally

here, and that moment when you hold her for the

very first time is certain to exceed any expectations

you might have had. You'll very soon get to know

her, what she looks like, and what she can do—and

understand what she needs to thrive.

WHAT YOUR BABY LOOKS LIKE

Throughout your pregnancy, you're bound to have wondered what your baby will look like. Will she have a lot of hair and what color will it be? Will she be long and lean or petite and plump? Will she look like you? Well, now you can check her out from head to toe.

As you hold your beautiful baby and begin to examine her every inch, she might not look quite like the little cherub you imagined. Exactly how your newborn will look depends on how she was positioned in your uterus, her genetic make up, and what sort of delivery she had. Cesarean babies, for

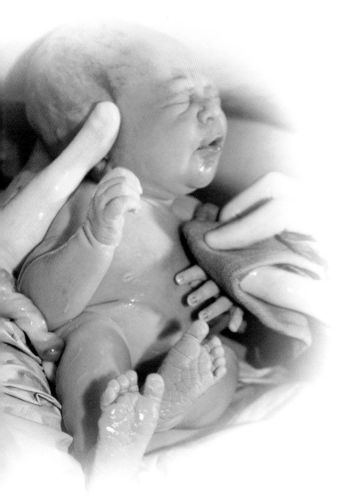

example, who haven't had to squeeze down the birth canal, may have more normal-shaped skulls and less squashed faces than babies who have had a vaginal birth. It's not unusual for a mother to feel a little let-down by her baby's appearance immediately after the birth, and, if you do, don't worry. In a very short time, all those newborn features will fade, and she'll look as beautiful as you could wish. In the meantime, here are some of things you may notice about your baby.

TYPICAL NEWBORN CHARACTERISTICS
All newborns share certain features that can be a surprise to some parents. Make sure you take the opportunity to ask your healthcare providers any questions you have about your baby's appearance. Draw on their professional knowledge, too, to acquire the skills to take care of her basic needs.

An elongated, swollen, and bruised head
Your baby's skull bones are soft at birth to allow her head to pass through the birth canal. As she's squeezed and pushed out into the world, her head bones are molded, which can leave her head with a conical, pointed shape. Even some babies who are delivered by cesarean section have a degree of head molding, because they have spent the last few weeks upside down, wedged tight in their mother's uterus. Either way, the molding doesn't last long and you'll notice that your baby's head starts to become rounder within a few days.

Your baby may have a blister-like swelling on her head known as a caput. This can be caused by her head pressing against the dilating cervix during contractions or by the suction of a vacuum delivery (see page 229). This harmless swelling should disappear in a matter of days. Also, your baby's head may look bruised, especially if she was delivered by forceps or had a fetal scalp electrode (see page 217) attached during labor. This bruising generally gets better within a week or so.

Fontanels

You also may notice a soft, pulsating spot on the top of your baby's head. This is called the anterior fontanel, and is one of six your baby has on her head altogether. They're simply gaps where the bones of your baby's skull haven't yet fused, and they are there to allow her head to grow quickly during her first year. They act also as a cushion, protecting her head from injury. By the time your baby is about 2 years old, the fontanels will have closed.

Although these soft fontanels look like they're very vulnerable, they're actually covered by tough, fibrous tissue, so you won't hurt your baby if you touch the area gently. You can comb the hair over the soft spot without any problem.

A squashed face

Looking straight at your baby's face, you may notice that her nose looks a little flattened, maybe even pushed to the side. Your baby's eyes may look bloodshot and her eyelids puffy. She may even have some trouble opening up one eye or the other at first. Again, these are caused by your baby's position in the uterus and the tight trip down the birth canal. All these effects should improve quickly over a day or two. If your baby is reluctant to open her eyes at first, don't try to force them open. If you like, you can encourage your baby to open her eyes naturally simply by lifting her above you with her head higher than yours.

While you look at her eyes, notice the color. Many babies are born with dark blue eyes, because melanin, the body's natural pigment, is not present in the irises at birth. The color of babies' eyes often alters as the pigmentation increases, and any changes are usually complete by 12 months of age.

Some babies are born with a common condition called "sticky eye." If your baby has this, you'll probably notice it as a yellow discharge around the eyelids (see page 365). Although this isn't serious, it should be treated by a doctor.

Vernix and hair

At birth, most babies are covered with blood and mucus, as well as a protective layer of thick, white grease, called vernix. This develops during the last trimester of pregnancy and protects a baby's skin from becoming waterlogged. Babies born prematurely have a lot of vernix on their skin, while overdue babies have virtually none at all. In some hospitals the vernix is washed off, while in others it's left to wear off naturally, usually within a few days.

Many babies—and particularly those who are born a bit early—have a layer of fine, downy hair over their skin called lanugo. Nobody knows for sure why lanugo is there, but it's thought that it might help keep the vernix in place and regulate your baby's body temperature. Most of this hair will fall out by itself during the first few months.

Your baby may have been born with a thick head of hair or almost no hair at all. If she has hair, it will mostly be replaced by new growth over the next few months, and her hair color and texture may change quite a lot from what you see at birth.

DID YOU KNOW...

Most estimates of birth weight are inaccurate
Ultrasound scans can be a couple of pounds off and manual palpation is unreliable. But researchers in California have now come up with an equation that predicts birth weight more accurately, using factors like the baby's sex, the parents' height, and weight gain in the third trimester. Even altitude was taken into account—people who live up mountains have, on average, smaller babies. This development allows women expecting large babies to plan an early induction or cesarean.

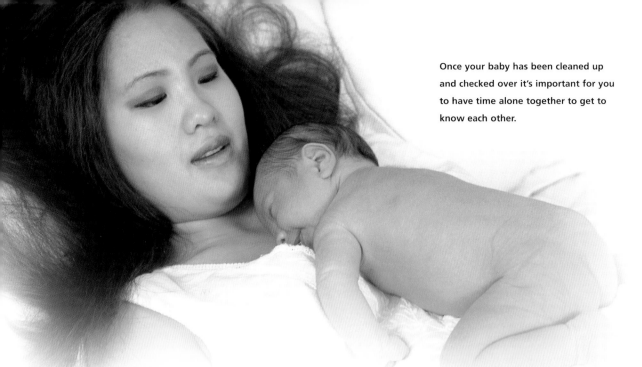

Once your baby has been cleaned up and checked over it's important for you to have time alone together to get to know each other.

Blue hands and feet and long nails

Your newborn's hands and feet may have a bluish tinge during the first few days. This phenomenon, known as acrocyanosis and caused by poor circulation, is normal and will improve as she gets older. The rest of her body should be nice and pink.

Your baby's fingernails may be long, especially if she was born late, but they are very delicate, and it's best not to cut them at this stage. You can file them gently or your healthcare provider may put scratch mitts on your baby's hands if it's thought that she might scratch herself.

Swollen breasts

You may notice that your baby's breasts are slightly swollen. In some newborns it's even possible to see a milky white discharge. This is perfectly normal in both boys and girls. Both the swelling and the discharge are caused by pregnancy hormones remaining in your baby's body. The swelling and discharge will disappear in a few days.

Swollen genitals

If your baby is a boy, you may notice that his scrotum (the sack that surrounds his testicles) is somewhat swollen. This swelling, known as a hydrocele, is caused by fluid surrounding the testicles and usually goes down within a few months. If it doesn't, then speak to your healthcare provider, as surgery may be required. Also, some baby boys are born with a condition known as undescended testicles, which means that their testicles have not yet moved outside the body. If your baby has this condition, your healthcare provider will keep a check on it (see page 378).

If your baby is a girl, she may have slightly swollen genitals and a white vaginal discharge. When she is between a few days and a couple of weeks old she also may have a very small amount of vaginal bleeding. Both the discharge and the bleeding are caused by pregnancy hormones remaining in her body and will cease as the hormone levels drop.

The umbilical cord

Shortly after the birth, the umbilical cord is clamped and then cut (see page 225). However, a small stump will remain, which will have a clamp on it to prevent bleeding. Within a few hours, the cord will dry out and go from being soft and spongy to dry and black. The cord will fall off by itself, usually within one to two weeks. Before this you should treat the cord gently, particularly when washing your baby (see page 312).

Dry skin and spots

Once your baby has had her first bath, her skin may appear dry and cracked. This is a result of the time that she's spent immersed in liquid. Dry skin is often more noticeable in babies born a bit after their due dates, because all the vernix will have worn off, leaving the skin unprotected. Any dry patches should get better within a few weeks. In the meantime, it's fine to apply a very mild moisturizer to any dry patches on her arms and legs. Make sure this doesn't contain any added perfumes, as these might irritate her delicate skin.

During the first few days, your baby is likely to have a rash or two. There are several common rashes among newborns, for example:

◆ *Erythema toxicum* This consists of red, blotchy spots with white heads in the middle and appears mostly on a baby's trunk. Its causes are unknown.

◆ *Milia* Also known as "milk rash," this appears as whitish-yellow dots on a baby's face, especially on the nose, and, less commonly, on the roof of her mouth. This is caused by enlarged oily glands in your baby's skin.

◆ *Pustular melanosis* This usually starts as small, white dots that then break and become scaly, brown rings. Its causes are unknown.

All of these rashes are harmless and will disappear by themselves during the first couple of weeks. However, always get a rash checked by your baby's healthcare provider. Very occasionally, rashes are an early sign of infection that will require medical treatment (see page 364).

Identifying your baby's birthmarks

These are very common and are usually harmless. But your baby's healthcare provider may want to check them as your baby grows.

Stork bites These collections of dilated blood vessels appear as a red mark on the back of a baby's neck. Stork bites may not go away but are soon covered by hair.

Salmon patches These are similar to stork bites but appear on the forehead **1**, over the eyelids, or under the nose. Unlike stork bites, salmon patches fade with time.

Strawberry marks These raised, red marks **2** are collections of blood capillaries. They may grow during the first year, but almost all fade by the age of 9 if left untreated.

Mongolian spots These are common on dark-skinned babies and appear as bruise-like, flat, bluish-gray patches around a baby's bottom **3**, shoulders, back, and arms. They are caused by clusters of pigment cells in the skin and usually fade within a year.

Port wine stains These red or purple marks, usually on the face, head, or neck, are rare. They don't fade but may be treatable with plastic surgery.

Café-au-lait patches Small, flat, brown or coffee-colored oval patches are very common. They are usually permanent.

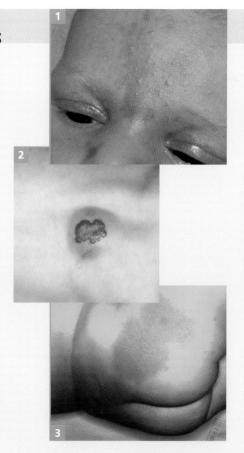

YOUR BABY'S POSTPARTUM CARE

After you and your baby have spent some time getting to know each other, your baby will probably be taken to the nursery for a bath, a pediatric exam, and some routine procedures. If you have the birth at home these will be carried out by your healthcare provider.

Following a vaginal birth in hospital, most women stay in hospital for a couple of days; after a cesarean section, the stay is usually at least three to four days. If both you and your baby are doing well and you are keen to get back to the comfort of your own home, you may ask for an early discharge. In this case, you may need to arrange for a nurse to visit you at home—in some areas you automatically get a visit—or plan a visit to the doctor after a few days.

If you stay in hospital to recover, you may have your baby in the room with you or your baby may stay in the hospital nursery. Having your baby room in with you is a great opportunity to get to know your baby and his needs. However, if he stays in the nursery it can give you time to rest and recover. If you have the option, you may prefer to do a mixture of both: Have your baby with you during the day but not at night; or spend your first night alone and then have your baby with you after that.

Medical attention for your baby

Your baby will receive a considerable amount of medical care immediately after his birth and during his first few days to make sure that all is well.

A full physical exam At 1 and 5 minute intervals after the birth, hospital staff will perform the Apgar test (see box, opposite). Then, at some stage during the first few days, your baby's features, spine, anus, fingers, and toes will be checked, he'll be weighed, and his head and length may be measured **1**. His hips will be checked for proper movement and placement **2**.

Eye ointment Just after birth, your baby will be given antibiotic eye ointment to help prevent infections.

Vitamin K shot At many hospitals, babies receive an injection or drops of Vitamin K shortly after birth. This is because newborns often have low levels of this vitamin, which is necessary for the process of normal blood clotting.

Heel stick After the first 24 hours, your baby may have a blood sample taken from his heel. This blood can be used to check the baby's thyroid function, as well as test for a rare metabolic disorder called phenylketonuria. If there is a family history of any conditions, a test may be done for it. The tests offered vary among healthcare providers and hospitals, so it's important to discuss which ones your baby is being given.

Hepatitis B shot Before you're discharged from hospital, your baby may receive the hepatitis B vaccine to prevent an infection of the liver,

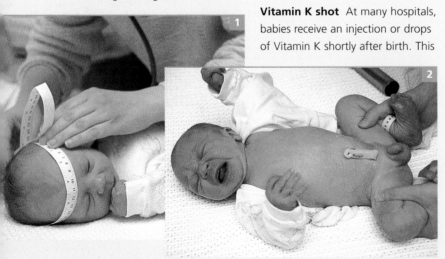

Learning to care for your baby

If you haven't already attended parenting classes (see page 172), your hospital stay can be a useful time to learn how to take care of your baby with the help and support of expert staff. They will be able to show you how to change a diaper, give him a bath, and take care of the cord, as well as answering any queries you have about feeding. Many hospitals organize short classes, in which you can learn about caring for your baby. These classes also give you the chance to meet other new parents going through exactly the same experience as you. This should help you be as relaxed as possible about looking after your baby on your own. Of course, worries and concerns may crop up once you're home, but your baby's healthcare provider will be happy to speak with you or see the baby, if necessary. For information about what you'll need on the journey home, see page 206.

If you're not having your baby in a hospital, speak to your healthcare provider to find out about classes you can attend in your area.

although not all hospitals do this. If given, the course will be completed in three doses by the time your baby's a year old.

Bodily functions After your baby's birth it's a good idea to keep track of how much and how often he is feeding, as well as noting the frequency and appearance of his stools and urine.

Weight Your baby will probably be weighed regularly in his first few days. Don't be alarmed if his weight drops at first; it's normal for babies to lose up to 10 percent of their birth weight in the first few days. He should begin to gain by the time he's 1 week old.

MORE **ABOUT** | the Apgar score

This test was developed by Dr. Virginia Apgar to allow a quick assessment of a newborn's health. The word "Apgar" stands also for the signs that the doctors and nurses are looking at. For each of these, your baby will be given a score of 0, 1, or 2. Babies rarely receive a total score of 10, but a score above 6 is usually fine. If your baby receives a low score, don't worry—it simply means he needs some temporary medical help and close monitoring. It's not an indicator of his future health.

SIGN	POINTS		
	0	1	2
Appearance	Pale or blue	Body pink, extremities blue	Pink
Pulse	Not detectable	Below 100	Over 100
Grimace (reflexes)	No response to stimulation	Grimace	Lusty cry, cough, or sneeze
Activity (muscle tone)	Flaccid (no or weak activity)	Some movement of extremities	A lot of activity
Respiration	None	Slow, irregular	Good, crying

WHAT YOUR BABY CAN DO

Your baby might seem helpless at birth, but, in fact, she has capabilities and a personality. Over the following weeks and months, she'll be adding to her store of knowledge very rapidly, as this is what she is programmed to do.

From the moment your baby is born, her senses are flooded with information, activating her brain into a surge of development. Neurons (nerve cells) start to work overtime, creating thousands of connections with other cells. The brain's structure is stimulated and physically changed by the types of messages it receives. If your baby's brain doesn't receive enough information, development in one area may be arrested or impaired—for example, if a squint is left uncorrected for too long, the brain will learn to look through one eye, and that habit can't be corrected, even with glasses. On the other hand, if you talk, sing, and play with your baby from very early on, you will be actively encouraging the neural pathways to form.

You can't get your baby to do something before the appropriate brain pathways have been established, but she will get there in her own time and at her own developmental rate. In fact, your baby's brain will more than double in size during the first year after birth, and to maintain this tremendous growth, her brain will use 60 percent of the energy she gets from food. But, because this process takes some time, your baby will already have some bodily functions in place and certain reflexes that help her survive (see below).

BREATHE, FEED, AND DIGEST
Perhaps the most miraculous skill your baby acquires is the art of breathing independently. While she was in the uterus, her lungs weren't needed, as the placenta provided her with oxygen from her mother's blood. The moment she's born, she has to switch to using her lungs to obtain vital oxygen for life. As she takes a breath, contact with the outside air results in the lungs expanding, and blood passing directly to the lungs, instead of to the placenta. Your baby may follow her first breath with a bout of coughing to clear her airways, but as soon as she begins to breathe normally, she will most likely cry.

Your newborn may hiccup quite a lot at first, but these bouts of hiccups won't upset her. They are caused by the sudden, irregular contractions of the immature diaphragm, which hasn't quite got breathing in and breathing out into steady rhythm. As the muscles involved become stronger, your baby will hiccup less.

Your newborn is also perfectly equipped to feed and digest food. Put a newborn baby to her mother's breast and she'll probably take to it right away, because of her strongly developed sucking reflex.

TUNE INTO HER ENVIRONMENT
At birth, all of your baby's senses are intact and ready to be used. She can already see, albeit fuzzily; she can hear, she can taste, she can smell, and she can sense touch.

Your baby's sight
Immediately after birth, you may notice your baby staring at you. She can see you quite well, but focuses best at 8 to 12 inches (20 to 25 cm) away from something. Interestingly, this is the approximate distance between you and your baby's face when you're holding her at your breast. Your baby will enjoying watching you and will track your movement for short periods. Sometimes you might notice her eyes crossing, which is normal and is a result of her lack of control over her eye muscles. As she gets used to seeing, this should disappear within a few weeks—if not, speak to your doctor.

Your baby's hearing
Babies hear very well when they're born, too. You may notice your baby turning toward you when you speak, and she'll have a definite preference for the

voices she heard while she was still in the uterus. You may notice that your baby seems to brighten when she hears your voice—this is a useful natural reaction, as you are vital to her survival.

Your baby won't like loud voices or noises, which will startle her and may even make her cry. If she's crying or fretful, white noise—the low-pitched sound of the washing machine or the dishwasher, for example—may have a miraculous calming effect. This is probably because they remind your baby of the type of noises she heard while in the uterus. Likewise, if you sang a particular song to your baby while you were pregnant, singing it again after the birth may bring about a delighted reaction.

Your baby's sense of taste

Babies seem to be able to distinguish certain flavors right from birth, and many experts believe that they, in fact, have a more delicate sense of taste than adults. Research has shown that if a baby is given bottles containing water with subtly different degrees of sweetness, she'll spend more time sucking on the bottle that contains the sweetest water.

Your baby's sense of smell

Newborns have surprisingly pronounced smell preferences. A baby can distinguish her own mother's breast milk from another mother's, and responds better to her own mother's milk. She may

HOW TO bond with your baby

A baby is usually very aware of her surroundings right from birth, which is why the time you spend together in the first few hours and days will be important for you both. Immediately after the birth, hold her close to you and look into her face. Babies have an inborn ability to distinguish people from other objects, and your baby will want to look at your face rather than anything else. Look into her eyes and smile to encourage this attachment.

Communicate your strong feelings for your baby through close physical contact. During her initial alert period after the birth, hold her naked against your skin so that she becomes familiar with how you feel and smell. Also talk to her in a quiet soothing voice—she'll recognize your voice from before she was born. As she gets older your baby will try to copy the noises you make

to her and will want to imitate your facial expressions. Through bonding in this way, your baby will begin to get to know you, learn to rely on you, and trust you. Make sure your partner has plenty of contact with her, too, so that your baby can develop an attachment to both of you. The early stages of your relationship with your baby can have an impact on her future, and knowing that she can depend on you both will give her the courage to venture out and actively explore her world as she gets older and becomes independent.

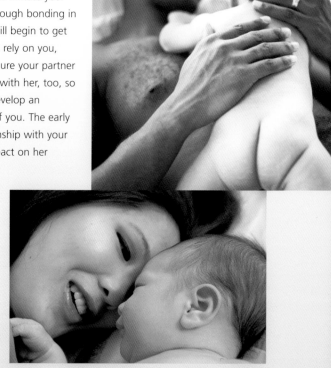

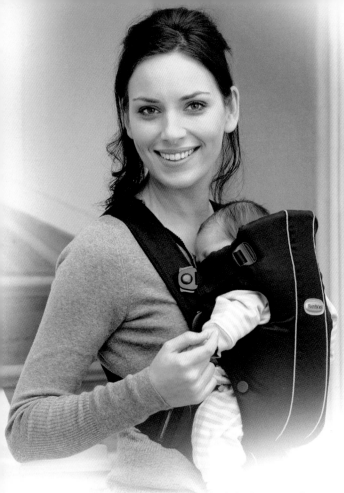

If your baby is fretful, carrying her in a
baby carrier so that she is held close to
your body will soothe her.

even use smell to help her find the breast. Babies
also seem to show preferences for certain smells,
being repelled by those she finds unpleasant, and
attracted by others that she finds pleasant.

Your baby's sense of touch

All babies love the feeling of being cuddled and held
close, which usually calms and reassures them. Your
baby will be soothed by the sound of your beating
heart and the secure, warm pressure of your body.
It's been found that premature babies, in particular,
thrive on skin-to-skin contact, or "kangaroo care" as
it's also called. Research has shown that removing a
preterm baby from her incubator and placing her
against her mother's skin for just a short spell every
day frequently leads to quicker weight gain and
more rapid development.

It used to be thought that babies were
developmentally too immature to feel pain, but a
relatively recent discovery is that they experience it

in the same way we do, if not more. Even in the
uterus, a baby will move away from external pressure
during examinations.

YOUR BABY'S PERSONALITY

Your baby has her own individual personality from
the moment she's born. She has her likes and
dislikes and reacts in her own unique way to you
and her environment.

One of the most exciting aspects of parenting is
getting to know your baby's patterns of behavior the
way no one else can. As a newborn, your baby has
very limited ways of communicating with you. But
through observation, you'll gradually learn the
details of your baby's personality, and the more you
interact and play with her, the easier it will be for
you to know what she wants.

Getting to know your baby

Some babies like to be rocked, while others enjoy
being still. Some babies like to be swaddled tightly,
while others prefer to have their hands and legs free.
Some babies quickly become uncomfortable in a wet
diaper, others don't seem to mind it at all. Babies'
behavior patterns are influenced by their
temperaments. You'll soon get to know your baby's
temperament, but in the early days you may find
yourself trying several strategies for caring for her
(see page 306) to find out what suits her best.

Understanding your baby's temperament

If your baby cries a lot, it may mean that she's
highly sensitive to stimulation. Sensitive babies
sometimes have trouble settling into a regular
sleeping pattern or feeding schedule. If your baby
has this type of temperament, she may respond best
to peace and quiet, rather than bright lights and lots
of stimulation. Introduce her to new people and
situations slowly to give her plenty of time to adjust.

Your baby's reflexes

Your baby is born with a number of important ingrained behaviors. These are automatic responses that are thought to help babies with basic needs. Many of these early reflexes will slowly disappear over the first 6 months.

The sucking reflex This is your baby's natural instinct to suck on whatever is put in her mouth. She'll suck readily on your nipple, on the nipple of a bottle, or on your finger. This reflex is crucial for survival, and a strong suck is a sign of a healthy baby. Your baby may also suck her fingers or thumb to soothe herself.

The rooting reflex This occurs if you tickle the side of your baby's cheek: She'll turn toward you and try to suck on your finger **1**. This

reflex helps a baby find food. It can help to tickle your baby's lips when you're encouraging her to feed.

The grasping reflex If you place your finger in your baby's hand. she'll grasp it tightly, and this grasp can be so strong that you could almost lift her up by her arms **2**. When you try to remove your finger, her grip will get tighter.

The moro reflex Also known as the startle reflex, this occurs when your baby hears a loud noise or is moved suddenly. During the startle, your baby's hands will suddenly go out to her sides with her fingers spread **3**. Then she'll bring her arms back into her chest with clenched fists, and probably end this with a crying episode.

The walking reflex Also called the stepping reflex, this occurs if you hold your baby upright under her arms and let her feet touch a

flat surface. She'll naturally make stepping movements and try to move forward **4**.

Diving reflex Although you should never leave your baby to swim under water, if you place your newborn under water for a short while, she'll swim happily without any problem. This is because her lungs automatically seal off once she hits the water.

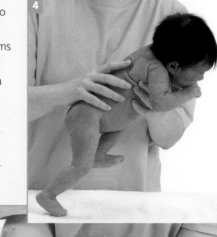

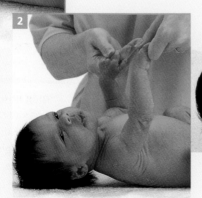

An easygoing baby will adapt to new people and places easily and have few sleeping and eating problems. However, if your baby's like this, it's possible for her to become overstimulated, because she's so easy to have around. If your baby averts her gaze rather than showing interest or if she suddenly falls asleep, it may be time to give her a break.

How your baby communicates
Initially, crying is your baby's only means of communicating her needs to you. Learning to understand her cries can be difficult at first, but with observation, patience, and the experience of trying different things to comfort her, you can learn a lot about what your baby is trying tell you.

All babies have different crying patterns. Some babies cry some of the time, and others cry very little, while others cry a great deal. Some babies are easy to calm, while others are harder to soothe. Sometimes a baby cries for no apparent reason and nothing seems to console her. The way that babies cry can differ too—some may cry intensely, others may only whimper. The one common factor is that babies cry because they need something and they are asking for a response to this need (see page 346).

YOUR BABY'S GROWTH
Your baby develops at an astounding rate over the first 3 months. Although most babies lose a small amount of weight after birth, they quickly regain this (see page 295). Once their original birth weight is achieved they gain, on average, ½ to 1 oz (15 to 30 g) each day for the first 6 months.

Although it may be hard for you to appreciate the daily change, friends who just saw your baby at birth may now marvel at her growth. Visits to the doctor will confirm this change, and allow you to see how much she has grown.

In addition to gaining weight, your baby will be developing her muscle strength. At birth, she will barely have been able to lift her head. By 4 weeks of age, she'll be able to lift her head up and turn it from side to side, although she'll still need you to support her head when you hold her upright. Just one month later, at 8 weeks of age, your baby will be able to lift her head and chest up when she's lying down on her front. Then, before you know it, at about 12 weeks, she'll be able to bring her chest up with her arms straight out.

By 4 or 5 months your baby will have developed some hand control and will be able to grasp objects. She will use her mouth to explore an item in her

DID YOU KNOW...

Newborn babies don't produce tears Although they spend a lot of time crying, babies can't actually produce tears until they're about 3 to 12 weeks old. This is because the tear duct is very efficient at removing any excess fluid from the tear glands before they overflow.

hand by gumming and sucking. By the age of around 6 months she will be rolling over and she will probably have learned to control her neck and head and will be beginning to try to sit upright.

Socially, your baby will become more and more interactive. When you first saw her at birth, she probably stared at you with a serious expression. Merely 4 to 8 weeks later, there'll be an unforgettable moment when she looks at you and smiles—her first signal of sociability. At the same time, her schedule will be becoming more predictable and you may have an easier time interpreting her moods and needs.

She'll begin also to make cooing noises at about 8 weeks, the beginnings of her speech development. By 4 months your baby understands all the basic sounds that make up her language. Between 4 and 6 months she discovers how to make different sounds and starts to "babble." Babbling usually involves practicing vowel sounds over and over again. But at this age she'll still communicate by crying.

14

CHAPTER

TAKING CARE OF YOUR BABY

Now there's a new baby—but also some new

parents. You have an awesome responsibility; this

tiny being is utterly dependent on you for

everything. Don't worry—every new parent wonders

whether he or she will do a good job, but you'll be

amazed at how soon you'll be comfortable with your

parenting skills.

FEEDING BASICS

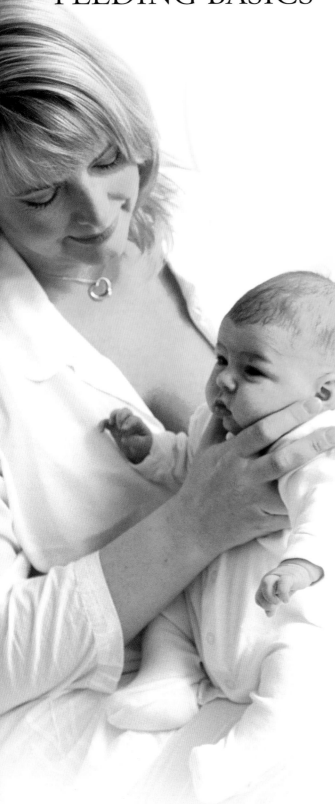

For the first few weeks, you'll probably find that feeding takes precedence over everything else. It may take a while to settle into a comfortable routine, but having some support at home— someone to keep an eye on your well-being—can make the process swifter and more successful.

You'll probably have decided already whether you want to breastfeed or bottlefeed your baby (see page 190), but there are now other things to consider, such as how often and who should feed him. Initially, you may be concerned about whether you're doing the right thing and whether he's getting enough nourishment, but, as you see your baby grow and thrive, you'll gradually relax and learn to trust your own judgment.

HOW OFTEN SHOULD YOU FEED?

Not so long ago, babies were fed on a rigid four-hourly schedule, regardless of whether they were screaming with hunger before the clock said it was time to feed them. Today, most health professionals recommend a more flexible schedule—that is, to feed your baby when he appears hungry. It's normal for a baby to want to feed frequently for the first few weeks, so if you accept that in the early days your breastfed baby may need nursing every two hours or your bottlefed baby every three hours, you can plan your day accordingly.

It may seem that you're doing nothing but feeding at first, but this period won't last forever— think of each feeding session as an opportunity for you to sit and rest. As your baby grows over the next few weeks, you'll probably find that the in-between periods get longer, and that your baby settles to a four-hourly routine of his own accord. Babies do vary in their ability to settle, however, so don't worry if your friend's baby seems to settle before yours.

Occasionally, smaller babies or babies who are sleepy—perhaps from drugs you were given during labor—don't always indicate when they need feeding. In this case, don't let your new baby go for longer than five to six hours without offering him your breast or the bottle.

HOW MUCH DOES HE NEED?

The needs of individual babies vary considerably, and you'll probably find that your baby sometimes takes more milk and sometimes a little less. Let his appetite be your main guide, but as a general idea: If you're breastfeeding, your baby will take as much as he needs from your breast; if you're bottlefeeding, your baby will need 2½ to 3½ oz (75 to 100 ml) of formula for each pound (0.5 kg) of body weight. Most bottlefed babies need six to eight feeds each day, so for a 7-pound baby, this would mean you need to give him 14 to 21 oz (415 to 620 ml) of formula in a 24-hour period.

Does my baby need water as well?

Breast milk contains enough water for your baby, so even in the hottest climate, if you're breastfeeding there's no need to give him supplementary drinks. Doing so could confuse him while he's trying to learn how to feed from your nipple. It also could overfill his tiny tummy, which may, in turn, interfere with his appetite.

If you're bottlefeeding your baby, you can give him a little extra water if it's very hot and humid and he's dehydrated or feverish. However, don't give him too much water or too often, as it may interfere with his appetite. If you do give your baby water, make sure that it's boiled then cooled, until your baby is 6 months old.

Signs of a thriving baby

Whether you're breast- or bottlefeeding, you'll want to be reassured that your baby is thriving. One of the best ways to do this is to make sure that your baby is regularly seen by his healthcare providers. They will weigh your baby and plot his weight on a centile chart (a chart that compares your baby's

DID YOU KNOW...

Babies have growth spurts If your baby was satisfied with the feeding routine, but then starts to be unsettled or demands milk more frequently, he may be having a "growth spurt" and need more milk. This usually happens at around the age of 5 to 6 weeks and again at 3 months, but can occur as early as 3 weeks of age. Breastfeeding more frequently for a day or two will increase your milk supply to meet the increased demand, and your baby will settle back into a routine again.

weight gain to national averages). If you have any concerns about feeding, you will also be able to discuss them. However, you'll get an idea whether your baby is thriving if:

- He's gaining weight steadily.
- He has a good skin color.
- He's lively, with bright eyes and firm muscle tone.
- He's contented, and seems satisfied after feeding.
- He has six or more wet diapers in 24 hours.
- He's passing soft stools.

PREVENTING GAS

All babies take in some air when they feed, but some seem to suffer from excess air more than others. If your bottlefed baby suffers from a lot of gas—you'll know because he'll seem upset and unsettled after his bottle—check that the holes of the nipples are the right size. To test this, hold a bottle upside down and watch how the formula drips out—it should be at a steady flow of one drop per second. If the formula flow is slower than this, the hole is too small and your baby is having to suck hard to obtain the formula. This can mean that when your baby feeds he takes in too much air along with his formula. On the other hand, if your baby tends to gulp from the bottle, check that the holes of the nipples aren't too large.

Make sure, too, that the bottle is always tilted enough when you feed your baby—the liquid should always completely cover the top of the bottle and the nipple area.

If you're nursing, excess air may be due to the fact that your baby isn't latching on properly (see page 301). It also may be due to irregular flow. If your milk tends to gush out before you put your baby to your breast, try expressing a little milk (see page 302) before you start to feed your baby.

Try also not to let your baby wait too long between feeding times. If he's hungry, he may cry too much and swallow a lot of air just before you feed him. He may also gulp down the milk too quickly, again causing gas.

Burping your baby

Some experts recommend you burp your baby after each meal to get rid of excess air; other experts maintain that it's not always necessary, particularly with breastfed babies. Babies have their own preferences about being burped, and your baby may like to nurse or take the bottle without stopping, and will scream indignantly if you try to burp him halfway through. Or he may need to stop in the middle to give a big burp. You'll soon get to know what your baby likes to do.

If your baby does have some discomfort from gas and is unable to bring it up by himself, sit him on your lap, leaning him forward slightly and supporting his head by placing your hand under his chin (see picture, page 294). Alternatively, hold your baby upright against your shoulder. Have a clean towel at hand or draped over your clothing in case he brings up any milk. Also, it may be helpful to gently pat or rub your baby's back. If your baby can't bring up gas in these positions, try laying him face down across your lap and rubbing his back.

If your baby often has gas and finds it difficult to bring it up, you might like to learn some baby massage techniques from a health professional. One simple massage technique that can help with excess gas is called "tiger in the tree" and is illustrated on page 346. Some mothers find that giving their babies colic drops can ease excess air, as this medication contains simethicone, a chemical that helps disperse trapped gas bubbles; other mothers find that these make no difference.

If your baby doesn't seem to suffer from gas, don't spend hours trying to get him to burp—some babies just don't. Or he may prefer to wait for an hour or so, before giving a big burp by himself.

SPITTING

Most babies spit up small amounts of milk occasionally, usually when they're being burped or are lying down. This may simply be a result of physical immaturity: The muscles between the stomach and the esophagus (the tube connecting the mouth to the stomach) lack coordination in some newborns. In other cases, babies may gulp a lot of air when they feed, and then when they burp afterward, they simply spit up a little bit of their meal with it. As long as your baby is well, is putting on weight, and the vomiting isn't forceful, spitting is usually nothing to worry about. You can try to help prevent it by burping your baby or by sitting him up in a baby chair straight after you feed him. You'll probably find that spitting problems resolve once your baby is 6 months old, is onto a more solid diet, and is drinking less milk.

If your baby is spitting up frequently or forcefully or appears to be in pain, he may be suffering something more serious, such as a gastric infection or disorder (see page 362). Contact your baby's pediatrician for a check-up and further advice.

STARTING TO BREASTFEED

During pregnancy your body will have prepared for nursing your baby, and there's no doubt that nature's way gives your baby the best possible start.

Nursing is a skill that has to be learned, just like riding a bike or driving a car, and it comes easier to some mothers and babies than others. But mothers who experience minor difficulties at first usually find that these can be overcome easily with patience and perseverance. If necessary, ask for help from your healthcare provider or contact a mothers' support organization like the La Leche League to find out about lactation counselors in your area.

THE FIRST TWO DAYS
Unless there have been any difficulties, such as an emergency cesarean, you'll usually be encouraged to nurse your baby very soon after the birth. Many babies take to the breast immediately and begin to suck away happily without any problems. However, some aren't quite ready—for example, if the birth has been difficult or the baby is premature. If this is the case for you, you can still stroke your baby and get to know each other until she's ready to nurse.

Initially, it's also not unusual for babies to have a 6- to 8-hour gap between each feeding session. Don't worry that she's not getting enough food—babies don't need a lot in the first few days.

PRODUCING BREAST MILK
Understanding the milk production process can help you breastfeed successfully. Each of your breasts is divided into 15 to 20 compartments called lobes. Within each lobe are several smaller compartments called lobules. These contain alveoli, which are grapelike clusters of cells that produce and store breast milk. Milk travels from the alveoli through the milk ducts. These ducts broaden out beneath the areola (the dark area around your nipple) to form milk sinuses, which release milk through the 15 to 20 openings in your nipple.

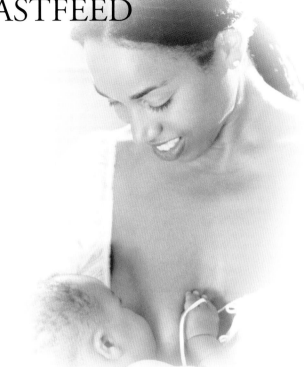

If practical, wear clothes that allow you to expose your breast easily, such as a loose top with a drawstring neck.

As your baby sucks, the nerve endings in your nipple and areola are stimulated and send signals to the brain telling it to release two hormones, oxytocin and prolactin. Oxytocin triggers your milk to flow, a process known as the letdown reflex (see below). Prolactin stimulates further production of milk in the alveoli, meaning your milk supply works on a supply-and-demand basis: The more your baby feeds, the more milk is produced.

The letdown reflex
When oxytocin flows into the blood vessels in your breasts, it causes the alveoli to contract, squeezing milk through the ducts, into the sinuses, and out through the nipple.

Some women experience this letdown reflex—also called the "milk-ejection" reflex—as a sharp, needlelike sensation in the breasts, and their milk spurts out in jets. Other women simply feel a tingling or warm sensation and the milk drips out. The letdown reflex may also be triggered in response to the baby crying or during sex. Some women who breastfeed never feel the letdown reflex at all, but this doesn't mean that it isn't working.

THE STRUCTURE OF THE BREAST

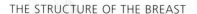

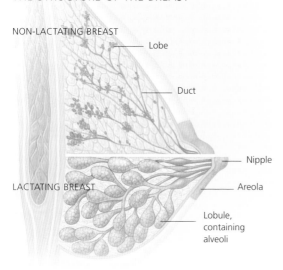

NON-LACTATING BREAST

Lobe

Duct

Nipple

LACTATING BREAST

Areola

Lobule, containing alveoli

If you find that your breasts leak milk when you're due to nurse or when your baby starts crying, you may find it useful to wear breast pads inside your bra. If your milk starts leaking when you're not ready to nurse, try pressing firmly on your nipples with the heels of your hands or your forearms to slow down the flow.

CHANGES TO YOUR BREAST MILK

Unlike formula milk, the nutritional composition of breast milk changes—both during nursing and over the weeks that you feed. This ensures that your breast milk contains all the food and water your baby needs for at least the first 4 to 6 months of life.

Colostrum

The first food your baby receives from your breasts is colostrum. This is manufactured during late pregnancy in response to the hormones estrogen and progesterone. It's a rich, golden-yellowish looking substance, which is produced for about two to three days. Although there's only a small amount of colostrum, it's a unique and valuable food for your baby. It contains a larger amount of protein than mature breast milk and all the minerals, fats, and vitamins your baby needs in the first few days of life. Colostrum is rich also in antibodies, which help protect your baby from infections and build a strong immune system. Colostrum works as a laxative, too, clearing out the meconium (the first dark green stools) from the bowels. Even if you don't intend to breastfeed for very long, it's worth offering your baby the valuable colostrum for the first few days.

Transitional and mature breast milk

After two to three days, colostrum gradually becomes transitional milk. You might notice this change as a feeling of fullness in your breasts. You may experience this "milk coming in" whether or not you nurse your baby. Transitional milk, which is thinner and whiter than colostrum, is a mixture of colostrum and mature milk.

After about two to three weeks, mature breast milk starts to come through. It has a watery, almost blue appearance when the milk starts to flow and changes to white as the fat content rises.

Foremilk and hindmilk

The changing appearance of mature breast milk reflects the fact that it is composed of two types of milk: foremilk and hindmilk. Foremilk is produced when you begin to nurse your baby. It looks thin and watery, because it's low in calories and fat and quenches your baby's thirst before she starts to feed.

As your baby continues to suck, the letdown reflex releases the hindmilk. This is rich in fat, energy, and nutrients, and although there is less of it than foremilk, it's the hindmilk that satisfies your baby's hunger and gives her the energy to grow. The time taken for the hindmilk to flow may vary from day to day. Sometimes it may take half a minute; at other times several minutes. You can make sure that your baby has enough of the rich hindmilk by ensuring that she latches on properly and that she empties the first breast before you offer the other.

MAINTAINING A GOOD MILK SUPPLY

The production of breast milk is stimulated by the hormone prolactin, which responds to the touch of your baby's mouth on your nipple. So, if you feed your baby whenever she appears to be hungry or when your breasts feel full, you'll naturally produce all the milk your baby needs.

Some women are concerned that their supplies of milk are inadequate and try to "build up" their reserves by restricting the amount of times that they nurse their babies. However, this can actually be counterproductive, as it reduces milk supply. If you worry that your baby seems hungry again shortly after feeding her, the solution may be as simple as feeding her more often and checking that she's latching on properly each time.

AVOIDING PROBLEMS

Sore nipples and engorgement are commonly present during the early days, but try not to let either problem discourage you from nursing. Nursing your baby on demand will help, as will correct positioning. Other, less common problems, are discussed on page 357.

Sore nipples

Many women experience tenderness when they begin to breastfeed, and this may be accompanied by a pinching or burning sensation. In most cases, soreness can be cured simply by trying a different feeding position, perhaps changing it each time you nurse your baby. You also may have to make several attempts to get your baby to latch on correctly. If you want to change position, remember to break the suction with your finger before removing your baby from the breast—pulling your baby away from your nipple will aggravate soreness.

Consider your nipple care, too. Very moist or very dry skin can cause soreness, so leave your bra off for a few minutes after nursing to allow air to your skin, and make sure you wear bras made from natural fibers, such as cotton, that let your nipples "breathe." Rubbing a little breast milk into your nipple after you finish feeding or placing cool wet teabags on your nipples also can relieve tenderness.

If at any stage your nipples become red and shiny or you experience shooting pains in your breasts, consult your healthcare provider. You may have an infection such as thrush (see page 358).

5 ways to boost your milk supply

1   To ensure that your baby gets enough nutrients, try to eat the same kind of balanced diet you were eating during pregnancy, making sure that it includes sufficient protein and calcium.

2   Your energy needs while nursing are higher than during pregnancy—you require an extra 500 calories a day above your pre-pregnancy diet.

3   You may feel more thirsty than usual, so take frequent sips of water. However, don't force yourself to drink large quantities (see page 332).

4   Keep your intake of caffeinated and alcoholic drinks low. What you eat and drink will pass through to your baby in your milk.

5   Watch your baby's reactions. If a food you normally eat seems to upset your baby, she simply may not enjoy it. Try replacing this food for another of similar nutritional value for a week.

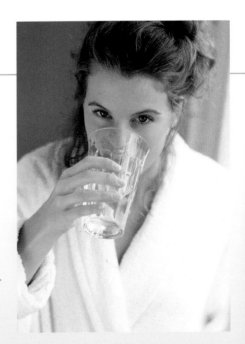

Successful breastfeeding

Before starting to nurse your baby, whether you're at home or in the hospital, try to make the atmosphere as calm as possible so that you can be as relaxed as you can. If necessary, take the phone off the hook or put a notice on the door asking not to be disturbed. Have a drink nearby to keep up your fluid intake.

GETTING COMFORTABLE

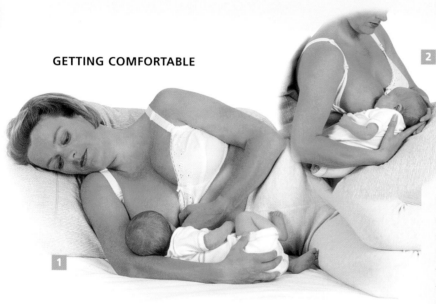

A comfortable nursing position can be the key to successful feeding, so try out a few to see which work best. Generally, most women nurse sitting upright on a chair, often with their feet raised and a pillow on their lap, but other positions can be adopted in certain circumstances. Lying on your side **1** can be useful if you're tired or if you find it uncomfortable to sit—perhaps if you've had an episiotomy. Make sure that you have plenty of pillows to support you. Lay your baby facing you with her mouth in line with your breast and your arm supporting her head. If you've had a cesarean or if your baby wriggles or arches her back, bend your knees and support your back with a pillow. Lay your baby on your lap **2**, with a pillow to raise her, if necessary. Support her head with your hand.

Whichever position you choose, your baby should be held close to you with her whole body facing your breast, her chest next to your chest. You should be able to bring her to your breast easily.

Your baby's mouth needs to form a tight seal over most of your areola. If this "latching on" isn't achieved, your baby will chew or suck on your nipple, which can lead to problems such as nipple soreness (see page 299) or cracked nipples (see page 358). Some women find it difficult to get their babies to latch on at first. It often needs practice and patience in the early days.

Position your baby

Before you begin feeding, make sure that you and your baby are both comfortable. If you're sitting upright you can either support her head and shoulders on your forearm or hold her head and shoulders with your free hand. Her head should be at the same level as your nipple and she should be able to reach your breast without any effort. For alternative positions see box, left.

You may find it helpful to cup your breast with your hand **3** or to support your breast by placing your fingers against your ribs just underneath it. Try not to place two fingers in a "scissors grip" around your nipple, as it can prevent your baby feeding properly. Nor do you need to press your breast away from her nose to help her breathe— her flared nostrils allow her to breathe and feed simultaneously.

Your baby may instinctively start to suck as soon as she feels your breast against her cheek, or you can brush your baby's lips against your nipple to trigger her rooting reflex. Once she opens her mouth wide, draw her quickly to your breast.

Check that she has latched on
Your baby needs as much of your breast in her mouth as possible. If she's properly positioned **4**, she'll have a mouthful of breast, including your nipple and much of the underside of the areola, and her bottom lip should be curled back. Her jaw muscles will work rhythmically, as far back as her ears. If your baby's cheeks cave in when she's sucking, she isn't latched on properly. In this case, you'll need to reposition your baby and try again. You can break the suction by inserting your little finger in the corner of her mouth **5**.

Change breasts if necessary Your baby's sucking pattern will alter while she feeds, from short sucks to longer bursts, with pauses in between. She'll let you know when your breast is empty by playing with it, falling asleep, or letting your nipple slide out of her mouth. You can then offer her the other breast.

When you need to remove her from your breast, break the suction with your finger (as above). Don't worry if she refuses the second breast, but start with it the next time. It's important that your baby empties one breast before you offer her the other, because the last milk she'll get from your breast is calorie-packed hindmilk.

Engorgement

A few days after the birth, when the milk comes in, many women's breasts become engorged, feeling swollen, hard, and painful with the accumulation of blood and milk. If this occurs, nursing can become difficult, sometimes painful. Nursing frequently—perhaps eight times or more in 24 hours—can help you avoid engorgement. But if your breasts do feel full, try expressing a little milk before you start to nurse. Placing a cloth dipped in warm water on the areola before you begin to nurse, and using a cold compress after you finish can help, too. Some women find that chilled cabbage leaves can offer relief: Wash the outer leaves of a cabbage and place them on each breast for 10 to 20 minutes. Breast massage is another solution (see page 323).

COMBINING BREAST WITH BOTTLE

There may be occasions—such as when you return to work—when you want to give your baby breast milk from a bottle or intersperse breast milk with formula. Try to avoid this in the early days if you can, as your baby will probably need time to get used to feeding from your breast—to feed from a bottle she'll need to learn a new sucking action. But once you've established a successful routine, you can try expressing your milk (see below). If your baby is reluctant to feed from the bottle at first, you may find that it's easier to let someone else give her the bottle when you're out of the room. Alternatively, try feeding your baby from a dropper or spoon.

If you want to stop nursing altogether, it's best to do so gradually, interspersing breast milk with formula in a bottle. Not only will your baby need time to get used to feeding from a bottle, but your body also needs time to readjust. If you stop suddenly, there's a chance that you may develop problems such as engorgement (see above).

HOW TO express your breast milk

At times, you may want spare breast milk, if, for example, your partner is taking a turn at feeding, or you're going out for a while. You can express milk using your hands or a pump.

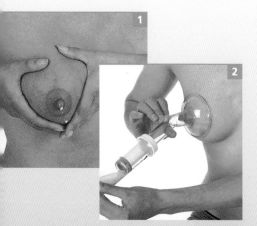

Your milk should be expressed straight into a sterile bottle, sterile plastic container, or breast-milk freezer bag. You can store the expressed milk in the fridge for 24 hours, or freeze and use it within three months.

To express milk by hand **1**, stimulate your milk flow by gently stroking downward from the top of your breast toward the areola. Then place both your thumbs above the areola and your fingers below, and begin rhythmically squeezing the lower part of your breast while pressing toward your breastbone.

Many women find a hand pump or an electric pump quicker, more effective, and easier than expressing milk by hand. For example, to use a syringe-style hand pump, simply place the funnel over your nipple, forming an airtight seal **2**, and then draw the cylinder in and out a few times. This sucks the milk out of your breast. You may need to try several pumps to find out what suits you, so see if you can borrow or rent a pump before buying.

BOTTLEFEEDING YOUR BABY

Feeding your baby with infant formula milk from a bottle is a safe alternative to breastfeeding, as long as you maintain good hygiene and follow the manufacturer's instructions carefully.

Once you've made the decision to bottlefeed your baby, you'll quickly establish your own routine of cleaning and sterilizing the equipment, preparing the formula, and giving the bottle. It may seem like a lot of work, but all these processes have become much quicker and easier than they were in the past. If you haven't already bought all of your feeding, cleaning, and sterilizing equipment, see page 198 for some advice. There also are many different formulas on the market to suit individual parents' and babies' needs. Whichever you use, always keep in mind that bottlefed babies may be more prone to infections than breastfed babies, so you'll need to pay particular attention to hygiene.

TYPES OF FORMULA

The US Food and Drug Administration (FDA), advises that babies who aren't breastfed should be given iron-fortified formula until they're one year old. Baby formulas are carefully produced under government guidelines so that they replicate human milk as closely as possible and contain the proper amounts of fat, protein, and vitamins.

Babies under the age of one year shouldn't be given ordinary cow's milk, because it contains high levels of protein and minerals, which can put a strain on a baby's immature kidneys and cause dehydration. Cow's milk also doesn't contain sufficient iron for young babies. Goat's milk and condensed milk are also unsuitable for young babies.

If you're unsure as to which formula is best for your baby, your healthcare provider will be able to give you guidance. You can buy formula in powder, liquid concentrate, and ready-to-feed forms at most grocery and drug stores. Powdered formulas are usually the cheapest of these, while ready-to-feed

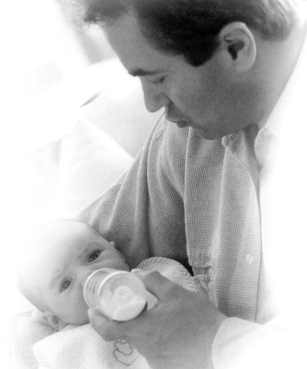

Keep your baby in a semi-upright position as he feeds. It will help him swallow the formula more easily.

forms are the most expensive but can be useful in the first few weeks, while you're getting used to feeding or if you're short of time.

There are two basic types of formula: those based on modified cow's milk and specialized formulas, usually based on soy milk.

Modified cow's milk

Most bottlefed babies are fed with a formula based on modified cow's milk, and if your baby has been fed on this while in the hospital without any problems, there's no reason to change when you get home. If you're concerned that your baby isn't putting on enough weight or still seems hungry after you've given him his bottle, consider changing to another brand or type. However, always ask a health professional's advice before you do this—the

Preparing a healthy formula

In contrast to breast milk, which is always clean, it's possible for bacteria to get into baby formula and give a baby an upset stomach. To avoid this, thoroughly clean and sterilize all equipment before you make up a bottle.

STERILIZING THE EQUIPMENT

Feeding equipment can be washed and sterilized in a dishwasher or by doing the following:

Wash all equipment Fill the sink with hot, soapy water. Then clean the bottles, nipples, rings, discs, and

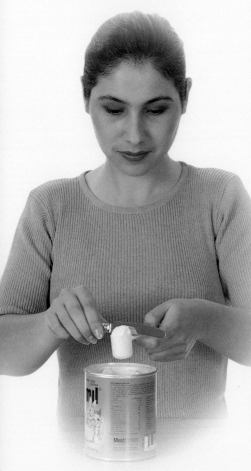

caps individually, removing stubborn milk deposits. Use a bottlebrush to wash bottles, particularly around the thread at the top. Turn the nipples inside out, scrub them with a nipple brush, and squirt water through the holes to check for blockages. Finally, rinse everything thoroughly in warm, running water.

Sterilize all equipment If using a chemical sterilizer, empty the chemicals into the unit according to the manufacturer's instructions. Then immerse everything fully in the solution for the recommended length of time. If you're not using the items immediately, you can keep them in the sterilizer for up to 24 hours. Rinse with cooled, boiled water before use.

Alternatively, you can use a microwave or stove-top steam sterilizer or boil most of the items in a covered pan for 10 minutes—nipples need only 3 minutes.

MAKING UP A FORMULA

Preparing formula correctly is vital for your baby's health and well-being. Begin by getting everything together, then wash your hands.

Boil some water Bring some fresh or filtered water to the boil and simmer for 1 to 2 minutes. Let it cool. Avoid using bottled water, softened water, or repeatedly boiled water, as it may contain high levels of mineral salts. If your tap water contains high levels of lead, consider buying a water filter.

Combine the formula Add the correct amount of cooled, boiled water to each bottle, then add the correct number of scoops of formula, leveling each scoop with a knife. Always use the scoop provided, and add only the recommended number of scoops per ounces (or milliliters) of water. Replace the discs and rings, and shake vigorously.

Add the nipples and store Remove the discs and rings, then place the nipples upside down in the bottles—they shouldn't touch the formula. Replace the discs and rings and cover the bottles with the caps. If not using the bottles immediately, store them upright inside the fridge.

SAFETY FIRST

Measurements Never heap or pack a scoop of formula or add an extra one, and make certain the amount of water is correct. If the formula is overconcentrated it may make your baby dehydrated, but if it's too weak, your baby won't get enough nourishment. To make extra formula, add more water and powder in the correct proportions.

problem may not lie with the formula, but may be due to feeding techniques or an intolerance to a particular formula; or it may be caused by a medical condition that requires further investigation.

Specialized formula milk

For full-term, bottlefed babies who are diagnosed as intolerant to lactose or protein in cow's milk, or who have other feeding or medical problems, a range of specialized formulas is available. These formulas will be prescribed by your healthcare provider, if necessary. These include hypoallergenic formulas and soya milks, which have been formulated to provide babies with all the nutrients they need.

FEEDING YOUR BABY

In the first few weeks, it can be a useful practice to prepare batches of formula in advance. Store prepared formula in the fridge for up to 24 hours, but keep bottles in the main body of the fridge, as it is slightly cooler than the door. You then can feed your baby as soon as he's hungry and he won't get upset while he's waiting, and then refuse to feed. Also, avoid too many different people feeding him at first, but let him get used to you and your partner. Feeding times should soon become a relaxing and enjoyable occasion, and you can help this by holding him close to you and maintaining eye contact with him (see page 345). By the time your baby is 3 months old, you'll see him starting to get excited when he knows his bottle is on its way.

Temperature of the milk

Although it's traditional to warm a baby's bottle to body temperature, most babies don't mind taking formula that's slightly colder, as long as it's at least at room temperature. You can use an electric bottle warmer, or you can place the bottle in a jug of hot, but not boiling, water for a few minutes. Don't use a microwave to heat formula, as the bottle may feel cool, but the formula, which continues heating after removal, may be very hot and scald your baby's mouth. Always test the temperature before you give your baby the bottle by letting a couple of drops fall on the inside of your wrist—it should be just warm.

Once you've heated the bottle, feed your baby right away. Never keep formula warm for longer than an hour, and always throw away unfinished formula. Germs can breed rapidly in warm formula and could result in your baby getting a stomach infection. If you're going out with your baby, take bottles of prepared formula in a cool box and warm them for your baby when he's hungry.

SAFETY FIRST

Choking Even when you're baby gets older, don't leave him on his own to feed from a propped-up bottle—there's always the risk that he could choke. You should inspect bottle nipples each time you wash them to ensure that they're not worn or damaged. If fragments break off in your baby's mouth it can be dangerous.

Giving the bottle

Make yourself and your baby comfortable before you start, and give him all your attention. Hold him securely in your lap with his head in the crook of your elbow and his back supported along your forearm (see page 303). Encourage the rooting reflex by touching your baby's lips with the nipple of the bottle. When he's ready, insert the nipple into his mouth. Keep checking that it doesn't slip out, as this may prevent him from sucking properly. While he feeds, keep the bottle tilted at an angle of about 45 degrees, so the top is full of formula and not air. If the nipple becomes flattened, gently remove it from your baby's mouth to allow the air back in.

To help your baby relax, cuddle him close and talk or sing to him. Watch him all the time and respond to his demands. Some babies like to pause for air or to bring up some gas; others prefer to keep on feeding until all the formula has gone.

MEETING YOUR BABY'S NEEDS

Keeping an infant healthy and happy is a simple matter of meeting all of her daily needs. Besides feeding, she requires love, comfort, security, warmth, and protection against infection.

As you get to know your baby, you'll start to recognize what's needed or wanted. Changing your baby's diapers or giving your baby a bath can be a little daunting at first, but using the following guidelines will make you an expert in no time at all.

PROVIDING COMFORT

All babies cry at times, as it's their only means of telling their parents what they want. If your baby cries, it may be an indication that she's hungry, has a wet diaper, is overtired, or is too hot or cold. Attend to these things first, but if your baby is still crying, try the following to soothe her distress:

- *Holding* Pick up your baby and hold her close against you or carry her in a sling and talk, sing, sway, or gently dance.
- *Movement* Take your baby for a car ride or a walk in her stroller, put her in a baby bouncing chair, or sit in a rocking chair and gently rock her on your knee. But don't overdo it—too much jiggling can make a crying baby feel worse.
- *Noise* Music or sounds from machines, such as the vacuum cleaner or washing machine, can calm some babies, as can a musical toy.
- *Bathing* If your baby enjoys it, give her a warm bath. Once she's 2 months old, you can try adding one or two drops of essential lavender oil—it may have a calming and soothing effect.
- *Swaddling* Fold down the top-right corner of a light cotton blanket about 6 inches (15 cm). Lay your baby on her back with her head on the fold.

Pull the left-hand corner across your baby's body and tuck it under her back. Bring the bottom corner up under her chin. Finally, bring the right-hand corner across her body and tuck it under her back. The blanket should be secure but not tight, and you can leave your baby's arms free if she prefers. Feel the back of your baby's neck regularly to check that she doesn't get too hot.

- *Massage* Lay your baby on her front across your knees and stroke her gently down her back and legs. Alternatively, hold her in the "tiger in the tree" position (see page 346). To learn more techniques try attending a class in your area.
- *Pacifier* If your baby likes to suck, a pacifier can work wonders. Check with your pediatrician what type to use and clean it between each use.

If your baby doesn't stop crying no matter what you do, consult your doctor; persistent crying may be due to a number of causes. But if your pediatrician

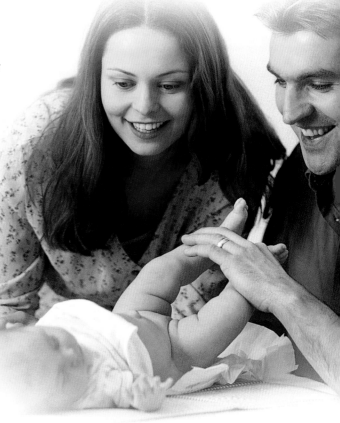

Involving your partner in the day-to-day care will give him an opportunity to get to know his baby.

SAFETY FIRST

Shaking your baby A constantly crying baby can invoke powerful emotions in some parents. But whatever you may feel, always handle your baby gently. Shaking can cause brain damage or even death. If you're frustrated by your baby's cries, contact a your doctor or parents' support group.

pronounces your baby fit and well, don't blame yourself for the crying. Some babies will cry whatever you do and may just need to "cry it out."

CHANGING A DIAPER

Newborn babies have very small bladders, so they can urinate up to 20 times a day in the first few weeks. Some babies also pass stools after every meal, so diaper-changing is going to take up a big part of your early days as a parent.

Choosing diapers

The type of diapers you choose will depend on what you prefer and what suits your lifestyle. Keep in mind that you don't have to stick with one type, but you can mix and match to suit your needs.

Disposables are popular with many parents, because they're more convenient, labor-saving, and easy to use. You don't have to wash and dry them or worry about buying separate plastic pants, diaper liners, or pins or clips. For these reasons, disposables can be particularly useful if you're out for the day or

traveling. Advances in design have meant that disposables today are also very good at drawing moisture away from your baby's skin, helping prevent skin irritations and diaper rash.

However, disposables can end up being very costly if you rely on them all the time. They're also thought to be harmful for the environment, because they're usually made from wood pulp treated with chemicals, and most end up in landfill sites, where they take hundreds of years to decompose. If you do choose disposables, non-chlorine bleached diapers are more environmentally friendly. Also, never flush them down the toilet. Disposables come in a range of sizes and styles, so you may need to try out a few brands to find diapers that fit your baby well.

Cloth diapers may eventually be cheaper than disposables, as they are a once-only purchase. They can even be used for another child. Reusable diapers have come a long way in the last decade: Many are now shaped so that they're easy to change, and some

MORE **ABOUT** | your baby's excretions

One strange thing about becoming a mother is that you become obsessed with the contents of your baby's diaper. In fact, this is perfectly sensible, as they can tell you about your baby's health. In the first couple of days your baby will pass meconium. This sticky, greeny-black substance is left over from the amniotic fluid your baby swallowed in the uterus. Your baby's stools will then change, depending on how she's fed: If she's breastfed, they will be yellowy-orange and loose, and won't smell very strong; if she's bottlefed, her stools will be pale brown, firmer, and smell noticeably.

Immediately after the birth, your baby's diaper may also be stained dark pink or red. This is normal and a result of urates in her urine. If you're concerned about any change in the frequency, color, or consistency of her stools or urination patterns, tell your healthcare provider. Stools streaked with blood or frequent, pale, watery stools will need to be investigated.

have attached Velcro fastenings to replace pins or clips. Some incorporate a waterproof layer, which helps with both diaper-changing and cleaning. If the ones that you buy don't have this layer, you'll need to buy some plastic pants to put on top to make them waterproof. Consider getting diaper liners, too. These can draw moisture away from your baby's skin and prevent staining of the diapers.

Washing cloth diapers

Thorough washing, disinfecting, and drying of cloth diapers takes time but is necessary to prevent your baby from getting an infection. You can wash diapers at home or there may be a diaper-washing service in your area, which is an environmentally friendly alternative to individual washing.

KEEPING YOUR BABY CLEAN

Your newborn has very sensitive skin and a limited potential for getting dirty, which means that on a daily basis you'll need to wash only her face, neck, hands, bottom, and feet. This can be done with a sponge bath (see page 312). After a week or two, you can start to bath your baby. However, at this stage, you'll need to bath her only once or twice a week at most. No soaps, lotions, creams, or oils are needed when washing or changing your baby, as some products may dry your baby's skin or cause diaper rash. Cooled, boiled water will be fine.

When cleaning your baby, you'll need to take particular care when cleaning around the cord stump and, if your baby boy has been circumcised, you'll need to take care around his genitals.

HOW TO treat skin irritations

Babies' skins are very sensitive and most experience minor irritations, such as diaper rash or cradle cap at some stage. You can successfully prevent and treat both these conditions at home by taking the following advice.

The first signs of diaper rash may be a mild red patch or small bumps on the buttocks. The skin may be angry-looking and moist, with open spots or blisters around your baby's buttocks or between the legs.

As diaper rash is mainly caused by prolonged contact with urine and feces, the best way to prevent it is to change your baby's diaper as soon as it's wet or soiled. If your baby does have a rash, clean the area gently but thoroughly and apply a light diaper rash cream. Exposing your baby's bottom to the air for a while—perhaps after you've removed a soiled diaper—will help the rash heal. If the rash doesn't clear up with ordinary

creams, and the skin is bright red with white or red pimples in the folds, it may be infected with thrush (see page 364). In this case, consult your healthcare provider.

Cradle cap is a common and harmless condition that appears as greasy white or yellowish scales on a baby's scalp **1**. Cradle cap clears up of its own accord with time, but it can be unsightly. If you want to get rid of

the scales, try massaging aqueous cream or warmed baby oil into your baby's scalp. Leave the cream or oil on overnight, then brush **2** or wash it out. Never try to pick off the scales because you could cause an infection.

In severe or persistent cases of cradle cap, see your healthcare provider, as the cause of the skin problem may be a condition such as eczema (see page 364).

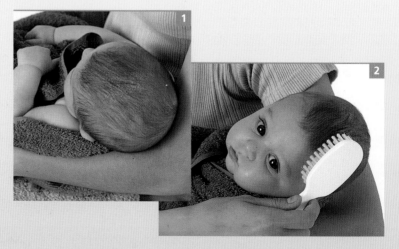

Care of the cord

Your baby's cord stump will turn black, shrivel up, and fall off—normally within about 5 to 10 days. In the meantime, keep it clean and dry, using cooled, boiled water, surgical wipes, or antiseptic powder, depending on what your healthcare provider advises. Leaving the stump exposed to the air as much as possible will help it heal quickly.

DRESSING YOUR BABY

The best clothes for your baby will be easy to put on, machine washable, and made of natural fibers, such as cotton or wool, which are warm, but allow your baby's skin to breathe. For further information on the clothes your baby will need see page 200.

When dressing your baby, remember that the objective is to keep her warm, not hot. For the first week or so after birth, she won't be able to regulate her body temperature, so it's important not to overdress or underdress her. Unless your home is very cold, your baby generally won't need to be dressed in more than a diaper and nightgown at night, and an undershirt, diaper, and stretch suit during the day—or an undershirt and diaper in warm weather. Outdoors, according to the season, add a sweater and socks or bootees to this, and, in very cold weather, a bunting bag, mittens, and a hat. Take care that your baby doesn't overheat if you're out shopping; in the car or in a store, remove her hat, mittens, and outdoor clothing.

To help protect your baby's delicate skin, wash her clothes using nonbiological washing products designed for sensitive skins. Avoid fabric conditioner and bleach, as these have a potential to cause skin irritation. If your baby develops any rash or redness that you think may be related to the washing products, try running her washed clothes through an extra rinse cycle to remove any traces of soap or detergent. If the problem continues, talk to your healthcare provider.

PROVIDING A SAFE PLACE TO SLEEP

For the first few weeks of her life your baby will sleep and wake at random. In these early days, you can choose to take your baby out with you in the

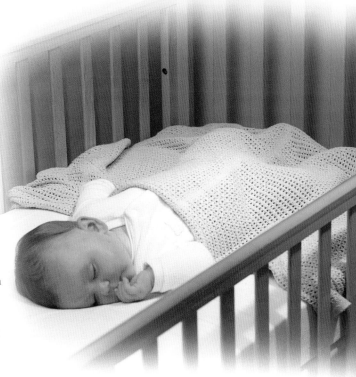

The feet-to-foot sleeping position, in which your baby's feet are at the bottom of the foot of the crib, allows her to move without getting tangled in the blankets.

evening or keep her up until you go to bed. Or, you may prefer to establish a regular bedtime routine from the beginning (see page 348).

Whatever routine you decide, the way that you put your baby down to sleep is important. Most parents worry about sudden infant death syndrome (SIDS)—also called crib death—which happens when a baby dies suddenly, without any apparent explanation. Fortunately, crib deaths are rare, and research has found that you can significantly minimize the risks by checking that your baby sleeps in the correct position and conditions:

- *Always put her to sleep on her back* This is the safest sleeping position unless the pediatrician has advised you otherwise. While your baby's awake, however, she should have time on her tummy to develop her neck, shoulder, and arm muscles.
- *Tuck in any blankets and sheets* If there are coverings in your baby's crib tuck them in around the mattress so that her face can't become

covered. Also, place her in the "feet-to-foot" position (see page 309) so that her feet reach the end of the crib, with the blankets tucked under the mattress and reaching up only as far as her chest. Alternatively, dress your baby in warm sleep clothing and don't use any coverings.

- *Check that the crib conforms to safety standards* And don't let her sleep on soft items such as a sofa, armchair, water bed, beanbag, or cushion.
- *Don't overheat the room* And don't let your baby get too hot. The room should feel comfortable for a lightly clothed adult—a room temperature of 61 to 68°F (16 to 20°C) is ideal.
- *Avoid placing soft items in your baby's crib* This includes items such as quilts, pillows, comforters, sleeping bags, sheepskins, and soft toys.
- *Make sure your baby's mattress is clean* Keep the mattress, dry, firm, and well aired.
- *Take care if you share your bed* If you want to share your bed with your baby, make sure that she doesn't sleep on soft surfaces and can't get buried under any loose coverings. Also, don't share your bed with your baby if you smoke or have drunk alcohol or taken illegal drugs, as these can all increase the risks of SIDS.
- *Don't fall asleep nursing your baby* Or while holding her on a sofa or armchair.
- *Let your baby sleep in the same room as you* Having your baby close is best for the first six months, or you can use a baby monitor.
- *Don't smoke* And always keep your baby out of smoky atmospheres.
- *If your baby is unwell, seek advice promptly* For signs that your baby needs to be taken to the doctor, see box, right.

SAFEGUARDING YOUR BABY'S HEALTH

After your baby's birth, you'll be invited to take her to see a nurse or pediatrician for development checks at regular intervals. Your baby's first health check will be when she's around 2 weeks old, and then at 2, 4, 6, 9, and 12 months. At each visit your baby's weight, height, and head circumference will be measured to make sure she's growing properly. The purpose of the checks is to detect as early as possible any problems that may affect your child's health and development. They also provide an opportunity to discuss any concerns you may have about your baby's health and well-being.

At the age of 8 weeks, most babies start their routine immunization schedules. At this age, babies are usually given initial vaccines against diphtheria, tetanus, pertussis (whooping cough), polio, and one type of meningitis, caused by Haemophilus influenza type B (Hib). Subsequent doses and other vaccines are given at ages 4, 6, 12, and 18 months, as well as in later childhood. Your pediatrician will discuss any possible side effects of immunizations before they are given.

HEALTH FIRST

Symptoms Babies often have minor illnesses, and new parents sometimes find it hard to tell whether medical help is needed. Below are some guidelines for when to call the pediatrician—these are slightly different for newborns (see page 360)—but if you're ever in doubt, always err on the side of caution. Seek help if your baby:

- Has convulsions (fits) or is floppy.
- Has difficulty breathing, turns blue, or has stopped breathing.
- Cannot be wakened or is unusually drowsy or unresponsive.
- Has severe vomiting or diarrhea, appears to be in severe pain, or passes blood in her stools.
- Refuses to feed twice in a row.
- Develops a purple-red rash, similar to bruises, anywhere on the body.
- Has a high fever—a body temperature above 100.4°F (38°C).
- Has a high pitched or unusual cry, or screams or cries inconsolably.

PICKING UP YOUR BABY

It's natural to feel a little nervous when you first pick up your baby, but she's tougher than you think. You do, however, need to support her head.

Support your baby Slide one hand under her head **1** and the other beneath her back and bottom.

Bring her to your chest As you stand upright, bring your baby close **2**. Keep her head slightly raised.

Rest her in your arms Slide the hand under her bottom up to her head. Bend your other arm so that her head rests in your elbow **3**. Use your free hand for support.

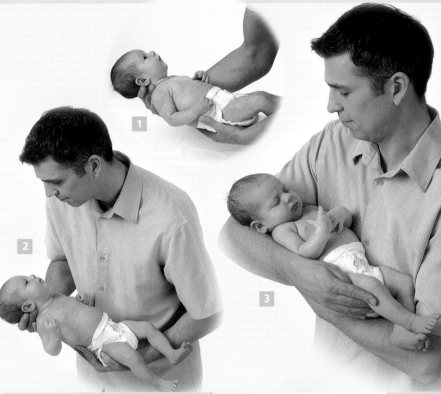

HOLDING YOUR BABY

Your young baby can appear fragile, but you shouldn't be afraid to hold her firmly. Babies like to feel secure when they are held and yours will enjoy the closeness and warmth of your body. As well as being cradled in your arms, she may enjoy these holds:

Face down Position your baby's head just over the crook of your elbow with your forearm supporting the length of her body **1**. Place your other hand between her legs so that you can support her tummy.

Against your shoulder Holding your baby upright allows her to feel and hear your heartbeat. Use one hand to take your baby's weight under her bottom **2**, and the other to support her head and neck.

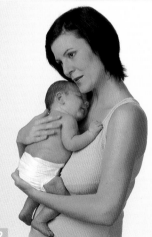

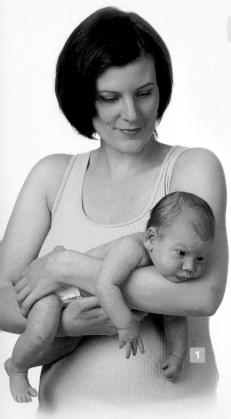

Until the cord stump falls off you only need to wash your newborn's face, neck, hands, feet, genitals, and bottom each day.

To give her a sponge bath, have on hand a bowl of cooled, boiled water, some cotton balls or a soft cloth, and a soft towel. To avoid the spread of infection, always use a fresh cotton ball or cloth for each part of your baby's body. If she gets cold, keep her diaper on while you clean her top half, then put an undershirt on her while you clean her bottom half.

CARE OF THE CORD

Until the cord stump falls off, wash it each day to prevent infection. Incorporate this into your sponge-bath routine. To clean the cord, dip a cotton ball into the cooled, boiled water, then wipe the stump and the area around it gently. Dry thoroughly with fresh cotton.

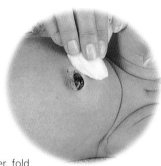

When putting on your baby's diaper, fold it back below the stump to keep it dry from urine. If the area around the stump is red or there is any discharge, consult your healthcare provider.

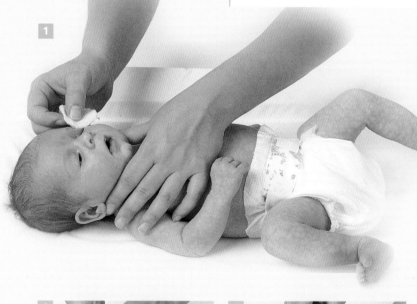

Clean your baby's face Dip a cotton ball in the water and wipe one of your baby's eyes, moving from the inner to the outer corner **1**. Using a fresh cotton ball or cloth, repeat on the other eye. Using more moistened cotton balls or cloths, wipe the rest of her face, including her nose and ears—but avoid wiping inside these sensitive areas. Clean in her neck creases, then gently pat her skin dry.

Clean your baby's hands and arms Gently unclench each of your baby's hands and wipe clean **2**, particularly between her fingers. Lift her arms and, using fresh cotton balls, wipe the armpit areas. Pat these areas dry with a cloth or towel.

Clean your baby's feet Use more moistened cotton balls to wipe the top and bottom of your baby's feet and between her toes **3**. Dry each foot carefully.

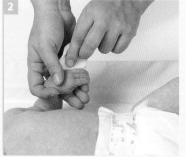

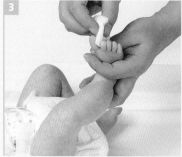

Remove your baby's diaper If your baby has had a bowel movement, take her diaper off slowly using the front to remove as much of the mess as possible **4**. Fold the diaper over, place in a plastic bag and put it aside for later disposal.

Clean her tummy and legs Holding your baby firmly but gently, moisten a cotton ball and wipe her tummy area. Using fresh cotton balls, clean along the folds of your baby's legs **5**. Wipe downward and away from her body to avoid transmitting any infections to her genital area.

CARING FOR A CIRCUMCISED BOY

If your baby boy has been circumcised, avoid giving him a bath until the wound has healed. If he has a dressing, you may need to apply a new one when you change his diaper for the first day or two. Use a light dressing such as gauze and put petroleum jelly on the gauze so that it won't stick to his skin.

It will probably take around 7 to 10 days for the wound to heal. During this time the tip of the penis may be red and raw, and there may also be a yellow secretion. It may even become ulcerated if it comes in contact with wet diapers. If there's persistent bleeding, fever, pus-filled blisters, or swelling, consult your baby's pediatrician.

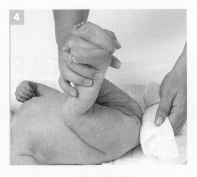
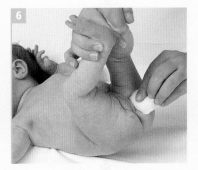
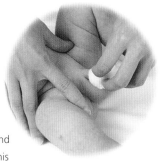

Clean her genitals and bottom
When cleaning a girl, hold her ankles gently with one hand, put your finger between her ankles, and lift her bottom slightly. Using fresh cotton balls, clean the outer lips of her vulva—but don't clean inside **6**. Always wipe downward when cleaning her genitals so that you don't transfer bacteria from her anus to her vagina. Then, keeping her bottom raised, clean her buttocks using fresh cotton balls. Clean the backs of her thighs and up her back if necessary. Dry the whole area thoroughly.

CLEANING A BABY BOY

Your baby boy may urinate when you remove his diaper, so do so slowly. Clean this area thoroughly. Dry.

Using fresh cotton, wipe his penis using a downward motion—don't pull the foreskin back. Clean around his testicles as well. Holding your baby's ankles, lift his bottom gently, and clean his anal area, and the backs of his thighs. Pat the whole area thoroughly dry.

GIVING A TUB BATH

Most babies love bath times but, as your baby won't be getting very dirty, she won't need a bath more than about once a week. As some babies do feel the cold, it's best to warm the room and have everything ready before you start. You'll need two soft towels, a bowl of cooled, boiled water for washing her face, cotton balls, non-sting baby shampoo, a plastic baby bathtub or basin, and a clean diaper and clothes.

FILL THE TUB AND TEST

Place the tub on a secure surface, and make sure that it won't slip. Try to keep the tub away from drafts.

To avoid scalding, always put cold water in the tub first then add the hot water. Mix thoroughly and check the water with your elbow or the inside of your wrist to make sure that it's comfortably warm—it should be about body temperature.

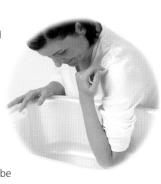

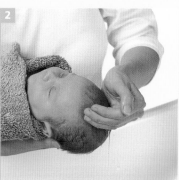

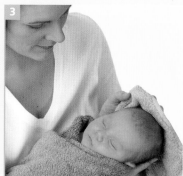

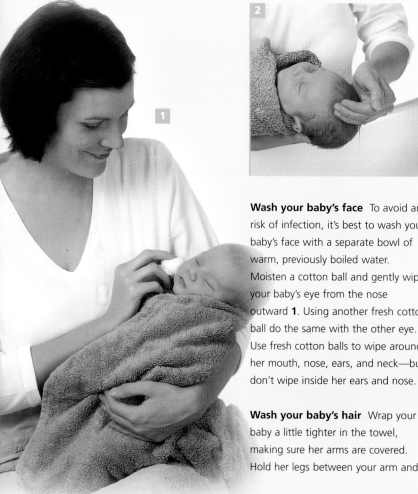

Wash your baby's face To avoid any risk of infection, it's best to wash your baby's face with a separate bowl of warm, previously boiled water. Moisten a cotton ball and gently wipe your baby's eye from the nose outward **1**. Using another fresh cotton ball do the same with the other eye. Use fresh cotton balls to wipe around her mouth, nose, ears, and neck—but don't wipe inside her ears and nose.

Wash your baby's hair Wrap your baby a little tighter in the towel, making sure her arms are covered. Hold her legs between your arm and side so you can grip them under your armpit. Support her body along the length of your forearm and her head with your hand. Bring her over to the bathtub or basin. Use your free hand to take some of the water over her hair. Gently apply some nonirritating baby shampoo to her scalp. Rinse it off with handfuls of water **2**.

Dry your baby's hair Pat—rather than rub—your baby's hair dry using the edge of another soft towel **3**. Don't press the soft fontanels too hard and avoid covering her face, as she might panic and cry.

SAFETY FIRST

SAFETY FIRST

Stay with your baby Bath your baby in a baby bathtub until she can sit up on her own. Never leave her alone, even for a minute—babies can drown in a couple of inches of water. If you have to leave the room, wrap your baby up and take her with you.

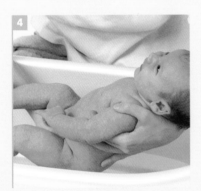

Place your baby in the tub Unwrap your baby. Place one arm behind her back and grip the arm farthest from you. Support her legs and bottom with your other hand and gently lower her into the tub **4**.

Wash your baby's body Supporting your baby's head and shoulders with one hand, wash her body with the other **5**. Pay particular attention to the areas under her arms and at the top of her legs. However, at this young age, she won't need much washing. As she gets older, you'll need to move her around a bit more to clean her more thoroughly.

Lift your baby out To remove your baby from the tub, keep one arm around her shoulder and slide the other hand under her bottom. Lift her out of the water in the same position as you put her in.

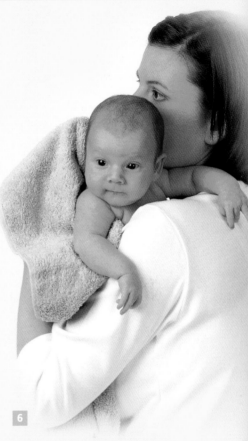

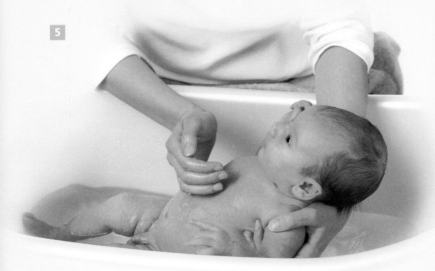

Dry your baby As soon as you've lifted your baby out of the tub, place her on a large, soft towel. Fold over one side and then the other, but avoid covering her face. Gently pat her dry **6**, paying particular attention to her neck, under her arms, and around her legs, genitals, and bottom.

Dress your baby Once your baby is dry, put on a clean diaper. Then dress her, while keeping exposed parts of her body covered with the towel.

PUTTING ON A DIAPER

To avoid diaper rash and to keep your baby comfortable, try to change her diaper as soon as it's wet or soiled. You can change your baby sitting down on the floor or on a changing table. If you use a table, always keep one hand on your baby, and never leave her alone.

When removing a soiled diaper, use the front to clean up as much mess as possible. Once it's off, clean your baby thoroughly as you would when giving her a sponge bath (see page 312).

Cloth diapers can be folded in a variety of ways to suit your baby; the rectangle fold outlined right is suitable for a newborn.

Fold the diaper Form a rectangle by folding the diaper in half. Fold one of the short sides a third of the way down. For a girl put this thicker area under the bottom **1**. For a boy, position the thicker part at the front. Align your baby's waist with the edge.

Fold the cloth between the legs Pull the corners of the diaper up between your baby's legs **2**.

Pin the sides Pin one side of the cloth, keeping one hand underneath the diaper to protect your baby's skin. Adjust the fit, then pin the other side **3**. As cloth diapers aren't waterproof, you'll need to fit plastic pants on top.

WASHING DIAPERS

Fill two buckets with sterilizing solution. Soak urine-soaked diapers in one and soiled diapers in the other. Leave to soak for at least 6 hours.

When you're ready to wash the diapers, remove them from the buckets using tongs. Rinse them and then wash in your washing machine, following the manufacturer's instructions. Dry them outdoors or tumble dry to keep them soft.

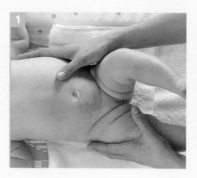
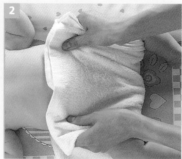
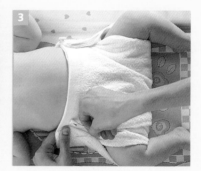

USING A DISPOSABLE DIAPER

Disposable diapers are quick and easy to fit. Although designs vary, most can be fitted in the following way.

Place the diaper under your baby Slide the opened diaper under your baby's body, lifting your baby's legs up by the ankles.

Fold and fasten Bring the front of the diaper up between the legs. Unpeel the tabs and bring the sides across to stick to the front.

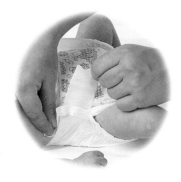

PUTTING ON AN UNDERSHIRT

Your baby will probably enjoy the contact she has with you while you dress her. If she's less enthusiastic, make dressing fun, with smiles and cuddles. Save time by gathering her clothes together before you start. When putting on an undershirt, try to keep the fabric clear of her face.

Open the neck Stretch the neck opening wide, and place the back of it at the crown of your baby's head **1**.

Pull it over your baby's head Gently pull the undershirt over her face, being careful not to pull her nose or ears. Adjust the fabric **2**.

Fit the sleeves Reach down through one sleeve. Hold your baby's wrist and guide it through the sleeve. Pull the sleeve down with the other hand **3**. Repeat with the other side, and pull down the undershirt.

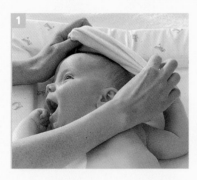
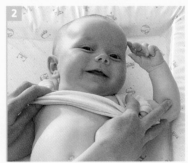
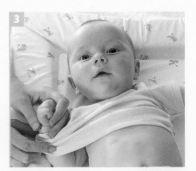

PUTTING ON A STRETCH SUIT

Open all the fasteners of the stretch suit before you start, then lay your baby on top of the opened suit.

Insert your baby's legs Gather the leg material and slide it over her foot **1**. Pull the material up her leg. Repeat with the other leg.

Insert your baby's arms Gather up one sleeve, and slide it over her wrist **2**. Repeat on the other side.

Fasten the suit Straighten the sides **3**, then do up the fasteners, starting from the bottom and working up.

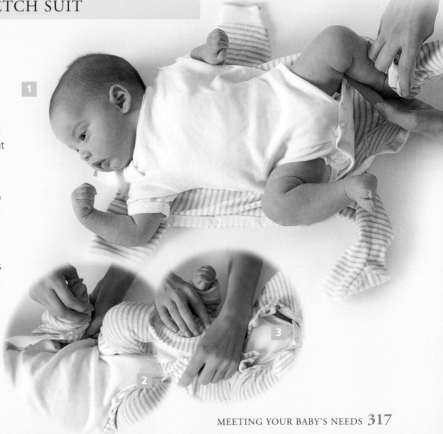

IN THE CAR

An infant car seat will provide the best protection for your baby when in a car. However, recent surveys have shown that the majority of car seats are wrongly fitted. Follow the manufacturer's instructions carefully, and make sure that the seat fits your make of car—some require a special anchorage system.

Fit the car seat Infant car seats are best placed on the rear seat, but some are suitable for the front passenger side, provided there is no air bag fitted. Your baby should face the rear until she's old enough and strong enough to control her neck, at about one year of age. Strap the seat in place, checking that the straps aren't twisted. The seat belt buckle must not rest on the frame. Check that the belts are tight enough to prevent excessive movement.

Strap your baby in the seat Place your baby in the seat and fasten the straps securely. As you're driving, keep checking your baby. If the infant seat is in the back, consider fitting a second mirror so that you can keep an eye on her without turning your head. The insides of cars can get very hot. Check your baby regularly for

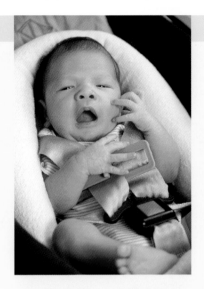

overheating and use a sun diffusion screen on the window, if necessary. Never leave your baby alone in a car.

USING A CARRIER

Until the age of 3 months, place your baby in a carrier facing your chest so that her head is supported and she can feel your heartbeat. An older baby will enjoy facing forward, looking out at new surroundings.

No matter how much support the carrier provides, always protect your baby's head with your hands when bending forward or to the side. Never leave your baby unattended in the carrier or use it as a crib.

Put on the carrier Strap yourself into the carrier, following the manufacturer's instructions **1**. Fasten one side.

Ease your baby inside Supporting your baby's head, lift her into the carrier. Support her weight on the open side with one hand while you ease her legs into the holes with your free hand. Fasten the straps and buckles, then adjust them so that your baby's weight is evenly supported **2**. When you've finished using the carrier, always take your baby out of it and put her down somewhere safe before you take off the carrier.

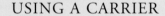

CHAPTER

15

LOOKING AFTER YOURSELF

Your baby's here at last and you're euphoric—if not a

little exhausted. You may be feeling unexpectedly

uncomfortable, perhaps even a little bit down. But

relaxation, a nutritious diet, and gentle exercise will

help your body readjust to its nonpregnant state and

give you the energy to focus on being a mom.

YOUR BODY AFTER THE BIRTH

You have, no doubt, become used to being pregnant over the past nine months and you may now feel slightly strange—both physically and emotionally. Take special care of yourself until you heal properly and then you can start concentrating on getting back to a fitter body.

The physical changes you experience after the birth can be a real shock; you'll have uterine contractions and heavy bleeding, probably accompanied by a sore, numb perineum, and rock-hard breasts. The sheer effort of giving birth can leave you feeling like you've just gone ten rounds with a heavyweight. Although you've lost quite a lot of your belly, it still may be a big disappointment—all saggy and baggy and you wonder how you'll ever firm up again. At the same time, plunging hormone levels—no longer needed to sustain the pregnancy—may make your emotional responses unpredictable. If you feel

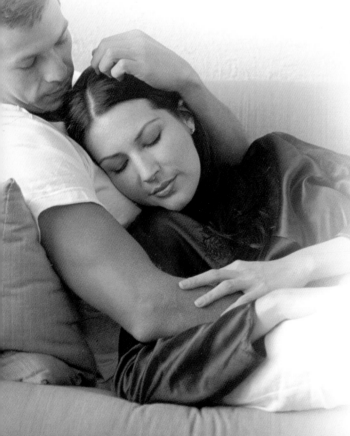

anxious and depressed, try to remember that all these symptoms will pass as your body recovers from the birth. However, it's vital to seek help if something doesn't feel right or is worrying you.

AFTERPAINS

Immediately after your baby is born, you'll experience strong pains in your abdomen, similar to period pains. Known as afterpains or postpartum uterine cramping, these are triggered by the release of oxytocin, the hormone that initiates your labor contractions, and works to contract and shrink your uterus and decrease bleeding.

A sign of a contracting uterus

Immediately after the placenta is delivered your uterus weighs about 2 lbs (1 kg). In six weeks' time it will be 95 percent lighter. If you breastfeed your baby, your uterus will shrink in size more rapidly, because more oxytocin is released during breastfeeding. By the end of the first week, the top of your uterus will be halfway between your belly button and the top of your pubic bone. Two weeks after the birth you shouldn't be able to feel the top of your uterus at all. It's an amazing process, considering how large your uterus was at the end of pregnancy when it contained your baby, placenta, and amniotic fluid. Your uterus will always remain larger than it was before your pregnancy, but once you have regained your abdominal strength, no one will know this—not even you.

Easing the pain

The discomfort from any postpartum contractions should decrease each day. If you feel you need to take some medication to alleviate the pain, ibuprofen or acetaminophen are safe, even if you're breastfeeding. Taking aspirin isn't recommended as it can increase bleeding—the drug also will pass into your breast milk and may harm your baby. If these medicines aren't helping your pain, you should notify your healthcare provider. Warm baths also can be soothing, but you may prefer to wait until any bleeding has decreased.

LOCHIA

After the birth, you will have a discharge made up of blood, mucus, and tissue from your uterus. Known as lochia, this discharge will be exceptionally heavy, since the bleeding is mainly coming from the site of the placenta. It will look dark red, be quite thick, and may contain large blood clots. It can be particularly heavy when you get out of bed.

Changes in flow

Lochia can last up to six weeks, but the flow will gradually become much lighter, while the color will change to a reddish-brown, through to a yellowish and then almost clear discharge. Use maternity pads (extra-large sanitary towels), not tampons, to absorb the discharge. At first you may have to change them every time you go to the bathroom.

Tell your healthcare provider immediately if the bleeding suddenly becomes heavier, turns bright red, contains unusually large clots, or smells very unpleasant. This could be a sign of postpartum hemorrhage (see page 356).

SORENESS AND SWELLING

After the birth, your genital area will be swollen, sore, and stretched. If you had a long, difficult labor, stitches, or an episiotomy, you'll have a lot of pain and discomfort, and the perineum (the area between the vagina and anus) may feel quite numb. Doing Kegels (see page 122), from as early as day one, will help you regain your muscle tone and promote healing by increasing the circulation in the area.

6 ways to ease perineal discomfort

1   Drink plenty of fluids to dilute your urine so that it doesn't burn as much, and empty your bladder regularly.

2   Try putting an ice pack or a small pack of frozen peas, wrapped in a soft cloth, on your perineum to decrease swelling and help relieve any discomfort. Do this for 5 minutes, every couple of hours during the first 24 hours.

3   Try squatting over the toilet rather than sitting down. Angle your buttocks so urine misses the tender spot.

4   Keep a jug of cool water in the bathroom and pour water between your legs as you pass urine and when you have finished so that there is no urine left on your skin.

5   Sitting in a sitz bath (a bowl filled with warm water) or applying warm compresses for about 20 minutes three times a day will ease discomfort.

6   Try soaking a sanitary pad in witch hazel. It will feel cool and can prevent blood from sticking to pubic hair.

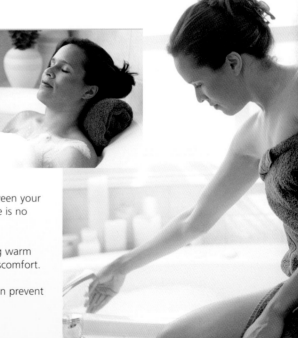

You may have some abrasions around the area of your urethra as a result of stretching during birth. These heal rapidly and don't usually require stitches, but they may sting when you urinate. If you had to have stitches after an episiotomy (see page 187) or a tear, they won't need to be removed but should dissolve within a few weeks. When you empty your bladder, urine passing over the area will sting.

Maintaining good hygiene

It's vital to keep your genital area scrupulously clean to avoid infection. When you wash your perineal area, or after you've been to the toilet, always wipe

---

HEALTH FIRST

Persistent swelling As your body get rids of excess fluid after the birth, pregnancy swelling should subside. However, if the swelling remains or if you experience bad headaches or pains in your legs, call your healthcare provider, as these are signs of high blood pressure (see page 253). If you experience swelling in one leg accompanied by severe pain, this could signal deep vein thrombosis (see page 252) so you must see your doctor.

---

from the front toward the back to prevent the transfer of bacteria from your rectum to your urethra. Change your sanitary pad every four to six hours, at least, to keep the area fresh and to check the amount of bleeding. Always wash your hands before and after you clean your perineal area and after changing a sanitary pad.

Difficulty passing water

You may experience problems urinating after the birth, especially during the first 24 hours. You may not feel the urge to go at all, or you may feel that you want to go but can't. It's essential that you empty your bladder within six to eight hours of delivery to avoid urinary tract infections (see page

259) and to prevent your bladder from becoming distended, which could cause a loss of muscle tone. Drinking plenty of fluids and getting up and walking about as soon after delivery as you are allowed will help get your bladder working. If you haven't urinated within eight hours of the birth your healthcare provider may suggest putting in a catheter (a tube inserted into your urethra) to empty the bladder. After 24 hours you will urinate frequently and copiously as the body fluids of pregnancy are expelled from your body.

Concern about bowel movements

Your first bowel movement after delivery may cause you some anxiety. If you have had stitches you may be concerned about splitting them open, or you may be worried about making hemorrhoids worse (see page 69). Your abdominal muscles, which you use to eliminate waste, may be temporarily ineffective because they have been stretched.

The more pressure you feel to have a bowel movement the less likely you are to perform. So the best thing you can do is not worry. Although your first few bowel movements are likely to cause discomfort, your stitches won't be affected, and you should be back to normal within a few days. Eating fiber—whole grains and fresh fruit and vegetables—and drinking fluids will help get your bowels moving again. Gentle exercise and Kegels will help ease any discomfort. However, if you are constipated your healthcare provider may suggest stool softeners or a laxative.

BREAST DISCOMFORT

Even if you choose not to breastfeed, the hormonal changes that prime the breasts for breastfeeding will still take place. The pituitary gland begins the process of lactation (milk production) by producing and releasing the hormone prolactin. Once this process has begun, your baby encourages the milk production by her frequent sucking. Whether you're breastfeeding or not, two to four days after the birth your breasts will become larger and firmer and may be painful as they prepare to provide milk. This is referred to as engorgement.

HOW TO massage your engorged breasts

If you're breastfeeding, your baby's frequent sucking will help diminish engorgement, but in some countries, women are encouraged to massage their breasts to relieve discomfort. Try this Japanese breast massage technique to ease any pain.

Start by massaging the base of your breasts. Cup your breasts, supporting them from below. Push your chest forward while pushing your breasts together with your hands. The flow of milk from the base of your breasts will be much freer.

Hold your left breast and gently move your hands on the breast, in a circular action around your nipple. Repeat on your right breast. Repeating this massage daily during the engorgement period should help alleviate discomfort. Other techniques are provided below.

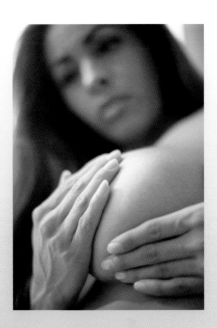

Easing breast discomfort

While your breasts are engorged, wearing a well-fitted, supportive bra will make you much more comfortable. Some experts recommend wearing a bra 24 hours a day during the engorgement period. Before breastfeeding, it may help to stand under a very warm shower or put warm compresses on your breasts. The moist heat will dilate the milk ducts and when your baby sucks, the milk will flow more freely, and your breasts will be relieved of pressure.

If you're not going to breastfeed, try putting a cool compress on your breasts and take an analgesic such as acetaminophen or ibuprofen. Don't stimulate your breasts or try to express milk to relieve pressure, as this will only cause your body to produce more milk. Engorgement lasts around two to five days—lack of stimulation by a sucking baby will gradually slow and then stop the production of milk. There's no need for special care for healthy breasts. Washing your breasts with mild soap and rinsing well is all that is necessary. If your breasts are inflamed, extremely uncomfortable, or if you have cracked nipples, see page 358 for care instructions.

WEIGHT LOSS

On average, giving birth results in a 12-lb (5-kg) weight loss, which sounds great, until you check your shape in the mirror to see huge breasts, a distended stomach, and sagging skin. However, this is exactly how a postpartum body should look. Your breasts are preparing to feed your baby; your stomach sticks out because of fluid retention and because your uterus hasn't yet contracted to its original size; the sagging is caused by overstretched skin and loss of muscle tone. Over time, your body will get closer to its pre-pregnancy shape. Your waist may be slightly bigger, but a healthy, nutritious diet and the right exercise regime will do wonders. However, now is definitely not the time to put yourself on a diet (see page 333).

SKIN CHANGES AND HAIR LOSS

Altered hormone levels after the birth can be hard on your skin, making it spottier, drier, and more sensitive. Skin pigmentation such as the linea nigra and chloasma (see page 66) should fade gradually, but some may never completely disappear. To

Recovering from a cesarean

A cesarean section is major abdominal surgery so it's inevitable that you'll experience some pain after delivery—you'll have discomfort from the incision as well as discomfort from after-birth contractions. Care following a cesarean differs slightly from that given for a natural birth.

When you can be moved, you'll be brought to the maternity unit. You may be encouraged to get up later that day, with assistance. Moving around will help you feel better and recover sooner.

Pain relief Medication will be offered to you after the surgery and for the next few days. Depending on the anesthesia program in the hospital, you may get continuous pain relief by a special intravenous (IV) line that you control, called patient controlled analgesia (PCA). Don't be afraid to give yourself adequate medication. Short-term

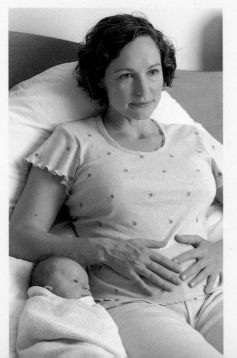

postpartum medications won't significantly affect your baby and the analgesia will help you move more and sooner, speeding up your recovery. Also, inadequate analgesia—and continued pain—can interfere with the letdown reflex if you're breastfeeding.

If you had an epidural or spinal, morphine analgesia can sometimes be given through the epidural catheter to carry you through the first 24 hours. You also could receive injections of a narcotic. After the first day, you may be given medication by mouth.

Eating and drinking For the first 24 hours you'll have an intravenous line through which fluids are given. You may have a liquid diet on your day of surgery and progress to solids, depending on your medical condition and healthcare provider.

Going to the toilet You may have a catheter inserted to drain your bladder. On the second or third day after surgery, you may find that you experience gas pains. This is because it usually takes a few days for your bowel to start functioning normally after abdominal surgery. This can add to your discomfort, but just walking around your room or the hallways can help your bowels start to work more quickly.

Care of the incision Using a pillow or abdominal binder can ease incisional discomfort. While walking, stand as straight as

possible and have someone with you in case you become dizzy. Supporting your abdomen with your hands can provide comfort.

The skin incision should heal within about a week. You or your partner should look at it daily to make sure it's healing properly. If you have inflammation or any pus-like drainage from the incision, consult your healthcare provider.

After the bandage is off, you can wash the area with mild soap, rinse well, and pat dry. For a few months after the wound has healed, you may experience a decrease in sensation on or near the scar. Most sensation will return and the scar will get less noticeable as your abdominal strength increases. It's also not unusual to experience a tingling sensation as the nerves in the skin begin to regenerate. It's generally believed that the internal uterine incision heals in six weeks.

Your healthcare provider will remove your stitches or staples before you go home or at an office visit, within four to seven days.

Returning home Most women stay in hospital for three to four days after cesarean birth. Once you're home, avoid heavy lifting or returning to work until you've had your check-up, usually in four to six weeks. You should plan to have help with other children, housekeeping, and cooking.

prevent dark areas from getting darker, avoid excessive sun exposure or protect your skin with a good sunscreen.

Stretch marks will fade in time. Retin-A cream or gel and laser treatment may slightly reduce their appearance, but before you embark on any treatment, make sure it's safe, if you're breastfeeding.

Excessive sweating

You can expect to sweat a lot after the birth as your body gets rid of the extra fluids accumulated during pregnancy. This can continue for up to six weeks. You'll perspire more if you're breastfeeding, as it speeds up your metabolic rate. Make sure you drink plenty of fluids to help accelerate the process. Wearing natural fibers, such as cotton and wool, will allow your skin to breathe. If you are concerned about your sweating take your temperature. If it's over 100°F (37.8°C), talk to your healthcare provider, as you may have an infection.

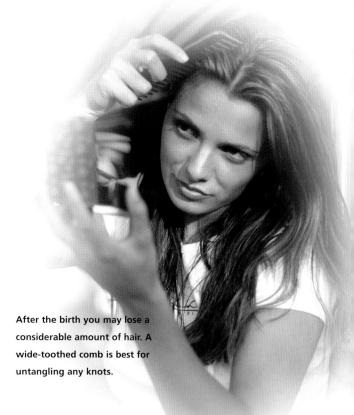

After the birth you may lose a considerable amount of hair. A wide-toothed comb is best for untangling any knots.

Shedding hair

Some women are alarmed to find their hair falling out in handfuls after the birth. This is perfectly normal and nothing to worry about. During pregnancy, hormones arrest the normal cycle of growth and loss. When hormone levels plummet after the birth, the resting phase goes into overdrive, resulting in what can seem like a massive loss of hair. However, this amount of hair is simply what you would have normally lost over nine months.

Within six months your hair should have resumed its normal pattern of growth and loss. In the meantime, eat healthily and handle your hair gently. Only wash your hair when necessary, using a mild shampoo and a nourishing conditioner. Don't use heated rollers, hair dryers, or straightening irons, as these may cause damage. It may be best to avoid chemical-based hair treatments, such as permanents or hair-relaxers, until your hair is back to normal.

BACK PAIN

This is very common after the birth and can last for months. During pregnancy your back has had to support the weight of your growing baby, as well as

compensate for weaker abdominal muscles. The presence of relaxin has made ligaments and joints looser, making you more prone to backache. Pregnancy also shifts your center of gravity, so you have a tendency to lean back and push your belly forward. Giving birth can exacerbate back problems, especially if labor is long and exhausting. If you had an epidural, you may experience pain in your lower back, where the anesthetic was injected. Once your baby's born, bending to pick him up or put him down, or sitting for long hours breastfeeding can make matters worse.

Aligning your spine

How long back pain lasts depends on your individual circumstances, but embarking on a gentle exercise program to build up muscle tone in your abdomen (see page 336) and back will alleviate a lot of problems. However, check with your healthcare provider or with a physical therapist when you can start to exercise. He or she may want to check that the pain doesn't stem from a more serious underlying condition such as a bruised or even broken tailbone.

To check your posture when standing, imagine that a wire is pulling your head toward the ceiling. Relax your shoulders so that your chest isn't too tight. Gently pull your abdomen in and lengthen your spine. If sitting down for long periods, make sure that your lower back is supported. Slowly roll your neck to the front and the side to relieve tension in your shoulders.

GETTING YOUR PERIODS BACK

If you aren't breastfeeding, your periods will probably start about four to six weeks after your baby is born. If you're breastfeeding, you may resume menstruation at around this time, or you may have irregular periods or not resume menstruation until you have stopped breastfeeding—all women are different. Like many women, you may find that your menstrual cramps are less severe than those you experienced before you were pregnant. It's unclear why this is but it's definitely a change for the better.

The amount of menstrual flow for the first few cycles can range from light to quite heavy, but should soon settle down into a more consistent pattern after that. You may find it helpful to mark on a calendar when the flowing occurs and the type—heavy, light, or spotting—to show to your healthcare provider. You also should describe any cramping or discomfort that occurs.

Choosing birth control

You will begin to ovulate before you have your first period following childbirth, so having unprotected sex could result in another pregnancy. To prevent this, you'll need to use some form of contraception as soon as you start having sex again. If you're not breastfeeding, you can start taking birth control pills about six weeks after the birth. If you are breastfeeding, estrogen-based pills can affect milk production. In which case, you may be able to take a progesterone-only pill. Avoid pushing any barrier contraception inside you if you have had stitches or until your cervix is completely healed. Your healthcare provider will be able to advise you in detail about birth control.

POSTPARTUM CHECK-UPS

After you deliver your baby, you will want to schedule an appointment with your healthcare provider to make sure that you're recovering well. This is usually about four to six weeks after the birth, but you may want to see your healthcare provider earlier if you have any medical worries, are suffering from depression, or have had a cesarean and need to have stitches or staples removed.

What the visit will involve

The purpose of a postpartum check-up is to find out how you're getting on and to check on any physical changes. Your healthcare provider will check that your weight and blood pressure are normal and healthy. There will be a pelvic exam to see if your uterus has reduced close to its nonpregnant size. Any incisions—cesarean or episiotomy—will be checked to see if they are healing properly. Your healthcare provider will ask about your bowel and bladder function, breast changes, any pains you might be having, and how your baby is feeding.

Keep a list of questions to ask at your visit. This is also the time to talk about how you're getting on emotionally, especially if you're feeling unusually tired or sad, you've experienced a significant change in your appetite, or you're just not feeling the way you expected.

You also can discuss suitable contraception. This visit is another opportunity to get any unanswered questions resolved and talk again about your physical and emotional sense of well-being. Make the most of these visits, that's why they're there.

ENJOYING MOTHERHOOD

Being a mother is one of the most important roles you will have in life and is fulfilling in a way you probably couldn't even imagine before your baby was born. Although your new baby will take up a lot of your time and energy, you still need to make time for you.

A new baby is a 24-hour-a-day responsibility, which can be a bit of a shock at first. Many new mothers start to feel that they're losing their identity in the early weeks and just see themselves as an extension of this tiny, but extremely demanding new baby. But making time for you and your partner is important, too. So enjoy all the happiness that comes with motherhood, but don't allow being a mother to completely take over your life—remember you are still a person in your own right.

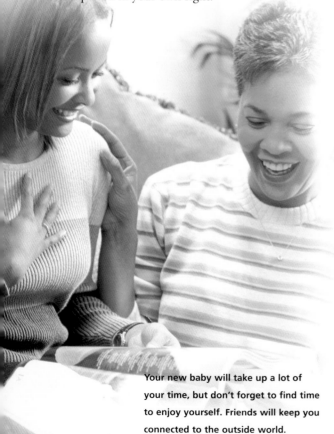

Your new baby will take up a lot of your time, but don't forget to find time to enjoy yourself. Friends will keep you connected to the outside world.

You may want to spend a few days after the birth alone with your new family before your mom and dad or other family members come for a visit. You and your partner are the best judges of your family dynamics, so talk about whether or not to have visitors, who they should be, how long they should stay, and how they can help. If you tell your family and friends what your feelings are before the birth and are very clear about what you want and need, the likelihood of rising tensions is reduced.

Your relatives and friends will all be eager to lend a hand as soon as the baby arrives and you may find their zeal a little overwhelming. Let them help you with some of the babycare chores, but don't be obliged to "play hostess"—you should be resting as much as possible. You could arrange for your mom or a friend to come in for an hour or two during the first few days to help with other household chores such as laundry, cleaning, and cooking. Or you could employ a postpartum doula (see page 184).

Don't try to force your baby to fit into your schedule—you'll find it far less frustrating to stick to hers, at least for the first few weeks. Try to sleep when she does so that you don't get overtired.

LEARN TO RELAX

As you try to determine what will help you relax, don't forget what worked for you during your pregnancy—massage, meditation, or breathing, for example (see page 124). You can modify such techniques to work for you now—choose a different mantra to fit in with the way you're feeling, such as "silence" or "energy."

Exercising on a regular basis will help you relax more easily. But don't do anything too energetic just before you go to bed—you may find it difficult to get to sleep. You'll still need to hold on to your strength for your baby, so don't choose an exercise routine that takes too much of your energy. Use this time to focus away from your daily chores and concentrate on you and the way you are feeling.

HEALTH FIRST

Postpartum depression If you are suffering from PPD it is important for the sake of your baby to get help. Many studies have been carried out into the effects of PPD on babies. In the short-term, some babies become withdrawn and stop expecting or demanding attention from their mothers. Others try harder and harder to get attention, crying incessantly and displaying anger at being neglected. More serious long-term effects include difficult and insecure relationship between mother and child and the child having behavioural problems later in life. There is also thought to be a link between PPD and lower IQ, which seems to affect boys more than girls.

Build up relationships

Another way to relax is to nurture your relationships. Your time and energy will be limited, so this may not be the best time to work on developing new friendships, but you could re-establish contact with old friends. Don't try to do too much—concentrate on the relationship, not activities. This may mean calling more often, writing letters, or inviting old friends over for a snack and a chat. Enjoying loving relationships will help you get through times of stress.

You may prefer not to leave your new baby with sitters for long periods, but as she grows stronger and breastfeeding becomes less frequent, it can be good for you and your partner to get out of the house for a short time. Find ways to fit fun excursions between feeding times, like a trip to the coffee shop or a lazy walk through the park—you can always keep in contact with your babysitter at home via a cell phone so that you don't worry.

DEPRESSION AFTER THE BIRTH

Postpartum blues, also called "baby blues," and postpartum depression (PPD) aren't the same—one is common and short-lived, the other may be emotionally debilitating and can have lasting effects on both mother and child. Being able to distinguish between them is vital.

Up to 85 percent of mothers suffer from the baby blues and it's considered by many to be normal. The symptoms can include mood changes, irritability, anxiety, confusion, crying spells, and appetite disturbances that occur a day or two after birth and last for about 10 to 14 days. Although it's not known what causes the baby blues, rapid hormone shifts and sleep deprivation are commonly suspected—all the more reason why you should nap whenever you can and try some relaxation techniques. As your baby gets a little older and establishes a feeding routine, she'll drink more and sleep a little longer at a time.

Recognizing postpartum depression

After 10 to 20 percent of all births, baby blues evolves into postpartum depression. In more than half of these cases it begins within the first six weeks and peaks at ten weeks after the birth. Common symptoms of postpartum depression (PPD) include loss of interest in usual activities, difficulty concentrating or making decisions, fatigue, feelings of worthlessness or guilt, recurrent thoughts of death or suicide, significant weight gain or loss, changes in appetite or sleep patterns, and excessive anxiety about your child's health.

PPD is often not identified by healthcare providers because, beyond six weeks after an uncomplicated birth, you don't usually see your healthcare provider on a regular basis—you're more likely to visit your baby's pediatrician. There's a new move to educate pediatricians and family practitioners about the importance of their role in identifying PPD. Don't hesitate to talk to your baby's doctor if you think you are depressed because not only are you at risk of recurrent depression later in life, but your condition may have long-term effects on your child's development and behavior.

CHECK IF YOU HAVE POSTPARTUM DEPRESSION

You may feel uncertain about whether you're depressed or not. Answer the following questions from the Edinburgh postpartum depression scale, a questionnaire especially devised to detect PPD. It's best to do this at about six to eight weeks after the birth of your child. In the past week:

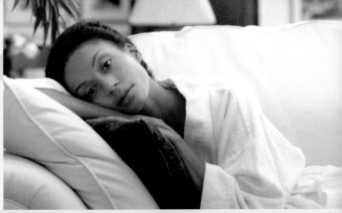

1 **I have been able to laugh and see the funny side of things.**
As much as I always could.
Not quite so much now.
Definitely not so much now.
Not at all.

6 **Things have been getting on top of me.**
No, I have been coping as well as ever.
No, most of the time I have coped quite well.
Sometimes I haven't been coping as well as usual.
Yes, most of the time I haven't been coping at all.

2 **I have looked forward with enjoyment to things.**
As much as I ever did.
Rather less than I used to.
Definitely less than I used to.
Hardly at all.

7 **I have been so unhappy that I have had difficulty sleeping.**
No, not at all.
Not very often.
Yes, sometimes.
Yes, most of the time.

3 **I have blamed myself unnecessarily when things went wrong.**
No, never.
Not very often.
Yes, some of the time.
Yes, most of the time.

8 **I have felt sad or miserable.**
No, not at all.
Not very often.
Yes, quite often.
Yes, most of the time.

4 **I have been anxious or worried for no good reason.**
No, not at all.
Hardly ever.
Yes, sometimes.
Yes, very often.

9 **I have been so unhappy that I have been crying.**
No, never.
Only occasionally.
Yes, quite often.
Yes, most of the time.

5 **I have felt scared or panicky for no very good reason.**
No, not at all.
No, not much.
Yes, sometimes.
Yes, quite a lot.

10 **The thought of harming myself has occurred to me.**
Never.
Hardly ever.
Sometimes.
Yes, quite often.

The four possible answer choices are scored 0, 1, 2, and 3 according to increased severity of the symptom. If you choose the first answer, give yourself 0 points; the last scores 3 points. Add the scores together for each of the ten questions—if your score is 12 or over, there's a strong possibility that you're suffering from depression, and you should talk to your healthcare provider as soon as possible.

What causes PPD?

Several theories exist about the causes of postpartum depression. Fluctuation in hormone levels after pregnancy is one of the most common. As yet, no one has identified a biological basis, but women can experience thyroid changes during pregnancy that, if treated, will help their depression. Your healthcare provider may suggest a thyroid test if he or she suspects PPD. You're at higher risk of PPD if you have a family history of depression or if you had PPD after a previous birth and stress from external sources, such as financial problems or lack of family support. This is important information to give to your healthcare provider—identifying the symptoms allows for early treatment, which can help shorten the course of this illness.

What treatments are available?

You may find it difficult to talk about your feelings with your healthcare provider or even a family member, particularly because there is an assumption that new mothers should be happy. Don't be embarrassed, PPD is an illness—let your healthcare provider know. He or she may suggest counseling and medications. Be certain to let your healthcare provider know if you're breastfeeding, to ensure that safe medications are prescribed. Sometimes counseling or medication can be used alone, but most frequently a combination is recommended.

9 ways to help yourself overcome PPD

1 Try not to feel guilty or inadequate. There is no such thing as a perfect parent—or a perfect child. Like all mothers, you will learn as you go along and even once you learn, don't expect perfection.

2 Eat heathily and avoid sugar, chocolate, and alcohol, as it's thought that these can all act as depressants.

3 Make time for things that make you laugh such as watching your favorite comedies. Laughter is a great way to relieve depression.

4 Try meditation or other relaxation techniques (see page 124).

5 Pay attention to your appearance. If you look good you will probably feel better about yourself.

6 Get out and about. Take the baby for a walk, or get your partner to look after the baby while you go out with a friend.

7 Join a new mothers' support group or a postpartum exercise class. Sharing experiences may help lift your spirits.

8 Don't force yourself to do things that you do not really want to do or which upset you. Treat yourself with a little kindness, and be occupied doing things which do not cause you anxiety.

9 Don't shut your partner out. Communication is very important for you both during the immediate postpartum period. If he understands how you feel he will be able to help and support you.

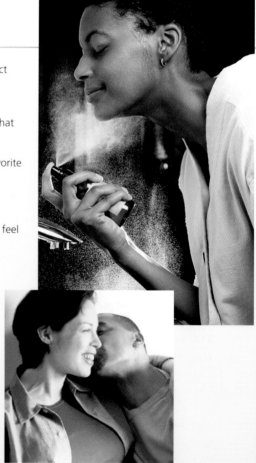

A HEALTHY POSTPARTUM DIET

You need to continue to eat well and healthily after pregnancy. It's vital to restore your nutritional status and boost your general health and well-being—this is particularly important if you're breastfeeding your baby.

Unless you've been eating exceptionally well during pregnancy, the demands of labor and birth are likely to leave you short on nutrients. You may have undergone a particularly long labor or you might have lost a lot of blood. A balanced diet is vital to maintain your health and give you the energy you need to care for your new baby.

However, the demands of your new baby may mean that you have little time to cook or to eat as healthily as you did during pregnancy. If this is the case, keep some healthy snacks on hand so that you can grab them when you get the chance (see box, page 332). Or when you do get the chance to cook, make enough for several nights and freeze the surplus, so that you can just defrost meals when you need to. It may be worth considering topping up with a broad based, well balanced multivitamin and mineral supplement, too.

NUTRITION FOR BREASTFEEDING MOMS

If you're breastfeeding, you're probably aware what a demanding activity this is. Your diet, through your milk, has to provide sufficient energy to supply the needs of your growing baby. In addition, your diet will need to contain enough vitamins and minerals to ensure your and your baby's well-being.

Your energy requirements

During pregnancy, most women build up a store of about 4½ to 9 lbs (2 to 4 kg) of body fat as a support for the extra energy requirements of breastfeeding. Even taking that into account, an increase in your energy intake now will also be necessary during lactation. Your appetite during the first few weeks after birth will be your best guide to how much you should be eating, but it's likely to be in the region of an extra 500 calories on top of the basic 2000 to 2200 calories a day recommended for nonpregnant women.

Key breastfeeding vitamins

The concentration of vitamins in your breast milk is largely influenced by what you consume. The vitamins you should pay particular attention to are:

◆ *Vitamin A* As with most nutrients, the demand for vitamin A is increased during lactation to cover the amount you supply to your baby. Most people already have a relatively high intake of vitamin A, so you should not have to take a supplement, but do try to top up your dietary intake. Some good sources of vitamin A are: fish oils, dairy produce, egg yolk, and yellow and red fruits and vegetables.

DID YOU KNOW...

Carbohydrates aren't fattening Foods such as potatoes and pasta aren't intrinsically high in calories—it's the addition of fats such as butter, oil, and cream that can dramatically increase their calorie content. If you're trying to lose weight—while maintaining energy—unrefined carbohydrates will, in fact, be your best source of energy. For example, 6 oz (170 g) of potatoes, provide very different amounts of energy depending on how they're cooked: Boiled potatoes contain 130 calories, roasted potatoes contain 268 calories, and French fries contain 430 calories. Stick to the healthier—and less calorific—option and you'll lose the weight more quickly.

- *The B vitamins* This family of vitamins is water soluble, which means that your body doesn't store them, so you should aim to eat foods containing vitamin B every day. Good sources include: whole wheat bread and cereals, lean meats, fortified breakfast cereals, fish, and eggs.
- *Vitamin C* Like B vitamins, this nutrient is water soluble, so aim to eat vitamin-C rich foods regularly. These include: citrus fruit and juices, kiwi fruit, berry fruits, green vegetables, potatoes, and bell peppers.
- *Vitamin D* Since the main source of vitamin D is from the action of sunlight on the skin, it's not surprising that breastfed babies show a seasonal variation in vitamin D levels in their blood. For babies born in fall, the concentration can decline to very low levels because winter milk contains little vitamin D. Some experts recommend that babies are given vitamin D in addition to breast milk; in other cases, breastfeeding mothers are advised to take a vitamin D supplement.

6 nutrient-packed snacks

1 Ready-to-eat and dried fruits, such as figs, apricots, and currants, are a source of iron and a good source of energy.

2 Bananas are rich in potassium, which controls water balance within the body.

3 Cheese and milk—low-fat varieties if you prefer—will help you get your calcium levels back up to prime.

4 Fortified breakfast cereals are a good source of many B vitamins and sometimes iron.

5 Sunflower seeds contain zinc, a nutrient that will help you to heal.

6 Strips of bell pepper, florets of broccoli, and cherry tomatoes will boost your levels of vitamin C to help your body fight off any infections.

Key breastfeeding minerals

If your intake of some minerals—in particular iron and calcium—is low, your natural body stores will be used to maintain your breast-milk levels. This will, of course, draw on your own already depleted stores following pregnancy, so it's sensible to try to ensure that your intake of these minerals is adequate to keep you and your baby healthy.

Your increased needs can be provided by a well-balanced diet. Iron can be found in red meat, fish, egg yolks, wholegrain cereals, spinach, fortified breakfast cereals, and legumes. Calcium-rich foods include dairy products, tofu, and green leafy vegetables. If you're lactose intolerant, however, you should consider taking calcium supplements to help prevent losing calcium from your bones.

Keep up your fluid intake

Make sure that you drink plenty of liquids—six to ten 8-oz (250-ml) glasses a day. It's especially important to drink when you're breastfeeding, as you're supplying your baby with 1 to 1⅓ pints (0.5 to 0.6 liters) of fluid each day. Always have a glass of water beside you when you're nursing, and take frequent sips. However, don't force yourself to drink too much water—drinking more than 12 glasses of water a day will actually slow down your milk production.

Any alcohol you drink will pass into your breast milk. It will alter the smell of your milk and may upset your baby. Excessive alcohol consumption may cause drowsiness, irritability, and slow growth in your child. For these reasons, it's best to avoid alcohol while you're breastfeeding. If you drink any at all, limit your intake to one glass of wine per day after feeding times.

When you drink a cup of coffee or tea or cola, the caffeine level in your milk peaks one hour later. Your baby is less well able to eliminate caffeine than you are, so it may accumulate in his system. Poor sleeping patterns and irritability have been observed in nursing infants whose mothers consume even moderate levels of caffeine, so try to drink no more than one cup of coffee or tea a day, and always at least two hours before you breastfeed.

CUTTING BACK ON CALORIES

You're no doubt anxious to get your old figure back and be rid of those extra pounds, but don't be too hasty. Diving into a restricted or crash diet is not only unhealthy, particularly if you're breastfeeding, but is also likely to prove counterproductive. If you don't eat enough calories, you run the risk of not meeting your needs for vitamins and minerals.

If you're breastfeeding, severe calorie counting will compromise your ability to produce milk. Once breastfeeding is well established, you can start losing weight moderately since this probably won't hamper your milk output. But take things slowly and sensibly. Cut back to no fewer than 1800 calories a day, and not before six to eight weeks after the birth.

If you aren't breastfeeding, you'll still need to keep up your energy requirements, but you can start cutting back to your pre-pregnancy requirement of 2000 to 2200 calories a day. Do this gradually, however, over a period of some weeks, and don't be too strict with yourself too soon.

Even if you're not breastfeeding it's worth thinking about balancing your intake of vitamins and minerals to keep yourself fit and healthy for your new baby. Pregnancy will have depleted your body's stores of nutrients, so you'll need to eat a balanced diet rich in fresh foods, to restore your pre-pregnancy nutritional status. Watch your intake of fats, oils, and sugars, and fill up on fresh fruits and vegetables. Unrefined carbohydrates, such as brown rice and whole grain bread, cereals, and pasta will give you the energy to look after your new baby.

Menu planner for breastfeeding moms

Here are a few meal ideas for keeping up your essential breastfeeding vitamins and minerals, healthily and deliciously.

Breakfast

- Fortified breakfast cereal, topped with apricots and low-fat milk.
- Boiled egg with whole wheat toast and low-fat margarine.
- Glass of orange juice and a bowl of strawberries and banana.
- Waffles with maple syrup and chopped strawberries.

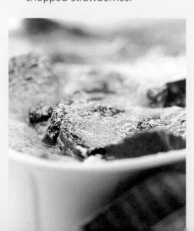

Lunch

- Baked potato with sardines and green leafy salad.
- Tuna and baby spinach sandwich with low-fat mayonnaise.
- Crêpes stuffed with avocado, red bell pepper, and feta cheese.
- Bagel with cream cheese and cos lettuce.

Dinner

- Grilled lamb steak with baby carrots and green beans tossed in olive oil.
- Steamed tofu in spaghetti with sugar snap peas and yellow bell peppers.
- White fish in a cheese sauce with new potatoes and broccoli.
- Chicken and seafood paella.

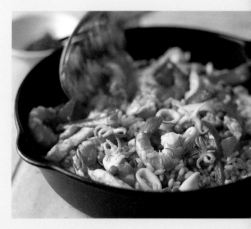

Desserts

- Kiwi fruit with yogurt.
- Blueberry frozen yogurt or sorbet.
- Meringue nests filled with apricots and half-fat cream.
- Bread and butter pudding made with panettone.

GETTING BACK INTO SHAPE

The key to regaining your pre-pregnancy figure is to combine healthy eating with a strengthening and toning exercise regime. But take it easy—your body has been through a tremendous upheaval and needs time to recover.

Some weight gain during pregnancy is healthy and necessary for the proper development of your baby. Your body will have deposited fat in response to primitive survival messages about being prepared, in case of famine, to cope with the demands of breastfeeding. Fortunately, famine is rare in developed countries and you will be more concerned after the birth of your baby with getting rid of the excess stored fat in a safe and healthy way. It's important to maintain a healthy, balanced diet (see page 331) and not start a drastic weight-reduction plan. However, excessive weight gain or prolonged retention of the extra weight after delivery can be harmful to your health.

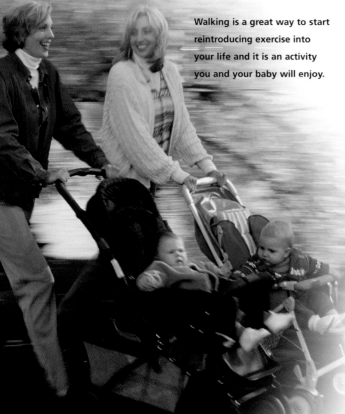

Walking is a great way to start reintroducing exercise into your life and it is an activity you and your baby will enjoy.

BEGIN GENTLY

If you're breastfeeding, your body is continuing to adjust to its new role. As a new mother your body already has many demands on it so guard against overexercising and getting dehydrated.

If you're still flowing from the delivery process, don't start a moderate exercise program until the bleeding subsides and you get the go-ahead from your healthcare provider, after your first postpartum check-up. Until then, if you feel up to it and had no complications during your delivery, you can start by taking your baby for a walk.

When you're feeling up to it, you can begin some simple exercises to target areas of your body that have become particularly weakened over the past nine months and need the most work to get back to the way they were. But remember to listen to your body—when you feel tired, rest.

Check that you're okay to exercise

Before embarking on any exercise program, you need to check that the pair of vertical muscles of your abdomen haven't separated during pregnancy. This common condition, called *diastasis recti*, occurs when the muscles of your abdominal wall separate down the middle during pregnancy to give your uterus room to expand. After your baby is born, the muscles are still quite stretched.

To check for separation, lie on your back with your knees bent. Place two fingers horizontally on your belly right below the navel. Take special care if you've had a cesarean. If you can move your fingers more than two fingers' width laterally, then you probably have separation. Recheck every three to five days until the separation has healed. If it doesn't heal within 12 weeks after the birth, contact your healthcare provider for a referral to a specialist.

Meanwhile use the "hug technique" to strengthen your abdominal muscles. Lie on your back with your knees bent and cross your arms at your waist as you raise your head and shoulders off the floor.

Exercising after a cesarean

While still in bed try making circles with your feet to keep leg muscles toned and prevent blood clots. Immediately after surgery you can begin isometric abdominal contractions. Practice holding in your abdomen, and combine with Kegel exercises for maximum effect, supporting your incision with your hands or a pillow. Avoid injuring the new incision with sit-ups or leg raises—you can begin doing more advanced exercises about four weeks later, if you are cleared by your healthcare provider.

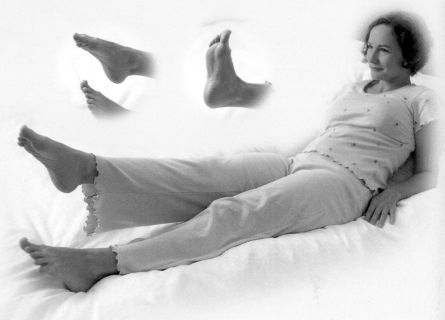

Another technique is to practice holding your abdominal muscles in during your everyday activities, such as doing laundry.

Modified sit-ups

It's important to exercise to regain abdominal muscle tone. This will improve your posture and decrease any risk of lower back pain. A little toning now can save a lot of problems later.

You can do this gentle exercise as early as the day after the birth. Lie on your back and slowly raise and then lower just your head, looking at the ceiling and keeping your shoulders on the floor. Don't do this from your bed, you need to lie on a firm surface. You also can try isometric exercise: contracting your abdominal muscles and then releasing. This exercise is recommended because it doesn't strain your muscles.

Pelvic-floor exercises

Your pelvic-floor muscles will probably be quite sore immediately after delivery, but as soon as you feel up to it you can start a few gentle exercises. The sooner you start, the sooner your vaginal muscles will be strengthened. Clench your pelvic-floor muscles ten times in succession. You'll find the exercise easier each time you do it. If you're experiencing perineal pain, clenching your pelvic floor and maintaining the clench as you sit down will make it more comfortable to sit. The sore perineal muscles will be drawn upward and inward, and the pressure of the chair or bed will be directed onto the muscles of your buttocks. Most of the swelling will go down within a few days and the soreness will subside in about a week.

Pelvic-floor exercises should become a part of your regular exercise program for the rest of your life—they will help decrease your risk of developing urinary incontinence now and in the future and will help maintain your vaginal tone after menopause.

RESUMING AN EXERCISE ROUTINE

After a straightforward, uncomplicated birth, you can usually start an aerobic exercise program in about six to ten weeks. If you had a cesarean section, you may need at least ten weeks to heal and not feel

Work out with your baby

These exercises will help you tone up the usual stubborn places and get your body on the road to recovery. However, don't do any that you think might cause you pain.

Remember to warm up with 5 minutes of gentle aerobic exercise, such as walking, before you work your muscles. Make sure that you breathe throughout each activity—don't hold your breath. And sip water before, during, and after your workout.

Arms Place your baby on the floor. Kneel in front of him, and place your hands on either side **1**. Keeping your abdominals pulled in, bend your elbows and slowly lower your face toward your baby **2**. Then straighten, without locking your elbows straight. Try doing ten at a time and then rest for a few minutes. Repeat your session of ten, two more times.

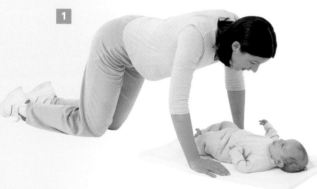

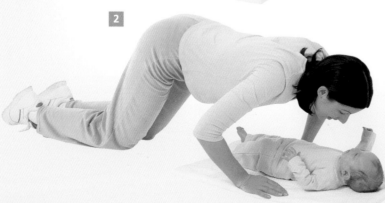

Buttocks Stand facing a wall and place your hands against it for support **1**. Squeeze your buttocks, then keeping your back straight and your abdominals tight, lift your right leg behind you slowly **2**. Hold briefly, then return to standing. Repeat until your buttocks start to get tired. Change legs.

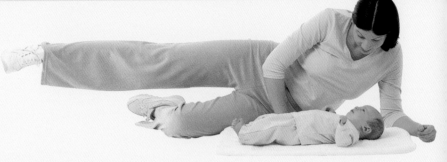

Thighs Lie on the floor on your side, beside your baby. You can then do leg extension exercises while your baby either sleeps or watches you. Lying on your left side with your legs straight, lift your right leg up a little, slowly, ten times. Repeat with your top leg bent and then switch sides.

Abdominals This is a great way to improve the strength in your abdominal muscles and your baby will enjoy the contact he has with you. Lie on your back, and place your baby carefully on your abdomen with your knees bent to support his head. Grab your thighs on either side of your baby and slowly raise your head and shoulders off the floor. Try to keep your neck straight and don't bring your chin into your chest. Repeat ten times, rest, and do two more sets of ten.

USING YOUR BABY AS A WEIGHT

This exercise works all the major leg and buttock muscles as well as working the arms and chest as you push your baby outward and back in toward you. Place one arm underneath your baby's bottom and through his legs, using your other arm to steady him **1**. Or hold your baby firmly under his arms and in close to your chest. Stand with your back straight and your feet hip-width apart **2**. Step forward with your right foot into a small lunge position. Then extend your arms out straight holding your baby **3**. Pull him back in and straighten up. Repeat ten times on each leg.

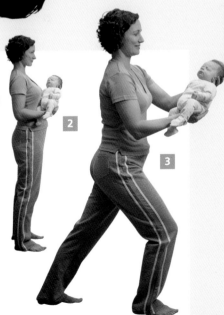

sore from the incision. When your healthcare provider thinks that you're ready, you can start your exercise program.

Remember to start slowly. You should wear a good support bra—not a sports bra, as this binds the breasts and may hinder lactation—or wear two bras so that your heavy, and possibly tender, breasts are supported during the activity. If you're breastfeeding, you may want to exercise after you feed your baby or after you express milk so that your breasts aren't full. Try not to do anything too strenuous until you've stopped breastfeeding completely because lactic acid—a by-product of exercise—can build up in your milk.

Warming up and cooling down

Don't forget that every aerobic activity must have a good 5- to 10-minute warm-up and cool-down, so you may have to adjust your total activity time accordingly. You can incorporate stretching and relaxation exercises as a warm-up and cool-down to muscular conditioning activities or to your aerobic conditioning work out.

Building strength and endurance

The advantage of muscle conditioning exercises is that they can be done in the privacy of your own home. Exercises that target particular areas of concern are provided on the following pages.

If you have a sitter, and have access to a fitness club, you may want to start a muscle-conditioning program at the gym. You may even be able to find a fitness club that offers childcare while you exercise, and some gyms have special postpartum exercise programs. If you prefer to start a weightlifting program, either with free weights or gym equipment, safety and proper technique are most important. Speak to a qualified instructor to find out exercises that will be safe for you to do. Keep the weights low—you should be able to lift them for two sets of 12 to 15 repetitions comfortably.

Improving your heart and lung fitness

As during pregnancy, you should use the FITT principle (see page 121) when you're considering your aerobic exercise program. Depending on how you're feeling and how much time you have, start by exercising three times a week. You can then slowly increase your schedule to a maximum of five times a week. If you find that you're getting too tired, decrease back to three times. You should exercise every other day to allow your body to recover after the workout, especially if you're breastfeeding. Remember to sip water before, during, and after activity—if you don't replenish your fluids, you may suffer from dehydration and be unable to produce as much breast milk.

Begin your first cardiovascular session with 15 minutes of activity at your target heart rate (see page 121). You can then increase your time by 5 minutes every week. Most people use 40 minutes to one hour as a maximum target time for working out. However, if you get tired or only have time for 20 minutes of activity at your target heart rate, work yourself up to that level and then maintain it.

When choosing your aerobic activity, you could pick up your favorite activity again or start a new one. You may want to start with an activity in which your body weight is supported, such as biking, swimming, or aquafit classes. However, don't get back in the water until lochia (see page 321) has stopped or until your cesarean incision has healed. Whatever aerobic activity you choose, don't attempt too much too soon—let your body be your guide.

SAFETY FIRST

Signs you should stop As with any exercise, you may experience some soreness until your conditioning returns. You shouldn't, however, experience any pain. If you do, or if you feel dizzy or faint, you should stop. If pain or dizziness persists, call your healthcare provider.

16 CHAPTER

ENJOYING PARENTHOOD

Becoming a parent affects you in ways you can't imagine, and the learning curve in the first few weeks is particularly steep, as you adjust to the realities of having a new baby at home. Everyone has to learn to be a parent, but if you stay as calm, cool, and collected as possible, you'll soon find you'll adopt the role with ease.

EARLY DAYS AS A PARENT

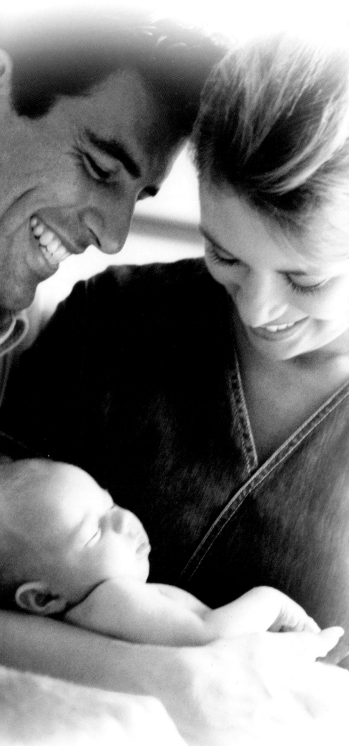

Adjusting to a new arrival might not always go according to plan—family life with a new baby takes a lot of getting used to, and there are no universal signposts for success.

On top of the physical after-effects of the birth, you're bound to experience a whole range of emotions—some of which may not be quite what you expected. Some parents, buoyed up by joyful emotions and an "easy" baby, launch into parenthood with great enthusiasm and ease, while others are more cautious now that the reality of being a parent is upon them. Everybody is different.

WHAT MIGHT THE EARLY DAYS BRING?

In addition to coping with physical discomforts, such as episiotomy stitches or a cesarean scar (see page 324), your regular routine will be affected immediately by the following:

- *A sense of responsibility* It suddenly dawns on you that you are now in charge of a helpless being who is totally dependent on you to feed her, change her, bath her, care for her, diagnose any problems, and love her.
- *A lack of routine* Your day was reasonably predictable before the birth, but now it's topsy-turvy, as you lurch from one feed or one diaper change to the next. You'll soon establish a new routine around your baby's needs but, in the meantime, accept that your life will be chaotic.
- *New demands* Looking after your new baby is extremely draining, both physically and mentally. Lack of your usual amount of sleep, the effort of learning new skills, and the new worries of parenthood, can put you and your partner under considerable physical and mental stress.
- *Visitors* Everyone wants to see the new arrival and you'll probably get terrific pleasure from showing her off to friends and relatives. However, this may mean that you have little free time to rest and to recharge your batteries.

- *A change of lifestyle* Perhaps you held down a full-time job before the birth, and maybe you and your partner often went out without planning ahead. You're now in a new phase, one in which you both have to sacrifice personal freedoms because there is an extra person to consider.
- *A period of adjustment* Like any parent you want to do a good job, to get things right for your baby. Be patient with yourself, however, and don't let the occasional minor upset rock your confidence in your abilities. You'll soon adapt to these changes in your life, and within a few weeks you'll wonder what you did with all that free time you used to have. The "downs" of parenthood will quickly be submerged by the "ups."

Highs and lows

One minute you may feel excited because your baby gulped down her milk without complaint, while the next you may be tearful because she is crying and you don't know what could be troubling her. At times, you might feel uncertain, vulnerable, even overwhelmed, but don't worry—minor mood swings like these are commonplace.

Small wonder, then, that almost four out of five women—and some men—have mild feelings of depression and anxiety in the first few weeks following their baby's birth. Known as the "baby blues" (see page 328), these emotions are so widespread that they are regarded as entirely normal. Depressed feelings may be connected to the huge drop in pregnancy hormones in your body following the birth, but they also are a predictable reaction to the huge responsibility of caring for a new baby, as well as the other changes to your body and lifestyle. Whatever the cause, the baby blues should soon pass as your confidence in yourself as a parent grows.

To help you cope with your fast-changing emotions, don't keep them bottled up, share your feelings with your partner or a close friend. Also, try to spend some time doing things that you enjoy,

such as watching a funny movie, reading a good book, having a friend to visit, or lazing in the bath and pampering yourself.

Reactions to the birth

Many women react to the birth itself in ways that they didn't expect. Some find that the experience didn't quite meet their expectations, and this response is often more marked when the birth didn't go exactly according to plan—for instance, because forceps had to be used. Any interruption to a smooth delivery can be traumatic—even when the baby arrives safe and well—and this can leave you feeling unsettled. Some women experience feelings

HEALTH FIRST

Postpartum depression (PPD) If you continue feeling depressed for more than a couple of weeks, it's important to talk to your healthcare provider, as it's possible that you may be suffering from PPD (see page 329). Other symptoms, which you might experience, include lethargy, difficulty sleeping, or feelings of panic, detachment, inability to cope, indifference toward your baby, or even a fear that you may harm your baby.

of failure when, for example, there was a need to use pain relief when they'd planned a "natural" delivery. These reactions to childbirth are normal and will soon pass. It may help to talk to your partner or other mothers about what you are feeling. If, however, you find that you can't stop thinking about the birth, then talk to your healthcare provider.

WHAT BEING A PARENT IS ALL ABOUT

Having a baby unleashes all kinds of new experiences, which is partly why it's so exciting to be a new parent. But alongside this exhilaration is the reality that the responsibility of caring for your new baby can be very daunting—restrictions on your time mean that you can't please yourself so easily. There are many daily decisions to be made about every aspect of your baby's life, ranging from the choice of stretch suits to the frequency of her feeds. Of course, there will be times when you're not sure what's the best thing to do, but the chances are that you'll get it right most of the time.

Parenthood is also about commitment. In these early months, your baby needs you to be there for her. Whether she's hungry, tired, bored, or sick, the fact that you're busy or exhausted makes no difference to her. Finding that extra strength to be able to care for her when she depends on you will encourage a strong emotional attachment between you and your child.

Amid the stresses and strains of new parenthood lie many moments of fun and fulfillment. Holding your clean, warm, satisfied-looking baby close to you, as she stares earnestly into your face, makes it all worthwhile. So will all the exciting new skills that she acquires over time. It's a lovely feeling to know that she's content.

You may be surprised to find that being a parent also involves discovering characteristics in yourself that you never knew you had. Many parents discover that they can do a lot more in a day than they previously thought, and that they possess a hidden strength and determination that had never surfaced before. They're often also surprised by the depth of love and protectiveness they feel for their new son or daughter.

Trusting in your partner

If you have another person in your life, then resist the temptation to keep everything to yourself. Initially, you may want to spend all of your time

5 ways for dad to get involved

1   Feed your baby. If she's breastfed, ask your partner to express some breast milk so that you can give your baby the occasional bottle.

2   Sing your baby a lullaby when you put her down for her afternoon nap or evening sleep.

3   Give her a bath. If you're anxious about holding her at first, bath her with your partner until you build up your confidence.

4   Take an interest in her playtime— sit down and have fun with her. The delighted expression on her face will be a lovely reward.

5   Dress her. Help out with getting your baby ready for the new day or for bed in the evenings. Change her diapers whenever you're around.

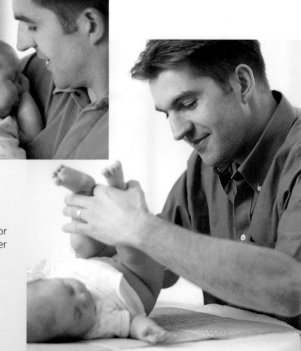

with your baby or you may feel that you are better at caring for her than your partner is, but you'll soon gain enough confidence to share the care of your baby without worrying about loss of control. Insisting that you do everything yourself can make your baby too dependent on your particular way. Bear in mind, too, that your baby learns different things from each of you. Whether your baby is breastfed or bottlefed, both partners can take a turn. Breast milk can be expressed, and both parents are equally capable of giving a bottle. The same applies to the routine caring tasks such as bathing, changing, and dressing. Your baby will enjoy love and attention from both of her parents—it doesn't have to be the same one each time.

KEEPING IN CONTROL

The reality of parenthood doesn't always match up to expectations, and you may find it more demanding than you'd anticipated. It can be hard always being on call to respond to your baby's needs—whether that's feeding, diaper changing, or cuddling. But you can be a responsive parent without losing control, without letting your baby take the upper hand.

To be in control, you should always have confidence in yourself and your ideas. This doesn't mean that you never have any doubts or that you'll never make any mistakes when looking after your baby. Of course you will—everybody has moments of uncertainty and at times wishes that he or she had done something differently. Don't let these occasional moments affect your self-confidence. You might think that every other parent is more capable than you, but you can reassure yourself that other parents have the same thoughts, too.

Always make a point of sharing your ideas and feelings with your partner or with a close friend. Explaining your ideas to someone else helps you clarify your thoughts, even if the listener doesn't offer any advice. And if advice is given, listen to what the person has to say and discuss the matter together. You may not change your mind at the end but you should feel more confident about the decisions you've made.

Making use of others' advice

Problems can arise, however, if you are showered with too many opinions—possibly conflicting—from well-intentioned relatives and friends, who are all convinced that their perspectives are best. They only want to help you, but too much advice can have the opposite effect and can totally confuse you. If you're struggling to make sense of all sorts of different babycare advice, it might be helpful to consider the following:

- *There's more than one "right" way to bring up your baby* While there are some principles of child-rearing that apply to every family—for instance, every baby should be loved—many issues come down to personal opinion. Feeding is one of these. Some parents stick to a rigid schedule while others prefer a less structured approach on this and many other matters.

- *What suits your friend's baby might not suit yours* Although your friend's baby falls asleep when driven about in a car for half an hour, the same strategy might not work with yours. Listen to suggestions from other parents, but don't automatically assume that their tips will have the same impact on your baby.

- *There are fashions in parenting* Years ago, parents believed that "children should be seen and not heard," whereas nowadays most encourage their children to express their views clearly and confidently. Views on parenting often change, and this could lead to conflict between you and your parents or in-laws. You might feel that your parents are criticizing you or worry that they will think you don't want their advice, so make sure you thank them for their help, but explain why that method doesn't suit you.

- *There's no point attempting to follow advice that you dislike* Suppose, for example, someone suggests that you should feed your baby every time she cries in order to get peace and quiet. This won't be right for you if you're the sort of person who likes to follow a more structured routine. You may follow it at first, but you won't stick with it for long. Only try techniques with which you feel comfortable.

The best strategy for coping with advice from friends and relatives—whether solicited or not—is to listen to the advice attentively, evaluate the suggestions very carefully, talk over the problem with your partner or a close friend, and then decide what you want to do.

Give something time to work

Once you've decided on a plan of action for looking after your baby, such as helping her sleep by singing her a lullaby, make sure you follow your plan through. If your strategy doesn't work first time, you may be tempted to give up and try something else. Stick with your initial idea for at least a few weeks before considering a change of tactic.

Accept that you're only human and that you won't always get it right the first time. This doesn't mean that you're a poor parent or that you won't ever get it right. What matters is that you learn from your experience. Make sure to applaud yourself when your efforts do succeed.

MAKE TIME FOR YOURSELF

Your new life can have plenty of free moments, if you know how to make them. The more you can plan, the better, so try to establish a basic routine for your days together, such as taking your baby out for a walk in the afternoons and giving her a bath or wash in the evenings.

Whenever you get a free moment take advantage of it. Relax and put your feet up—there's no law that says that you have to be on the go all the time. Make a point of having a 10 to 15 minute break a few times each day while your baby is asleep or while your partner cares for her. Use this time to do something you really enjoy. Or if your baby is settled after her feed and you feel like grabbing forty winks while she sleeps next to you, go right ahead— you'll feel much better for it. If you get a chance to practice some relaxation techniques (see page 124) in your free time, you'll feel even better.

Divide the chores

Following childbirth and with a newborn to care for, you'll probably find yourself less able to carry out household tasks that you previously tackled with vigor. Try not to take this as a sign that you can't cope. You and your partner may simply want to rethink chores and how you divide them up. Look at each of the following together and decide who will do them:

- Cooking.
- Shopping.
- Cleaning.
- Laundry.
- Ironing.
- Feeding your baby.
- Changing dirty diapers.
- Bathing your baby.
- Dressing your baby.
- Attending to your baby at night.
- Caring for older siblings.
- Doing yard work.
- Caring for pets.

If you find that you and your partner can't cope and you're feeling tired and stressed, consider enlisting some help. Don't be afraid to accept offers of help from friends or relatives—ask them to shop for groceries or iron a batch of clothes. Also consider hiring a nanny or a cleaner, even if only for a couple of hours a week. You could talk to other parents and find out how they sorted out the workload that comes with a new baby. And don't worry if you have to cut corners on the less essential household chores—no one will notice if you let the dust settle for a while—it's far more important for you and your partner to have time to relax into parenting.

OVERCOMING PROBLEMS

An infant will constantly challenge new-found parenting skills. Three areas however—feeding, crying, and sleeping—are of prime importance in your baby's life—and in yours—and most actual problems arise in these areas.

In the months leading up to the birth, you'll have been given a lot of information about different babycare methods, and some tried-and-tested techniques are provided in Chapter 14 (see page 293). However, you need to make sure that the methods you use are not only right for your baby but right for you, too. If it feels wrong, then it will become a source of anxiety for you, and, in turn, a source of anxiety for your baby. So go with your natural instincts. If you decide, for example, that you'd rather bottlefeed than breastfeed (see page 190), don't then become concerned that

bottlefeeding will have an effect on the emotional bond that you have with your baby—what matters is the sensation of relaxation and comfort that you create. Try to remember that feeding isn't just about physical nourishment, it's about emotional nourishment, too.

RELAX INTO FEEDING

Many feeding problems that parents experience in the first few months start off as very minor difficulties—perhaps the baby has trouble latching on or spits out some milk during a feed—but these can soon grow into major problems if they are fuelled by parental anxiety and tension.

Your baby is highly sensitive and will know if you are anxious—tension can cause your muscles to tighten, and if you're tense, your milk may flow less than when you're totally relaxed. This, in turn, can

HOW TO enjoy feeding time

If feeding isn't going as well as you'd like, your first priority is to trust yourself. Have confidence in your abilities, and tell yourself that minor difficulties aren't the end of the world—you'll soon establish a good feeding pattern.

Allow plenty of time for feeding so that you don't have to rush; don't schedule another task too soon after. Until you and your baby both get used to feeding, it may help to feed him in a quiet room where you won't be disturbed. Prepare yourself calmly and without hurrying, pick up your baby gently and softly. Then get comfortable in a position that suits you and your baby (see page 300).

Make sure that you connect with your baby during feeding by looking into his eyes, talking to him in a soothing voice, and holding him close against your body.

If your baby is taking his time to feed or won't latch on, take a break, and try again after 5 or 10 minutes— if you're getting stressed, it will give you both a chance to calm down. No matter how successful or fraught you find the feeding process, ask your partner to take a turn occasionally so that you can have a rest.

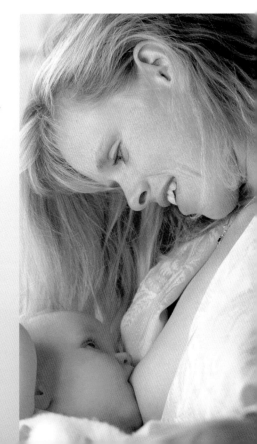

agitate your baby if he can't get enough milk and at the rate that he wants. This can set up a vicious circle, in which your and your baby's anxiety upset each other more and more, until you dread the prospect of feeding.

Assuming that your baby is in good health and that you've tried different practical strategies such as changing the feeding position or, if you're bottlefeeding, changing the formula—with the healthcare provider's approval—what can you do if feeding continues to be troublesome? Practical solutions won't work unless your whole approach to feeding is relaxed. If feeding times have evolved into a psychological struggle—because, for example, your baby feeds too slowly or feeds hurriedly then sleeps before finishing—then step back and have an objective look at the whole process.

Ask yourself the following questions: Do I look forward to feeding times? Do I enjoy holding my baby while I feed him? Does he look very settled and comfortable in my arms and when taking the breast or bottle? Does he seem satisfied when he's finished? If the answer to any of these questions is "no," it's time to consider the emotional dimension of feeding. The box on page 345 gives some ideas for creating a relaxed atmosphere and is useful for both breast- and bottlefeeding.

COPING WITH CRYING

A big challenge facing you in these early months is getting used to your baby's cries. You were so delighted to hear him cry moments after delivery, because that was the signal that he had arrived safely—but now that he's home, his crying can wear

Easing colic

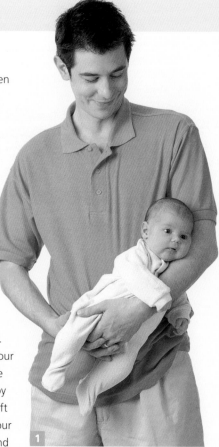
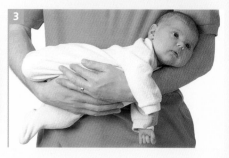
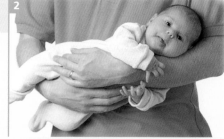

Colic is the term often used to describe piercing crying that often occurs at around the same time each evening, reaching its peak around 12 weeks old. Nobody knows for sure why a baby gets colic—explanations include poor feeding, milk allergies, weak digestion, excessive gas, and parental stress.

If your baby howls the place down and seems inconsolable, by all means call your doctor. But if you're told "he's just got colic," caring physical contact is still the best way to ease his distress.

A great way to help relieve your baby's anxiety is the "tiger in the tree" massage. Pick up your baby with his back to you and your left hand across his chest **1**. Bring your right hand between his knees and

place your palm flat on his tummy **2**. Tuck his foot under your arm and turn him over onto your hand **3**. With your right hand, gently knead his tummy.

you down. Try to bear in mind that crying is your baby's main way of communicating; it's his primary form of language and is a sign of healthy development. In fact, you'd be extremely worried if he didn't cry at all.

Your baby's crying is natural and doesn't mean that you're doing something wrong. Many parents experience guilt feelings when their babies cry, especially in the beginning, as though it's their fault their newborn is so tearful. Try to avoid such negative thoughts.

Learn to communicate

If your baby seems to be crying all the time, you can easily become overwrought and distressed yourself. In most instances, the main reason you become upset is that you don't know what your baby's crying means. You feel frustrated and worried watching his discomfort without knowing immediately what to do to help him settle. But, once you tune into his cries, you'll get to know what he's trying to tell you. Always look for an explanation—babies rarely cry just for the sake of it.

When your baby's screams pierce the air, think about what he might be trying to tell you and how you can respond:

- I'm hungry—feed him.
- I'm hot/cold—adjust his blanket or the room temperature.
- I'm uncomfortable—change his diaper.
- I'm bored—play with him.
- I'm lonely—give him some loving attention.
- I'm tired—rock him gently to help him sleep.
- I'm ill—take him to the doctor.

The common theme in all these suggested solutions is that he needs you. Of course, your being there won't stop him crying if, for example, he's hungry. But your loving, gentle touch should ease his discomfort until food arrives.

Be patient

Everyone has a favorite "recipe" for success on ways to soothe a crying baby, and some are given on page 306. It's far better to try out a new idea for soothing your sobbing baby than to sit helplessly with him.

DID YOU KNOW...

There are patterns of crying The peak period for crying is in the first three months of life, and babies cry most frequently when they are 6 or 7 weeks old. The typical baby cries heavily in the early evening, although he will also cry at other times of the day. Studies have found, too, that almost a quarter of all babies have periods of constant crying when there's no obvious reason for their tears. Finally, there are no gender differences when it comes to crying—boys and girls cry the same amount.

But whatever strategy you use, stick with it for a couple of weeks. Unless you're particularly lucky, a new method is unlikely to have an immediate effect. Only change tactics when you have seen no positive response after two or three weeks.

Your self-confidence as a parent plays its part, too. If you're tense and anxious when you pick up your crying baby—which you probably will be at first—he'll sense this and become even more tense himself. He'll cry more strongly, which will, in turn, increase your tension, and the spiral of parent–baby anxiety will escalate rapidly. That's why it's important that you try to take a relaxed approach when soothing your tearful baby. Remind yourself that his sobbing is just his way of telling you that he wants loving comfort from you. If you're becoming too tense, take a short break. Share the burden with your partner or a friend, where possible—a few minutes' respite may be all that's needed to put you in a more positive frame of mind.

If the crying occurs predictably at the same time each night, your baby may be suffering from colic (see box, opposite). However, if you're really worried about your baby's incessant distress, see your doctor.

Getting a good night's sleep

Between birth and the age of three months, your baby's sleeping habits change constantly. You'll probably long for those earlier pre-baby times when you could fall asleep at night with total confidence that you wouldn't wake until the alarm sounded the following morning. Those days are over, at least for the time being. For the first three months, your baby's sleep and your own sleep are less than predictable.

According to research, your new baby will result in your losing 400 to 750 hours of sleep in his first year. Up until his 5th month, you'll lose about two hours a night, gradually falling to about one hour a night until he's 2 years old.

Be philosophical and accept that lack of sleep is part of parenthood at this stage in your baby's life. You'll quickly learn to catnap yourself whenever you can; this can be a great way to recharge your batteries. If you have a partner, consider taking turns so that you comfort your baby one night and

your partner goes to him the next night—that way each of you gets some quality sleep at least every other night.

Your emotional and physical adjustment to this new state of affairs will be quicker if you understand that a great deal of your baby's changing sleep pattern is part of his natural development. When he's a couple of weeks old, he may only spend one or two hours awake each day; around the age of 3 months, he spends roughly 14 to 16 hours of his time asleep within 24 hours, but this is spread

evenly throughout the day and night—it's not until later that he'll start to sleep more during the night and less during the day. Not only that, research also reveals that he'll sleep for a maximum of only four hours at any one time.

This means that lots of his naps, and lots of waking periods, are scattered evenly throughout the day and night. The fact that you want him to sleep longer at night makes no difference to him.

Although they may not work immediately, you can take some positive steps to encourage your baby to sleep more soundly during the night. The following suggestions will help you create the best atmosphere for him to gently drift off to sleep:

Make him comfortable He's more likely to sleep when he's clean and dry with a fresh diaper, when his

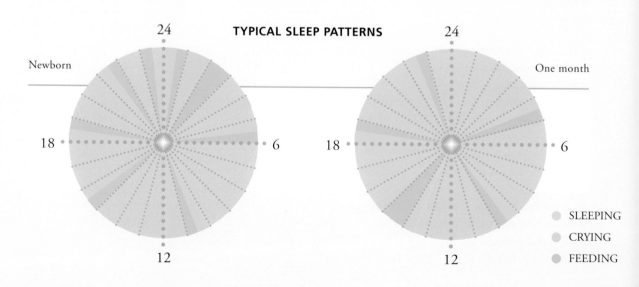

TYPICAL SLEEP PATTERNS

Newborn   One month

- SLEEPING
- CRYING
- FEEDING

RESPONDING TO YOUR BABY'S CRIES

There's considerable debate among psychologists about the best way to respond to a young baby who won't sleep. Some claim that a sleepless baby should be picked up and cuddled until he's relaxed enough to close his eyes. Others argue that picking him up each time will encourage him to stay awake the next time, as he'll quickly learn that this is the best way to get his parents' attention.

The challenge facing you is to make him feel relaxed and secure with you so that he's ready for sleep, but not so comfortable that he would rather stay awake in your company. If you pick him up every time he cries and refuses to sleep, he'll cry a lot more. Certainly, you need to soothe him when he wants to remain awake, but consider doing this without actually picking him up. The solution may be as simple as feeling the back of his neck to see if he's too hot and adjusting his blankets accordingly **1**, or relieving his loneliness by stroking his chest, forehead, and cheek **2**, playing with his mobile, or singing softly to him.

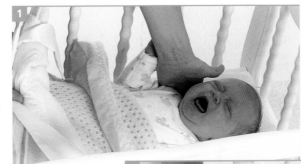

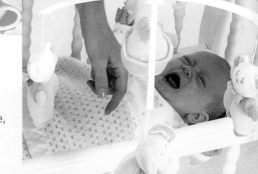

blankets are tucked securely around him, and when the bedroom is warm but not too hot—61 to 68°F (16 to 20°C) is ideal.

Provide a serene environment
He's much less inclined to fall asleep if there are loud, sporadic noises in your house. Although you don't need to tiptoe from room to room, aim for relative peace and quiet. A pleasant, peaceful bedroom atmosphere induces sleep.

Stick to a routine He may only be a few months old but he can respond to routine. Try to follow the same procedure each night before

putting him in his crib. For instance, feed him, bath him, cuddle him, and then read a story or sing a lullaby to him.

Try to be relaxed and calm This greatly increases the chances of achieving your goal. As you encourage him to nod off, your baby responds to your emotional state, either positively or negatively.

Consider feeding times Your baby will want to sleep soon after he has been fed at night. So think about feeding him after you've bathed him, changed him, and got him ready for bed.

Encourage comfort habits From very early on many babies begin to associate certain items or patterns with sleeping times. A musical mobile, pacifier, night light, or a special song played can become a signal that the baby is expected to sleep, and also provide comfort and security while he is alone.

SETTLING INTO FAMILY LIFE

Caring for your baby can be all-consuming, but it's important not to lose sight of yourself as an individual. It's also important, too, that other family relationships—between you and your partner and between your baby and the grandparents—are maintained.

Within a relatively short time, you may be eager to reestablish your own lifestyle, return to work, or pursue other interests. Don't feel guilty for thinking about yourself. Your partner or a trusted relative can look after your baby for a couple of hours so that you can spend time on your own, relaxing or going out with friends.

TO WORK OR NOT TO WORK?

Probably the biggest decision to make over the next few months is whether or not you'll return to work. Take your time thinking about this and move forward in a way that suits you and your partner.

Opting to stay at home

If you decide to care for your baby full time, this may well provide you with all the satisfaction you used to get from your job. Some women, however, worry that by staying home they will somehow lose their individuality. If you start to feel like this, focus on the fact that the job you have now—that of bringing up your baby—is equally, if not more, important than your previous one.

If you have the opportunity to stay at home, you may discover a whole new you. Many women point out how enjoyable it was discovering things with their babies and watching all the incredible changes they go through. And you can share all these with other new mothers who may become new friends.

Opting to go back

The first thing you'll have to consider if you decide to return to work is when. This will depend on how you're feeling and the arrangements you made for any maternity leave. Then, you must make your final decisions on childcare—whether a nanny or a nursery is necessary (see page 193).

When the time comes to return to work, it's the rare woman who doesn't feel a bit sad or guilty, thinking about the precious times she could be spending with her baby or wondering what will happen if she has an accident. Try not to let feelings such as these get you down. Concentrate on the notion that you'll feel more independent and fulfilled while working, and you'll pass on these qualities to her. Working will benefit your baby also by providing her with a stable financial background. And try to calm any worries that nobody can care for her as well as you can. If you've found a good caregiver, your baby will be fine.

Your baby should develop a close bond with her caregiver, but this won't affect the relationship she has with you. Of course, you need to find time to spend alone with her and build this into your routine. After you get home you can feed her, play with her, and then put her to bed—times that will be comforting for both of you.

Don't be surprised if you find returning to work very difficult at first. Many women today feel under pressure to be supermom, but accept that you will be tired and that it'll take time to get used to your workload and responsibilities at home. Now's not a good time to take on extra work or do overtime; decide what household chores you can delegate.

REMAINING A COUPLE

Amid the hubbub of this busier way of life, you need also to maintain your life together with your partner. After all, you're not just parents to your new baby—you both have your own emotional needs.

Living with a baby affects each partner in different ways. Maybe one of you now stays at home, whereas before you held down a full-time job, or maybe one partner resents the attention the other gives to your baby. Unexpressed, these concerns can create barriers between you. Honest communication is the best way to maintain a strong relationship, and for it to evolve as your family grows.

Reestablish your social life

Caring for your new baby normally leaves little energy for a social life, but make the effort anyway. When you feel ready, try leaving your baby with a reliable sitter. You don't need to go out for the entire evening at first; just taking in a movie or visiting some friends will provide a welcome break.

Be open with each other

Share your ideas about parenting with one another, as well as any concerns about your new role. Listen to your partner's hopes and fears, and make sure you voice your own. Bear in mind, too, that being a new mother is like falling in love all over again—except that the person you feel so passionate about is tiny and totally dependent on you. Even if your partner is also passionate about the baby, the apparent switch in your affections can make him feel hurt and left out—as if he no longer figures in this new relationship. The only way through this is to talk about it. Both of you should be honest—the worst thing you can do is pretend everything's fine.

Put sex back on the menu

Sex can become an issue in the early weeks. Exhausted, battered, and bruised from giving birth, it can be the last thing on your mind. Your partner, however, may feel quite differently and be very eager

HOW TO enjoy sex after the birth

If you've had stitches or are sore, the idea of penetrative sex can be disturbing. But there are plenty of other ways to express love. Kissing and cuddling sound obvious, but it's surprising how you can overlook each other's need for closeness when you're so focused on your newborn. Massage, mutual masturbation, and oral sex can be satisfying until you feel ready for penetration.

After the birth, when your estrogen and progesterone levels plummet, you may temporarily experience a loss of vaginal lubrication, as well as hot flushes and sweats. These may continue for some time. So, when you're ready for intercourse or want to try masturbation, use a water-based,

vaginal lubricant. Don't use petroleum jelly, because this is oil-based and can lead to an infection.

Make love in a position in which you can control the depth of penetration of your partner—with you on top or lying side to side—so that if the pressure becomes uncomfortable, you can ease away. Avoid the missionary position until you feel completely comfortable and pain-free.

If you have any worries or concerns about sex, don't be embarrassed to seek advice from experienced professionals—they'll be able to help you decide when you're ready to restart your sex life.

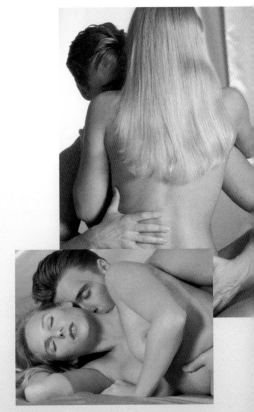

to get your sex life back to normal. Or you may feel eager to resume relations but your partner may be somewhat traumatized by what you went through to have your baby.

Although many healthcare providers advise waiting six weeks before having sex, it really depends on your individual circumstances and when you feel ready. If you had a relatively easy birth and don't have any discomfort, there's no reason to wait; if you had a difficult birth and had to have stitches, six weeks will seem way too soon. If you're unsure, your healthcare provider can help you decide.

When you do feel ready, take it at your own pace. When you're in bed together, tactfully explain what feels good and what doesn't. You don't have to go into graphic detail—gently moving your partner's hand to a particular spot may be all that's needed. If you're tense at the prospect of intercourse, you may just want to start by snuggling together—that's fine. You'll have more later on when you're ready.

Guard against feeling guilty if you don't want to make love. It's very common for your sex drive to decrease after childbirth, and not surprising when

DID YOU KNOW...

The age gap influences sibling rivalry Studies have found that if the gap is less than 18 months, your first child is unlikely to be jealous, because he won't fully understand what is happening. If the gap is around two years, sibling rivalry is often extreme. Your first child is old enough to know that a new baby affects him, and he may feel insecure. However, this age gap is healthier from a mother's point of view. With a gap of three or more years, feelings of jealousy are less likely. Your first child's life won't be significantly affected by the presence of a baby brother or sister and he'll probably be proud of the new family member.

your body's busy adapting to the physical readjustment and while you're experiencing exhaustion, lack of sleep, and the massive adaptation that a new baby demands. You may simply need to accept that with a baby needing room service 24/7, sex might not be as spontaneous as it was before.

Don't forget birth control
Ovulation can start even if you're breastfeeding and your periods haven't returned, so you need to use some form of contraception when you resume sex. Condoms are probably your best option at first. If you want to use other forms of birth control, you'll need to speak to your healthcare provider. You shouldn't take an estrogen-based pill if you're breastfeeding, as it can block your milk production (see page 326). However, it is usually safe for you to take the "mini-Pill," which contains progesterone only. If you want to have an IUD fitted, you'll need to wait until your cervix has recovered, which may take around six weeks. If you previously used a diaphragm, you'll need to get a new one fitted.

CONSIDERING EXISTING CHILDREN
If this is your second baby, the early weeks will be different from those with your firstborn. For one thing, you didn't already have another child to look after, and for another, you and probably your partner will already have experience of caring for a newborn. This will give you confidence, but bear in mind that you will feel more tired caring for two or more children.

Happy families?
With a second baby, the issue of sibling rivalry arises (see box, left). Jealousy between children in the same family is very common but it can be disruptive and cause havoc in family life. Fortunately, there are steps you can do to tackle the problem.

The first meeting of your existing child and the new arrival needs careful handling. Let your older child buy the baby a present and, when he visits you in the hospital, make a big fuss of him and try to make him feel important. Tell him how much the new baby loves him.

6 ways to encourage grandparents

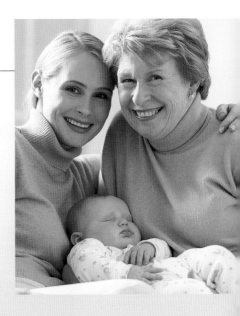

1. Some grandparents stay away from their grandchild, fearing that they'll be considered too dominant. A positive welcome will help put them at ease.

2. Involve them in your baby's care. If they are concerned that they're "out of practice," give them a simple task to start with, such as reading your baby a story. It will help them build their confidence.

3. Ask for their advice. Even though you may not agree with your parents' views about everything, they'll be flattered when you ask for their opinion.

4. Make them feel wanted. Tell them how fond of them their grandchild is and how you all look forward to their visits.

5. Don't make assumptions. It's easy to take it for granted that your parents will babysit for you at a moment's notice; they may need plenty of warning and they deserve thanks also when helping you out.

6. Conflicts frequently arise about discipline, with some grandparents being too lenient. So talk about discipline and make your expectations clear.

One strategy to encourage harmony when you're home is to get your older child involved in caring for the baby—this helps also to form a connection between them. How much your older child can do depends on his age, but you could ask him to fetch diapers, pick out clothes for the baby, or share toys. In addition, spend at least half an hour every day alone with your first child, perhaps when the baby is asleep. This special time boosts his self-esteem. Keep your older child's normal routine where possible— the less disruption, the better. And remember to continue taking days out together as a family.

INCLUDING THE GRANDPARENTS

Grandparents can be very important to a baby during her formative years. Although they are traditionally considered to spoil their grandchildren or to interfere with their upbringing, they can be ideal buffers between you and your children.

Today's grandparents are more likely to be active in later life and so can be more involved when their grandchild comes along. How much involvement your parents and in-laws have will be up to you— and it'll probably take some time before you're able to strike the right balance between accepting their help and discouraging any interference. Your baby's grandparents are probably aware of this, too, so try to discuss their level of help calmly and openly.

Grandparents as caregivers

If your parents or in-laws are willing and live close by, they may be able to help with childcare arrangements, which can be especially useful when considering a return to work. This option can save you a lot of money but does give them a huge responsibility, which can create family disharmony. You and your partner should sit down with your parents and discuss this fully as a family, sorting out as many potential problems as you can—such as how you prefer to feed your baby or put her to bed—before starting the arrangement.

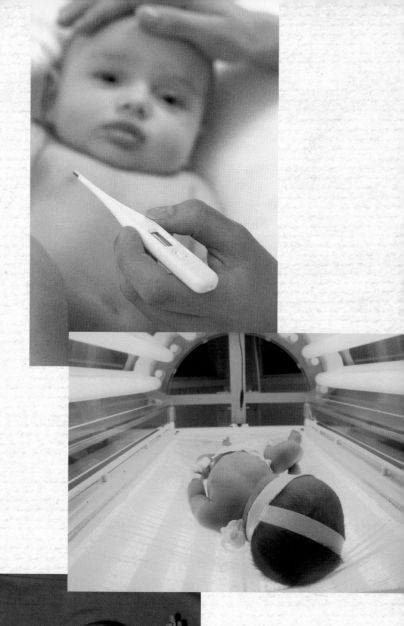

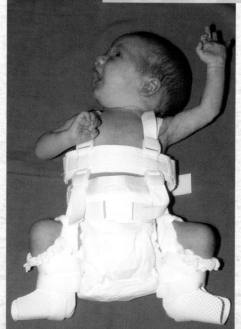

PART V

POSTPARTUM REFERENCE

MATERNAL COMPLAINTS AND TREATMENTS

After birth, many mothers experience some discomfort from stitches—if they've had an episiotomy or tear—and until breastfeeding is successfully established, breasts may be achy and tender. But major problems are normally rare. Always seek advice from your healthcare provider if you have any concerns.

COMPLICATIONS AFTER THE BIRTH

Postpartum infections

It's estimated that 1 to 8 percent of all births will be followed by an infection. Factors that increase the risk include: premature rupture of the membranes and prolonged labor, frequent internal exams, internal fetal monitoring, an infection already present during pregnancy, diabetes, and being overweight. The most common infection, endometritis, affects the endometrium (the lining of the uterus) but infections also can occur in the cervix, vagina, vulva, and perineum.

What to look out for
- Fever
- Abdominal pain
- Offensive vaginal discharge
- Inflammation, redness, and swelling

Treatment
Most infections that occur after a birth require medical treatment, usually with antibiotics. Endometritis may require hospital treatment, in which intravenous antibiotics will be given for two to seven days. Once treated it usually resolves within one to three days. Other infections may vary in their response to treatment, but most will clear up within seven to ten days. Breastfeeding can be continued during most treatments.

Postpartum hemorrhage

It's normal to have some vaginal bleeding, whether you had a vaginal birth or a cesarean, for several weeks after the birth (see page 321). Postpartum hemorrhage refers to excessive bleeding after delivery. There are many different causes of abnormal bleeding. The most common is that the uterus doesn't contract well. Other include retained placenta (where fragments of placental tissue have not been expelled) or unrecognized tears that occur in the cervix or vagina.

While postpartum hemorrhage usually occurs in the days following the birth, it also can develop several weeks later, if fragments of placenta remain attached or if an infection develops internally.

What to look out for
- Heavy, bright-red blood loss for 4 days or more
- Passing large numbers of clots
- Foul-smelling vaginal discharge
- Feeling faint, breathless, and lightheaded

Treatment
Some women are given medication for a day or two to help the uterus contract. Rest and drinking plenty of fluids also may be recommended. Anemia caused through loss of blood may be treated with iron supplements and a diet that includes iron-rich foods (see page 108).

Prolapse

During pregnancy and birth, the pelvic-floor muscles that support the pelvic organs can be weakened, leading to incontinence (see page 359) and, in extreme cases, prolapse, where organs in the lower abdomen drop downward. The most common form of prolapse is where the uterus descends into the vagina. If uterine prolapse is left untreated, it tends to worsen and a hysterectomy may be needed.

What to look out for

- Dragging sensation and feeling of heaviness in the lower abdomen
- Uncontrollable urge to urinate
- Leaking urine when coughing or sneezing
- Pain in the lower abdomen or back
- Uncomfortable or painful sex
- Constipation

Treatment

Starting pelvic-floor exercises (see page 122) as soon as possible after the birth can help prevent prolapse. Eating plenty of fiber will guard against constipation and therefore straining, which puts pressure on the pelvic floor. Mild to moderate uterine prolapse can be helped with ring pessaries —similar to the diaphragm contraceptive. If the prolapse causes discomfort or pain, various surgical procedures can be carried out, ranging from a vaginal repair to a hysterectomy.

Stitch complications

It is possible for episiotomy stitches to become infected, causing a great deal of discomfort. Bacteria can invade the site of a wound despite the best precautions and hygiene.

What to look out for

- Red, painful, swollen perineum
- Unpleasant odor from the area

Treatment

Infected stitches usually resolve with careful hygiene and frequent baths, but an infection of the perineum may require treatment with antibiotics, so you should seek advice from your healthcare provider. Occasionally, stitches come apart prematurely. Further stitches may be required, but simple hygiene procedures are often sufficient for healing to occur.

BREAST PROBLEMS
Blocked milk ducts

Anything that restricts milk flow in the breast can cause blocked ducts. They are commonly experienced by women who, for some reason, have a build up of milk. This may be caused by the production of excess milk or by a baby not latching on properly, not emptying the breast, or sleeping through and missing out being fed.

What to look out for

- Tenderness
- Redness, with or without heat
- Lumpiness, which reduces with massage or after feeding

Treatment

Apply heat, such as a wash cloth dipped in warm water and squeezed dry, to the affected area, along with massage before each nursing session to help

Pelvic-floor muscles, weakened by a rapid delivery, a long labor, or a large baby, can fail to support the uterus in its normal position so it drops down into the vagina. Other organs—the bladder, urethra, rectum, and abdominal lining— also can drop, put pressure on the vagina, and cause vaginal prolapse or vaginal wall descent. Different prolapses can occur in combination.

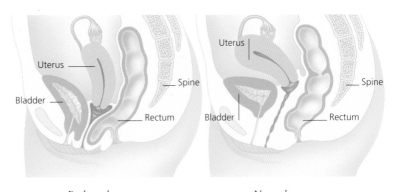

Prolapsed uterus *Normal uterus*

relieve the problem. Nurse frequently and use a breast pump at the end of a session if your breasts have not been completely emptied. Try different positions at each nursing session and make sure your baby is latched on correctly (see page 301).

Mastitis

If bacteria from your baby's mouth find their way into a blocked milk duct—often through a cracked nipple (see below)—the milk within may become infected, resulting in inflammation of the duct. This is called mastitis. The most usual site is the upper, outer segment of the breast. Women may be predisposed to mastitis by engorgement, stress, and a change in feeding patterns—for example, if your baby starts to nurse at longer intervals or is having occasional bottles.

What to look out for
- Inflamed, painful lump
- Shiny, red skin over affected area
- Feverish, flu-like muscle aches
- Nausea

Treatment
Mastitis requires treatment with antibiotics, analgesics, and the self-help measures given for blocked milk ducts. The medicines prescribed will be safe to use while nursing, because an important part of the treatment is continued breastfeeding. If there is no improvement after 24 hours of taking antibiotics, seek advice from your healthcare provider, as there is a risk of abscess formation.

Cracked nipples

While sensitive and sore nipples are very common during the first few days of breastfeeding, vigorous sucking, incorrect positioning, and milk left on the nipple can cause the nipple to crack. Cracked nipples are very painful and may become infected.

What to look out for
- Small cracks on the nipple, which may bleed
- Sharp, piercing pain during feeding
- Baby vomits blood or has blood in his diaper

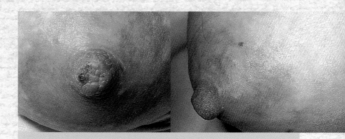

A cracked nipple (left) and mastitis (right) may make breastfeeding uncomfortable but neither condition precludes continuing to breastfeed. Cracked nipples are more common in fair-skinned women, although the reason for this is not known.

Treatment
Continue breastfeeding, making sure that your baby is latched on correctly (see page 301). Use a breast pump to empty your breasts if they still feel full when your baby has finished nursing. Expose your nipples to the air for a short while after each nursing session. Always wash your nipples with plain warm water—never use soaps or disinfectants—and gently pat dry. Clinical trials show that the many creams prescribed for cracked nipples are of little value in healing, although those that include lanolin are soothing. Breast shields may also help.

Thrush

Cracked nipples often become infected with the yeast *candida albicans* or bacteria *staphylococcus aureus*, resulting in thrush. Women who are prone to vaginal thrush yet have no problems with breastfeeding also can develop thrush on their breasts. Thrush also can be caused by antibiotics.

What to look out for
- Itchy, irritable, pink or red nipples
- Tiny white spots on nipples
- Stabbing pain deep in the affected breast

Treatment
Thrush can be passed between mother and baby, so both of you may need to be treated, usually

with an antifungal medication. Breastfeeding should continue during any treatment.

Letdown failure

If you are unable to produce adequate milk or if your milk does not flow freely, this is failure of the letdown reflex, usually a result of unrelieved breast engorgement in the first week after birth. Sometimes letdown failure occurs if a baby has problems immediately after birth and stays in the nursery, or is very small or premature and cannot or will not suck vigorously. Depression and emotional upset also can reduce milk production.

What to look out for

- Your breasts don't leak outside of nursing
- No letdown sensation (mild uterine contractions immediately after birth, then pins and needles in breast after two weeks)
- Baby seems unhappy and appears hungry
- Baby does not gain adequate weight
- Baby urinates infrequently

Treatment

Feed frequently in a quiet and relaxed place, sitting in a comfortable position with your baby correctly latched on (see page 301). Use a breast pump if your baby isn't providing adequate stimulation in terms of pressure or time at the breast. Discuss depression or emotional problems with your healthcare provider.

URINARY AND BOWEL PROBLEMS
Urinary incontinence

Physical changes that occur in the body during pregnancy—rather than weak pelvic-floor muscles, as was previously thought—are now believed to cause urinary incontinence. A common problem after a vaginal delivery, urinary incontinence may last for a few weeks or months.

Stress incontinence (a type of urinary incontinence caused by laughing, coughing, straining, or lifting something heavy) is very common and can last up to a year after delivery. It usually improves over time.

What to look out for

- Leaking small amounts of urine
- Feeling of fullness and an urgency to pass urine
- Inability to control urine flow

Treatment

Whatever the cause, regular pelvic-floor exercises (see page 122) are the best method of combating incontinence. It may take a few weeks before any improvement in bladder control is noticed, but you should persevere. Wear sanitary napkins or protective underwear to forestall leaks.

Fecal incontinence

A forceps delivery, severe tearing during delivery, or an episiotomy can damage the nerves and muscles of the anal sphincter, the muscles responsible for opening and closing the bowel. This can lead to loss of control over bowel movements. How long fecal incontinence lasts depends on how much damage has been done. Women who are affected can take anywhere from six weeks to four months and more to regain full control of their bowels after childbirth.

What to look out for

- Involuntary bowel movements
- Passing excessive gas

Treatment

Kegel exercises (see page 122) can strengthen your pelvic-floor muscles and increase blood flow to the perineum, which may help recovery. If the incontinence doesn't improve with these exercises, it's important to discuss the problem at your postpartum check-up. There's no need to feel embarrassed about it. It is far better to get the problem treated as soon as possible.

NEWBORN MEDICAL PROBLEMS

Most babies are born perfectly healthy, but problems occasionally arise and medical intervention is required. Although this can be upsetting, most problems can be treated successfully. Your healthcare providers will be able to explain any procedures that may be required.

INTESTINAL PROBLEMS

Constipation

This is the production of hard, dry stools, which may be passed less frequently than normal. It's very unusual for babies to be constipated in the first few weeks. If your newborn is constipated, vomits, or has abdominal distension, he may have a disorder of the digestive system.

What to look out for

- Hard, difficult-to-pass stools
- Less frequent stools
- Stools streaked with blood on the outside
- Abdominal pain or discomfort, leading to excessive crying and drawing up of knees

Treatment

A young baby with mild constipation should be offered plenty of extra fluids. Constipation that results from dietary changes, such as a different formula, usually resolves itself within a few days. More serious constipation, with hard, and painful-to-pass stools, requires medical treatment. Babies should never be given laxatives, unless they are prescribed by the doctor. Corn Syrup should not be given because of the risk of infant botulism, a severe infection that can damage your baby's nervous system. Sugared water should be avoided, as it can cause your baby to develop a sweet tooth.

Diarrhea

This is a sudden increase in the amount of stools, with looser, more watery stools than usual. The stools may be a greenish color and foul-smelling. Sometimes diarrhea is accompanied by vomiting.

The most common cause of diarrhea is a viral infection, although there are also bacterial causes, which can cause blood to appear in the stools. Diarrhea may also be associated with: a urinary infection; an upper respiratory tract infection,

WHEN TO SEE THE DOCTOR

Newborns can become unwell very quickly, so it is important to be aware of the symptoms that could indicate illness. If a baby develops any of the following, or appears unwell, urgent medical advice is required:

- Paleness or a bluish color around the mouth and on the face
- Fever with a temperature of 100.4°F (38°C) or more
- Body becomes floppy or stiff
- Eyes are pink, bloodshot, have a sticky white discharge, or eyelashes that stick together
- White patches in the mouth
- Redness or tenderness around the navel area
- Nose blocked by mucus, making it difficult for the baby to breathe while feeding
- Diarrhea—more than six to eight watery stools per day (see page 307)
- Forceful vomiting
- Vomiting that lasts for six hours or more, or is accompanied by fever and/or diarrhea
- Refusing to be fed
- Crying for unusually long periods
- Blood-streaked stools

RELIEVING ABDOMINAL DISCOMFORT

Massage can comfort a fretful baby. If you suspect your baby has bellyache, try the following procedure, making sure that room where you massage your baby is warm and draft-free.

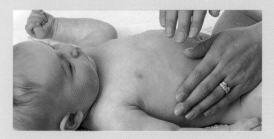

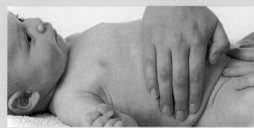

1 Massage hand-over-hand down the right side of the abdomen, from between the hip and the lower rib to below the navel. Repeat on the left side.

2 Cup your hand and gently knead the belly from side to side. Don't push downward as the baby will tense up. Keep it playful, so the belly remains soft.

3 Using your cupped hand, massage your baby's belly in a circular motion, clockwise from your left to your right. If your baby's belly is hard, gently tickle it before you begin so that it relaxes.

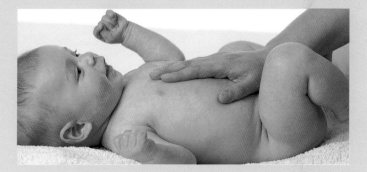

such as a cold or ear infection; or a more serious illness. In these cases it's often accompanied by a fever. Problems with feeding also can cause loose stools. Other causes of diarrhea in early infancy include an intolerance of a particular type of formula milk and the use of antibiotics.

What to look out for
- Very soft, watery, foul-smelling stools
- Vomiting
- Abdominal pain
- Fever
- Refusing to be fed
- Floppiness

Treatment
Avoid dehydration by offering more milk. You can give your baby cooled, boiled water between feeds. If he becomes dehydrated, he may require hospital treatment so that fluids can be given to replace the salt, electrolytes, and sugar that have been lost. If a bacterial infection is the cause, your baby may be put on antibiotics. If a milk allergy is suspected, a change of formula may be suggested.

Diarrhea caused by an infection usually gets better over a period of a week or so. Finding the right formula may require more time to resolve.

TAKING YOUR BABY'S TEMPERATURE

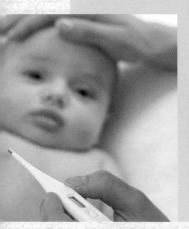

A young baby's temperature should be taken under his arm. If you're using a digital thermometer, wipe under your baby's arm to remove any sweat, then place the bulb into the fold of his armpit and hold his arm against his side to keep it in place. Leave for 3 to 4 minutes or until the thermometer beeps. Contact your healthcare provider if the temperature is raised to 100.4F (38°C) or more. Always mention that it is an axillary temperature (one taken under the arm), as this has a slightly lower reading.

Vomiting

Many babies spit up relatively small amounts of milk while or shortly after being fed, and if your baby is otherwise growing and doing well, any spitting is probably related to reflux of milk from the stomach, which will resolve itself in time. When a baby vomits, however, he forcefully throws up large amounts of milk, and he may do so quite suddenly. Vomiting can be the result of milk allergy. Anatomical abnormalities of the intestine, such as pyloric stenosis (see page 379) or a narrowed digestive tract prevent babies from keeping milk down. As with diarrhea, bacteria and viruses also can cause vomiting. If it is caused by an infection, your baby may also have a fever.

What to look out for
- Large amounts of milk being expelled
- Fever and/or diarrhea
- Persistent or forceful vomiting
- Blood in vomit

Treatment
You need to see your healthcare provider urgently if your baby has any of these symptoms so that the cause is identified quickly. If an infection is suspected, tests will be carried out and, if confirmed, antibiotics may be given. If the vomiting is related to a blockage in the intestine, an X-ray or ultrasound may be performed, and your baby may require surgery. Consult your healthcare provider immediately if your baby appears to be dehydrated, with a dry mouth and lips, lethargy, sunken fontanels (see page 283), or a dry or dark yellow-colored urine-stained diaper.

INFECTIONS AND SKIN DISORDERS
Fever

If your baby is under 3 months, most doctors would consider a temperature of more than 100.4°F (38°C) to be a fever. There are several reasons why a baby may develop a fever right after birth. The mother may have an infection that has been passed on to her baby. Even if the mother has a normal temperature, an infection can cause a fever in her baby. Less likely, a raised temperature can be related to the baby's environment: If the delivery room or nursery is too hot, a baby's temperature may increase.

What to look out for
- Skin that is warm to the touch
- Signs of a possible infection, such as a cold
- Lack of interest in feeding
- Lethargy

Treatment
No matter what the cause, an elevated temperature in a baby should never be ignored; it may be the first indication of a more serious problem. A raised temperature in a new baby usually indicates an infection of some kind. He may have caught a bacterial infection during birth or may have become infected with a cold virus from a visitor. Either way, a healthcare provider should always see a young baby with a suspected fever, as treatment may be required.

Colds

These are infections of the upper respiratory tract and are almost always caused by viruses. Colds are very common in babies. Some colds are mild and only last for a day or two; others are more severe, lasting for several weeks. Sometimes complications develop, such as an ear infection or a sore throat.

What to look out for
- Runny or blocked nose
- Clear, yellow, or green nasal discharge
- Sneezing
- Red, watery eyes
- Cough
- Fever
- Lack of appetite

Treatment

There is no cure for a cold. Antibiotics are ineffective against viral infections, although they may be used to treat any complications. A blocked nose makes sucking difficult, so encourage frequent breast- or bottlefeeding. Additional fluids should be given, as these will help loosen any congestion. Using a vaporizer or humidifier in the nursery may make your baby more comfortable. If he's having trouble breathing, his cold may have developed into a more serious problem, so contact your healthcare provider immediately.

Group B streptococcus (GBS)

Also known as Strep B, this is a very severe bacterial infection. The bacteria is found in the vaginas of approximately 25 percent of all women, but only a small percentage of the babies born to these mothers are infected. Many healthcare providers now check for the infection during pregnancy. In early-onset a baby becomes sick within hours after birth. In late-onset infection, which occurs a week or more after the birth, meningitis (see right) frequently ensues.

What to look out for
- Grunting noises
- Poor feeding
- Lethargy or irritability
- Abnormally high or low temperature
- Rapid heart rate
- Rapid breathing

Treatment

GBS is potentially fatal, so an infected baby will require urgent medical attention. If you tested positive during pregnancy, antibiotics will probably have been given during your delivery to decrease the risk to your baby. Late-onset Strep B requires immediate hospital treatment. With both types of infection, early intensive treatment could prevent potentially serious consequences.

Meningitis

This is an inflammation of the membranes that line the brain and spinal cord. It's usually caused by a viral or bacterial infection. Viral meningitis may be caused by a number of different viruses, and is commonly mild, with no long-term side effects. Very occasionally it can be severe and cause serious problems.

With a newborn, bacterial meningitis is usually caused by Group B streptoccocus. In babies over 3 months the three most common forms of meningitis are: hemophilus influenzae Type B (Hib); meningococcus Groups A, B, and C. Group B is the most common, but Group C is the most severe and can be fatal if not treated early.

What to look out for
- High-pitched crying
- Drowsiness or lethargy
- Bulging fontanel (soft spot) on the top of a baby's head
- Vomiting
- Refusal to feed
- Pale skin and cold limbs
- Sensitivity to light
- Fever and a blank, staring expression
- Stiffness of the neck
- Difficulty breathing
- A convulsion with stiffened body and shaking
- Reddish-purple spots that don't go away if

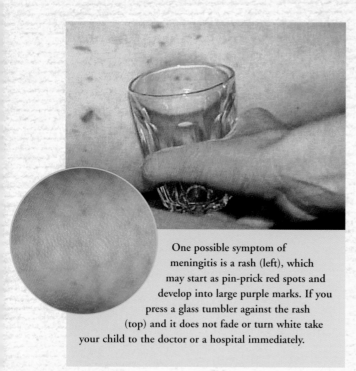

One possible symptom of meningitis is a rash (left), which may start as pin-prick red spots and develop into large purple marks. If you press a glass tumbler against the rash (top) and it does not fade or turn white take your child to the doctor or a hospital immediately.

pressed with a glass and that develop into bruises under the skin

Treatment

If you suspect meningitis, call your healthcare provider without delay or take your baby to the hospital for urgent evaluation. A lumbar puncture may be given to confirm any diagnosis. Antibiotics will be given if bacterial meningitis is suspected. A hearing test may be carried out after 4 weeks, as deafness is the most common side effect of bacterial meningitis. If the infection is viral, your baby should recover within a few days.

Oral thrush

Thrush is caused by a yeast (fungus) called *candida albicans*. This fungus also causes diaper rash. A baby may come into contact with the infection when he passes through the birth canal if his mother has a vaginal yeast infection.

What to look out for

- White patches on the tongue and the insides of the mouth

- Feeding is uncomfortable
- Severe diaper rash

Treatment

There are a number of oral medications that can treat thrush. If you are breastfeeding, you need to use anti-fungal cream on your nipples. All plastic nipples, pacifiers, and bottles should be thoroughly sterilized each time they are used.

Infantile eczema

Also known as atopic dermatitis, this is the most common form of eczema in babies under 12 months. Eczema is an allergic condition related to asthma and hayfever. It can be inherited but also can exist in isolation. It commonly appears on the face and scalp or behind the ears. Your baby may only have a few patches of dry skin; but if the eczema is severe, your baby's skin may become sore, inflamed, and weepy. This is unbearably itchy, so your baby will scratch continuously, leaving his skin open to infection.

What to look out for

- Severe itching
- Oozing, crusty patches of inflamed skin
- Patches of red, dry skin
- Flaking skin and occasional blisters

Treatment

Though it can only be managed, not cured, most children do grow out of atopic eczema. It is important to maintain a strict skin-care regime under medical supervision. Emollients will prevent your baby's skin from getting too dry and itchy. Steroid creams can reduce inflammation, but are generally only used if your baby's eczema hasn't responded to emollients. Antibiotics may be prescribed to clear up infection in severe cases.

Scratch mitts will help stop a baby from scratching. Breastfeeding for the first six months may give some protection against allergens.

EYE PROBLEMS

Blocked tear ducts

About 5 percent of babies are born with a blockage in their tear ducts. Many newborns have a partial blockage that gradually clears so, by the time they are 18 months old, the tear ducts are normal. Blocked tear ducts predispose your baby to eye infections.

What to look out for
- Weepy, constantly running eye
- Nostril remains dry when baby cries

Treatment
Keep your baby's eyes clean by wiping with cooled, boiled water using a fresh cotton ball for each eye. Massaging the area just under the eye right next to the nose where the duct is located will help. Antibiotics may be needed if there is an infection. Rarely, surgery is required to clean and dilate the ducts.

Conjunctivitis

An inflammation of the membrane covering the eyeball and the inside of eyelid, conjunctivitis—also known as sticky eye—is usually caused by a viral infection accompanying a cold. It also can be caused by a bacterial infection. Bacterial conjunctivitis occurs more commonly in babies with blocked tear ducts (see above). Rarely, conjunctivitis is a symptom of gonorrhoea or chlamydia infection, which has been passed from mother to baby.

What to look out for
- Mucus or "matter" in corner of eye
- Discolored—yellow or green—eye discharge
- Eyelids stuck together
- Dislike of bright lights
- Swollen, red eyelid

Treatment
Keep your baby's eyes clean by wiping away any sticky discharge with cooled, boiled water using a separate cotton ball for each wipe. Seek medical advice if the eyes remain red and swollen for longer than three days or the eyelids are stuck together. Antibiotics may be required.

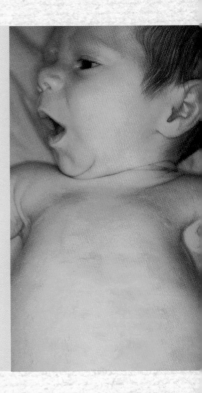

Eczema is diagnosed from your baby's inflamed, red scaly skin. The condition causes intense itching and constant scratching can lead to the skin being split, leaving it prone to infection. Commonly affected areas include the face, trunk, groin, knees, hands, and underarms.

BLOOD DISORDERS

Neonatal jaundice

Fifty percent of babies develop jaundice at birth. Usually this is because a baby's liver can't process bilirubin (a natural waste product of the baby's blood) fast enough, which results in a buildup of yellow pigment in the skin. The yellow color appears first on the head and passes down the body as the bilirubin level rises.

Babies who were bruised during birth are more inclined to have jaundice, because extra blood is broken down in the bruise and more bilirubin is formed. Premature babies also are likely to become jaundiced, because their livers haven't matured. Other less common causes of jaundice include infections and liver problems.

What to look out for
- Yellow tinge to skin
- Whites of eyes become yellow

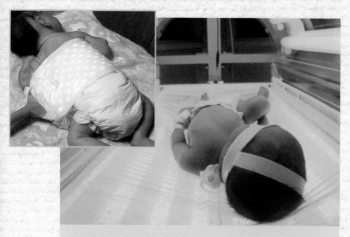

Jaundice may be treated with phototherapy while the baby is in an incubator (above). A new treatment is a bilirubin wrap (top left) where the baby can remain in a regular bassinet.

- Excessive weight loss
- Baby appears very sleepy and may have poor sucking ability

Treatment
Your baby's bilirubin levels will be monitored to make sure they don't become dangerously high, which can damage his nervous system. Blood can be drawn from your baby's vein or heel. Newer ways of checking bilirubin levels without drawing blood include a special light sensor that can be placed on the baby's skin.

Neonatal jaundice usually clears up by itself over a few days or weeks, but if bilirubin levels are high, phototherapy may be given. This is a very safe treatment, during which a baby is exposed to controlled amounts of ultraviolet (UV) light—not the kind that burns. The UV light breaks down excess bilirubin so that it can be disposed of through your baby's liver. Your baby will be placed in an incubator under lights for a couple of days, wearing just his diaper and with his eyes covered by a protective mask.

Newer bilirubin wraps or blankets allow a baby to sleep in a regular bassinet, stay in the hospital room with his mother, and avoid wearing an eye covering, since the light doesn't shine from above. In most cases, jaundice goes away for good.

Jaundice in infants after the early newborn period can be serious and of a different nature than newborn jaundice.

Hypoglycemia

This is a condition in which the amount of glucose (sugar) in the blood is lower than normal. Although reasonably common in newborn babies, there are certain babies who have a higher chance of having problems. Babies born to mothers who have diabetes during pregnancy may have problems controlling their blood sugar levels. Both particularly large babies and those who are small for their age also are more likely to have difficulties with blood sugar levels. Premature babies, babies who won't eat for long periods after birth, and those who have bacterial infections may also experience problems.

What to look out for
- Sweating
- Pale skin
- Rapid breathing
- Increased heart rate
- Jitteriness and jerky movements

Treatment
Simply feeding your baby may be all that is required to improve his blood sugar levels. Occasionally, if your baby doesn't respond, sugared water may be given intravenously to achieve adequate levels.

YOUR BABY'S HEALTH AND DEVELOPMENT

Through keeping a record of your baby's progress over the next few months you will be able to see how much she grows and develops during this period. You may also want to record the date of special milestones, such as a first smile or tooth, along with important medical information such as immunizations that have been given, and any illnesses she has had.

YOUR BABY'S GROWTH

Your baby's head circumference, weight, and height are a good indication of her general health and well-being during the first year. Although the range of "normal" at any age is very wide, there is an "average" range, into which most children fall (see page 368). Special allowances will be made if your baby is preterm.

At each check-up your baby will be measured, and her healthcare provider will plot the numbers on a chart of national averages for children of the same age and sex. You will then be told what percentile your child is in. For example, if your 2-month-old is in the 75th percentile for weight, that means that 75 percent of the 2-month-olds in the country are lighter and 25 percent are heavier.

Parents sometimes worry needlessly about these percentiles. Keep in mind that your child is an individual and will develop at her own pace. These measurements are only a general guide to assess your baby's developmental progress. The most important thing to watch for is that your baby is growing steadily.

How the measurements are taken

- *Head circumference* Unlike other vital organs, which are fully formed at birth, your baby's brain—and, therefore, her head—continues to grow during her first year. Your baby's healthcare provider will measure the size of her head by placing a flexible measuring tape just above her eyebrows and ears, and around the back of her head where it slopes up prominently from her neck.

- *Weight* After your baby is completely undressed she will be placed on a scale (either a traditional beam scale or an electronic model). Both types should be set to zero before the baby is laid down.

- *Length/height* Until your baby is old enough to stand still on her own, she'll be measured lying down. Sometimes a special device with a headboard and movable footboard is used to make sure the results are accurate.

Taking the measurements yourself

Your baby's healthcare provider may give you percentile charts to fill in at home. However, it is important to remember that your measurements may not be as accurate as when he or she takes them. Once you have plotted the measurements on the growth percentile charts you will be able to see how your baby is growing and how she compares to other babies of her age.

If you have concerns

Sometimes a baby has feeding problems, or you may be concerned that she is not getting enough milk at each feed. By weighing her regularly and plotting her weight gain on a percentile chart you will soon be able to see whether there is a problem. If you are concerned about any area of your baby's development you should discuss your worries with your child's healthcare provider.

CHARTING YOUR BABY'S GROWTH

The solid line in the middle of the colored band indicates the average growth rate in the first year. The colored band shows the range of normal measurements.

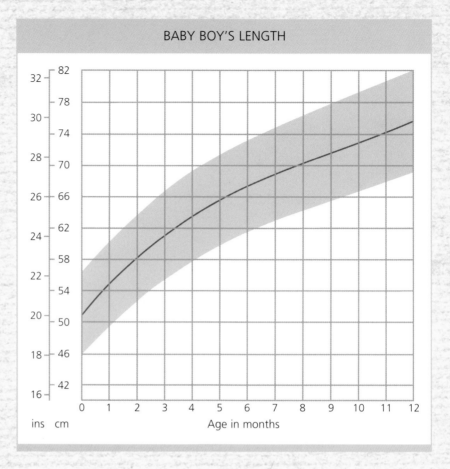

BABY BOY'S LENGTH

ins   cm

Age in months

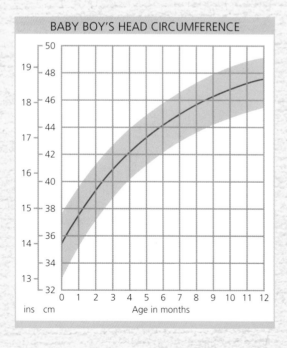

BABY BOY'S HEAD CIRCUMFERENCE

ins   cm

Age in months

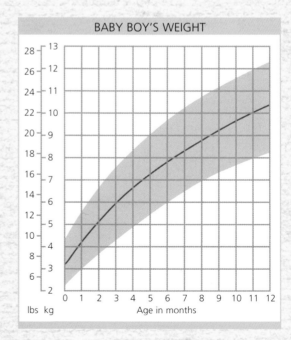

BABY BOY'S WEIGHT

lbs   kg

Age in months

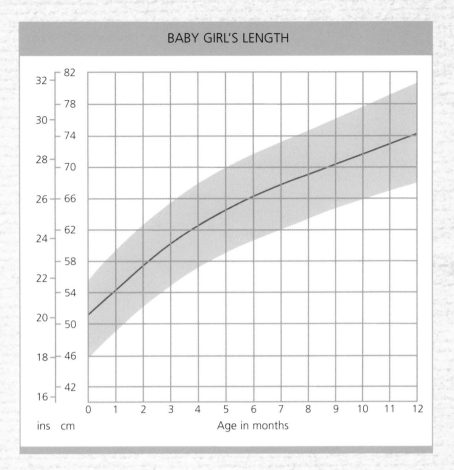

BABY GIRL'S LENGTH

Age in months

ins   cm

Your child's growth curves should fall somewhere in the colored band and should follow the shape of the curve of the solid line.

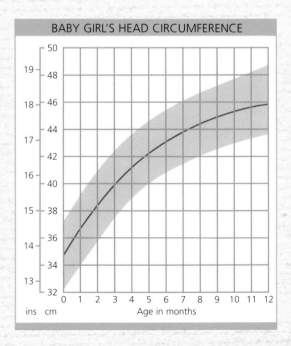

BABY GIRL'S HEAD CIRCUMFERENCE

ins   cm   Age in months

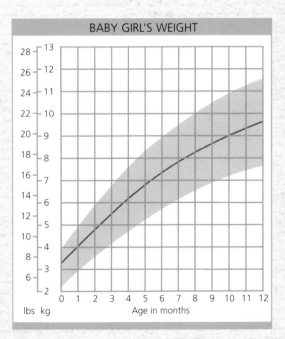

BABY GIRL'S WEIGHT

lbs   kg   Age in months

RECOMMENDED CHILDHOOD IMMUNIZATION SCHEDULE

This schedule is a general guideline only, and may vary depending on your state or province. Vaccination may be delayed if your child is sick with anything other than a mild cold or if her immune system is weakened by immune-suppressing medications.

AGE	VACCINE	HOW GIVEN
At 2, 4, and 6 months	Polio (third dose given between 6 and 18 months)	Injection
	Haemophilus influenzae Injection Type B (Hib disease)	Injection
	Diphtheria, Tetanus and Whooping cough (DTaP)	Combined injection
	Pneumoccocal (meningitis)	Injection
	Meniningococcal C (meningitis, Canada only)	Injection
	Hepatitis B (first dose sometimes given within 12 hours of birth)	Injection
Between 12 and 18 months	Measles, Mumps, and Rubella (MMR)	Combined injection
	Diphtheria, Tetanus and Whooping cough (DTaP)	Combined injection
	Varicellar (chickenpox)	Injection
	Pneumoccocal (meningitis)	Injection
	Meniningococcal C (meningitis, Canada only)	Injection
4 to 6 years	Measles, Mumps, and Rubella (MMR)	Combined injection
	Diphtheria, Tetanus and Whooping cough (DTaP)	Combined injection
	Polio	Injection
11 to 12 years	Tetanus and Diphtheria (Td)	Combined injection

GIVING PROTECTION FROM DISEASE

Immunization is one of the most important steps you can take to ensure your baby's current and future health. Since immunization was first invented, it has saved hundreds of thousands of children's lives. This simple procedure involves the use of vaccines, which protect children from serious, and sometimes fatal, infectious diseases by strengthening their immunity (the body's ability to fight off these diseases).

Natural immunity

Your baby is born with a degree of natural, inherited immunity, which she acquired before birth. That immunity is reinforced if you are breastfeeding, as breast milk is rich in antibodies, especially in the first few days after birth. But this type of passive, inherited immunity is only temporary—it wears off during your child's first year of life. This leaves her vulnerable to a host of serious diseases. Vaccinations give your child protective immunity against these diseases.

Generally, vaccines are safe and very effective. The benefits of immunization far outweigh any risks. Typical side effects may include a mild fever or slight rash, depending on the vaccine. More serious side effects are rare, but if other symptoms develop or fever is high, consult your child's healthcare provider.

Keeping an immunization record

It's a good idea to keep a record of the immunizations that your child receives. Record sheets are often provided by healthcare providers. They're valuable if you move or changes doctors, or if you need proof of your child's protection against certain infectious diseases, such as when you enrol your child in school. The immunization record should specify the types of vaccine, and be dated and signed by your child's healthcare provider each time an immunization is given.

HOW TO STOP AN INFANT FROM CHOKING

Infants usually choke because they have breathed in or swallowed a foreign object. If your baby can't cry or cough, something is probably blocking her airway and this will need to be removed immediately. If you suspect your baby is choking but she can still cry and cough, allow her to continue coughing, watch her carefully but do not pat her back or give her water.

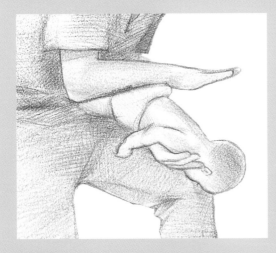

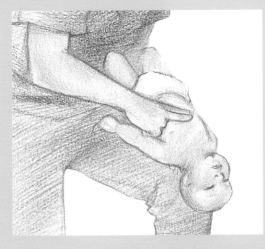

1 If she cannot cry, cough, or breathe, or if she is making high-pitched noises, stand up and lay her along your forearm on her tummy. Bend one knee and rest your forearm on your upper thigh with the infant's head extending past your bent knee. With the heel of your other hand, strike the infant between the shoulder blades five times. Each strike should be a separate attempt to dislodge the object.

2 If your baby is still choking, carefully turn her over and place two or three fingers in the center of the breastbone. Give five chest thrusts. Each thrust should be ½ to 1 inch (1 to 2 cm) deep, and should be a separate attempt to dislodge the object. Continue cycles of back blows and chest thrusts until the object is forced out and the infant begins to breathe on her own, or the infant becomes unconscious.

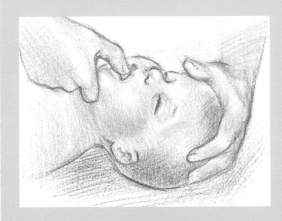

3 If your baby loses consciousness but is still breathing, place her on her back tilting her head back slightly and using a single finger, carefully feel and remove any obstruction from her mouth. If your baby remains unconscious and stops breathing, get help and start CPR (see page 372). If there is a pulse but no breathing, perform rescue breathing. To do this gently tilt her head back with one hand, and lift her chin with the other to open her airway, seal your lips over her mouth and nose and give one small breath every three seconds until she starts breathing on her own.

HOW TO CLEAR A BLOCKED AIRWAY AND GIVE CARDIOPULMONARY RESUSCITATION (CPR) TO INFANTS UNDER ONE YEAR OF AGE

It is always best to attend a first aid course to learn CPR and other life-saving techniques. The following steps should only be performed if your baby is not breathing. Always call, or get someone else to call, 911 after starting rescue efforts.

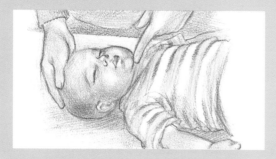

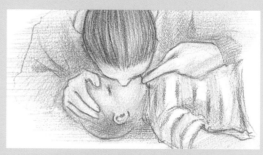

1 Lie the infant down on a firm flat surface such as the floor or a table, then gently tilt her head back with one hand, and lift her chin with the other to open her airway. It is important not to tilt her head back too far as this could kink her airway. Put your ear to her mouth and nose, and look, listen, and feel for breathing.

2 If she is not breathing, keep her airway open and place your mouth over the infant's nose and lips to form a seal and give two rescue breaths, each lasting about one second. Take a breath in between each rescue breath. A baby only needs tiny breaths as her lungs are very small; too much air in the lungs could damage them. Look for the chest to rise and fall with each breath to see if air goes in.

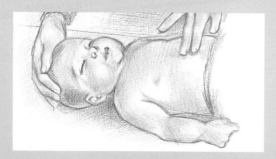

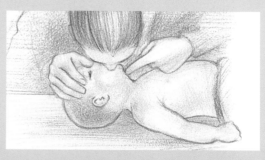

3 Check for a pulse by finding the baby's brachial artery on her inner upper arm with your index and middle fingers, and look for any signs of life, such as limb movement. If there are no signs of circulation, give chest compressions—imagine a line between the child's nipples, and place two fingers just below its center point. Apply ½ to 1 inch (1 to 2 cm) chest compressions in about three seconds.

4 After five compressions, seal your lips over your child's mouth and nose and give one breath. Repeat the cycle of five compressions and one breath nineteen more times and check for signs of circulation. If there are none, repeat the cycle of five compressions and one breath until help arrives or someone else takes over. Check for signs of circulation every few minutes.

BABIES NEEDING SPECIAL CARE

Most babies who are too small at birth—weighing less than 5½ lbs (2.5 kg) at birth—or are born too early will need some form of special care to enable them to catch up. A premature baby will most probably be treated in a neonatal intensive care unit (NICU).

Newborns are said to be premature if they're born before 37 weeks of age. Babies born after 24 to 25 weeks of gestation (pregnancy) may be mature enough to survive, but will be in intensive care for a while. Babies born at less than 23 weeks of gestation aren't usually mature enough to survive. Apart from age, other factors boost the outcome for a premature baby, including being female and African-American.

While premature babies face early difficulties, it is important to keep in mind that nearly two-thirds of premature babies who survive will either grow up to be completely normal or will have only mild or moderate problems.

THE CARE YOUR BABY WILL RECEIVE

A premature baby will need to be on a ventilator, as his lungs will not have matured. As infections often cause premature birth, your baby also will be given antibiotics and intravenous fluids, either through an IV or umbilical central line. A premature baby may be placed in a special bed with a radiant warmer to help maintain his body temperature, plus a cellophane wrapping to minimize the loss of heat and fluids through his thin skin. He also will probably be on a cardiorespiratory monitor with a pulse oximeter to measure the oxygen in his blood, and he may have a feeding tube if he is mature enough to eat.

Unless the baby is over 32 to 34 weeks, he probably won't be able to nurse or drink from a bottle but will have a tube in his mouth or nose that goes down to his stomach. A mother of a premature baby can express milk and store it at the NICU until her baby can take it.

Most premature babies are not ready to be discharged until some time around the date they were originally due. So for a baby born at 26 weeks, that can mean three months in the hospital. In general, a baby will need to be gaining weight, breathing well on his own—although he may need oxygen—and eating to be able to leave the NICU. After that his progress will be checked regularly by a team of specialist doctors.

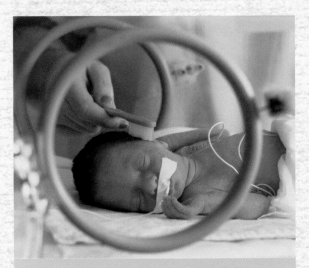

This premature baby, seen here in an incubator, is so tiny his hair is being brushed with a soft toothbrush. Electrodes have been attached to him to monitor his heartbeat and breathing.

BIRTH ABNORMALITIES

Although the great majority of babies are normal, about 1 percent will have some form of congenital defect. Babies can be affected by a large number of things during their development in the uterus, and many of the resulting defects can be treated before or after birth.

CONGENITAL HEART PROBLEMS

The heart is a complex organ and much of its structural development occurs between 3 and 7 weeks after conception. Congenital heart defects are the most common group of abnormalities, affecting nearly 1 in every 100 babies born. The range of defects is very wide.

A mother with a congenital heart defect, or who has had an affected child, has a slightly increased risk of having a baby with a heart problem. Many heart problems are also associated with other genetic problems such as Down syndrome (see page 249), and testing for such problems may be offered if a heart defect is found.

How heart defects are diagnosed
Most problems are detected on an ultrasound scan at 18 to 22 weeks. Many defects are not visible earlier than this. If there's a history of a heart problem, regular scanning may be carried out during pregnancy. However, some heart problems may not be seen at all on an ultrasound scan, even with experience; as many as 40 percent of problems can be missed.

Treatment
Intrauterine surgical techniques are being developed so that some defects can be treated before birth. After birth the management of a heart defect will depend on the severity of the diagnosis. For mild problems, a newborn baby can usually remain with his mother and will be assessed by a pediatrician in the hospital. More serious problems that can lead to a lack of oxygen will require specialist care. This means that the birth should take place where specialist care can be offered. Many heart problems are amenable to

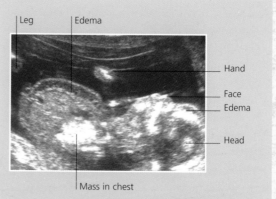

On an ultrasound scan for fetal hydrops, edema appears on the entire body, due to an accumulation of fluid in the tissues. In this case the edema is caused by a mass in the chest obstructing blood flow.

surgery, although there are some that will not allow the baby to survive outside the uterus.

Fetal hydrops
This is heart failure in the baby, and on a scan the skin appears swollen, and there is evidence of fluid within the chest and abdomen. The causes are many, including blood group incompatibility, which can be diagnosed in pregnancy.

How fetal hydrops is diagnosed
Through ultrasound scans

Treatment
Treatment will depend on the severity and cause of the condition. Some causes, such as anemia, can be treated, but others, such as those associated with severe heart defects, cannot. Babies with a blood group incompatibility may be treated with

intrauterine blood transfusions. Whether a baby diagnosed with hydrops will survive depends on the diagnosis, and how ill the baby is at the time of discovery. All babies who have reached this stage are very ill indeed, and many do not survive.

Septal defect
This is commonly known as a "hole in the heart." It may occur in the dividing tissue between the smaller or larger chambers of the heart. A small defect may not be detected and sometimes the condition only comes to light in later life. Septal defects that are diagnosed during pregnancy tend to be large, or are associated with other problems.

How a septal defect is diagnosed
Through ultrasound scans

Treatment
Small defects do not always require surgery. Larger defects are likely to require surgery.

Problems with flow of blood out of the heart
This can occur because the blood vessels have not joined up correctly or because the valves have not formed properly. Problems of this kind are often complex, and may be associated with septal defects (see above).

How blood flow problems are diagnosed
Through ultrasound scans

Treatment
Where connections are not in the right place, surgery is often successful. If the valves have not developed properly, surgery is more difficult and less likely to be successful in the long-term. Many of these conditions are extremely complicated. As with any abnormality in a baby it is important for parents to talk to a specialist in the condition during pregnancy to discuss what the best treatment will be for the baby.

PROBLEMS WITH THE SPINE OR HEAD
Neural tube defects
One of the most common developmental problems, a neural tube defect is the failure of the brain and spinal cord to develop properly during the first four weeks of pregnancy. This affects as many as 1 in 1160 live births in the United States, and results in varying degrees of damage to the baby. Many more pregnancies are thought to be affected, but because of the severity of the condition they result in miscarriage.

Spina bifida occulta is the mildest form, in which one or two vertebrae are malformed. In spina bifida occulta, the spinal cord is covered with skin, so it usually causes no problems. Sometimes it is only discovered as the result of an X-ray in later life. Occasionally, there may be a tuft of hair or skin dimple over the affected site.

Myelo-meningocele is a more severe form of spina bifida. This involves a lesion on the spine, which can somtimes be the size of an orange, where nerve tissue, muscles, and spinal fluid are exposed. The lesion can cause nerve damage leading to problems with muscular control and bladder and bowel control. Varying degrees of learning difficulty are other possible complications. Hydrocephalus is also a related condition (see page 376).

Anencephaly is the most severe neural tube defect. An opening at the upper end of the tube results in portions of the skull and brain not forming. Babies with this condition can't survive more than a few hours and are not conscious when they are born.

How neural tube defects are diagnosed
Spina bifida can be detected at 16 weeks by a blood test, called the maternal serum alpha-fetoprotein test (MSAFP). If the result of the test is high, the baby, and especially the spine and head, will be examined carefully by ultrasound. Sometimes it can be quite difficult to diagnose spina bifida, especially if the scan views are restricted. Other tests such as amniocentesis may also be used.

Treatment
The treatment given will depend on the size and type of the neural tube defect and its severity. This will be determined by ultrasound and magnetic resonance imaging (MRI) scanning after birth. If the baby has an open defect this will require an operation to close the spine. While this operation will close the defect, it cannot restore the nerves, which may have not developed properly. Hydrocephalus will also require an operation to relieve the condition after birth.

Prevention
Although the cause of neural tube defects is not clear, there is now good evidence that folic acid, a vitamin found in leafy vegetables, needs to be present in early pregnancy to allow the spine to close up properly. Because it is hard to achieve the recommended dose through diet alone, taking a folic acid supplement is now recommended three months before conception and up to the twelfth week of pregnancy. Experts have suggested that all women of child-bearing age should have 400 micrograms of folic acid each day. Mothers who have had a previous baby with spina bifida or anencephaly, or are on certain drugs such as those used to treat epilepsy, need to take a higher-dose of folic acid—5 mg. This can be prescribed by your healthcare provider, or obtained from pharmacies and many supermarkets.

Hydrocephalus
This is a build up of cerebrospinal fluid (CSF) in the head and is caused by an obstruction in the draining system around the brain. Usually the head of the baby becomes very large. Premature birth is the most common cause, because of a higher risk of bleeding into the brain, which may prevent absorption of CSF. It also can occur in babies with a congenital defect such as spina bifida; some cases are inherited, and some infections can have this effect. Babies known to have this condition may need to be delivered by cesarean. How the baby will be affected depends on the underlying cause. Some babies will grow up to have a normal intelligence, while others can be profoundly handicapped; however, this cannot be predicted before birth

How hydrocephalus is diagnosed
During pregnancy, hydrocephalus can be diagnosed by ultrasound scan. After birth, the head measurement carried out on every newborn can indicate whether the condition exists. Early diagnosis and treatment improves the outcome.

Treatment
After birth, an operation is usually carried out to allow the CSF to drain, via a shunt, into the bloodstream. The shunt remains in place for life. An operation to insert a temporary shunt may sometimes be carried out before birth. A permanent shunt is then inserted after the birth. Some recent surgical techniques, in which an opening in the skull is made, are suitable for some forms of hydrocephalus.

Cerebral palsy
This term is used to cover a group of disorders affecting movement and posture. There may be associated learning difficulties in about one in four of affected children. The cause can be abnormal development of the brain before birth, oxygen deprivation, infection, bleeding in the brain, or physical injury during birth. Physical symptoms range from weakness and floppiness of muscles to spasticity and rigidity.

How cerebral palsy is diagnosed
A reliable diagnosis cannot usually be made until a child is at least one year old, because many parts of the nervous system have not fully developed before then. Diagnostic tests may include EEG, MRI and CT scanning and vision and hearing tests. In some cases blood tests may also be used to evaluate inherited conditions.

Treatment
There is no cure for cerebral palsy, but there are treatments that will help minimize the effects and

help boost a child's abilities. These may include physical therapies, complementary therapies, and drug treatments. Surgery may sometimes be helpful in dealing with limb deformities.

GENITO-URINARY PROBLEMS
Urinary tract obstruction
This occurs when the flow of urine between the kidney and the bladder becomes partially or completely obstructed. A severe obstruction causing a complete blockage can lead to hydronephrosis (swelling of the kidney), which can cause loss of kidney function. This condition can be detected in a fetus as early as 15 weeks.

How urinary tract obstruction is diagnosed
Diagnosis during pregnancy is with ultrasound. In a newborn a renal scan, or a CT scan may be given. Other tests may be necessary, depending on the severity of the blockage.

Treatment
Fetal surgery may be considered in very severe cases, usually when both kidneys are affected. For this to be effective it must be done before there is substantial damage to the developing kidneys. Once the baby has been born, surgical treatment may be needed to relieve the blockage. Early treatment will help preserve kidney tissue and encourages the return of its function.

Kidney cysts
When the body of the kidney does not successfully fuse with the drainage system this can lead to a poorly or non-functioning kidney. Everyone can manage with only one functioning kidney, and to develop in the uterus a baby does not need to have any functional kidney at all, as the placenta removes waste products. However, once born, a baby needs kidney function. Sometimes abnormal development affects only one kidney, and the baby will usually have no serious problems, though sometimes the poorly functioning one has to be removed in childhood. Cysts can develop in the poorly functioning

kidney. But if both kidneys are affected, the amount of fluid around the baby will decrease, and the baby's lungs will not grow adequately. At birth the baby would have difficulty breathing, as well as poor kidney function.

There are other types of kidney cysts, for example a condition called adult polycystic kidney disease can occasionally be seen in the fetus. It does not cause problems until later in adult life. Usually one parent will have this condition, however, they may not know about it.

How kidney cysts are diagnosed
Diagnosis during pregnancy is with ultrasound. In a newborn a renal scan, or a CT scan may be used to check for kidney cysts.

Treatment
Depending on the severity of the problem, surgery may be required when the child is older. If there is a hereditary factor other tests may be done.

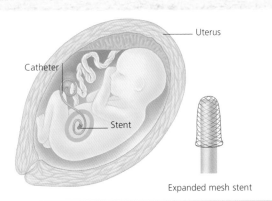

Uterus

Catheter

Stent

Expanded mesh stent

The latest treatment for urinary tract obstruction is carried out while the baby is in the uterus. A stent (right) is placed via a tiny hollow tube—catheter— through the mother's abdomen, into the fetal bladder to allow urine to escape.

Hypospadias

About 1 in 300 boys is born with this condition. The opening of the urethra, which is the tube bringing urine from the bladder to the outside, normally at the tip of the penis, develops in the wrong place, most commonly on the underside of the penis. This causes problems with urination and may also cause the penis to curve downward, which may affect sexual performance when adulthood is reached.

How hypospadias is diagnosed
- Inability to pass a normal stream of urine
- Curved penis
- Hooded foreskin

Treatment
In very mild cases, no action will be taken. In more severe cases, surgery will be needed to extend the urethra. Children with hypospadias shouldn't be circumcised, as the foreskin will probably be used as part of the repair surgery.

Undescended testicle

Normally, during fetal development, the testicles pass from the abdomen through a canal into the scrotum. In some cases this doesn't happen prior to birth, and the exact cause usually isn't known. The condition occurs relatively frequently in premature babies, while full-term healthy babies are much less likely to have this problem. The testes usually descend by the 28th week of pregnancy, so if a baby is born prior to this time, the testes may not have had time yet to descend. Sometimes only one testicle descends or the descent is incomplete.

What to look out for
- Scrotum appears small or unevenly developed
- Testes cannot be felt in scrotum

Treatment
Usually the testicles will descend on their own during the first year. Sometimes a testis, which is sitting in the inguinal canal, is not truly undescended, and will drop spontaneously. If a testicle remains undescended, hormones may be given to help it descend by itself or surgery may be required.

Left untreated, a baby will have a higher than average chance of being infertile, and of developing testicular cancer as an adult.

DIGESTIVE TRACT PROBLEMS
Intestinal obstruction

An obstruction can occur anywhere in the intestines, from the esophagus to the anus. Blockages at the top can lead to an accumulation of amniotic fluid, and are usually diagnosed during pregnancy. A blockage just below the stomach is known as a duodenal atresia. This type of blockage is commonly found in babies with Down syndrome (see page 249) and a test may be offered for this. Lower blockages may not be recognized until after birth.

How intestinal obstruction is diagnosed
Ultrasound scanning is used to identify the cause of the blockage.

Treatment
If a baby has an obstruction, surgery will be needed after birth to bypass the block to allow the baby to begin feeding.

Abdominal wall defects

These occur when part of the abdominal wall has failed to develop, leaving a hole. The contents of the abdomen can then escape outside the cavity. In some cases there is a membrane covering the contents. This is called an omphalocele or exomphalos and can be associated with other genetic problems in the baby, and testing may be offered. If the bowel is not covered, the condition is called a gastroschisis. This is not associated with any other developmental problems in the baby. If the baby remains healthy, a vaginal delivery should be possible. Sometimes, if the baby is unwell in other ways, or has a large exomphalos, a cesarean section may be offered.

How abdominal wall defects are diagnosed
A baby with one of these conditions is likely to
appear small, so close monitoring during
pregnancy will be required. Abdominal wall
defects can be picked up on ultrasound scanning.

Treatment
The baby will need an operation to close the
defect. Usually this can be done at a single
operation. Occasionally small amounts of bowel
will need to be removed if damaged or blocked.
Feeding is introduced slowly, and the baby will
need to spend quite a long time—two to four
weeks—in hospital until feeding is established.

Pyloric stenosis

This occurs when the pylorus (ring of muscle that
links the duodenum to the stomach), becomes so
enlarged with muscle that food can't pass.
Symptoms usually start between 3 and 12 weeks.
The condition is more common in boys and
seems to run in certain families.

How pyloric stenosis is diagnosed
A physical examination is given and ultrasound is
used to confirm the condition.

Treatment
The condition is treated with minor surgery,
where a small cut is made in the pylorus. After the
operation your baby will feed normally and weight
gain will be rapid.

Diaphragmatic hernia

The diaphragm is a muscle, which separates the
organs of the abdomen from those of the chest.
During the fetus' early development in the uterus,
there is a hole in the diaphragm, which usually
closes by the end of the third month. If the hole
stays open, the contents of the abdomen, such as
the intestines, can be pushed up into the chest
cavity. If this happens, these organs can displace
the heart and lungs and prevent them from
growing normally.

How it is diagnosed
This condition will be detected using ultrasound.
Babies with this condition frequently have
breathing problems once they are born.

Treatment
A baby born with a diaphragmatic hernia can have
an operation to have the defect in the diaphragm

The diaphragm keeps
the organs in the
abdomen from going
into the chest cavity
(far right). When there
is a hole in the
diaphragm, the
stomach and
sometimes the
intestines push up into
it, preventing the heart
and the lungs from
growing properly
(see right).

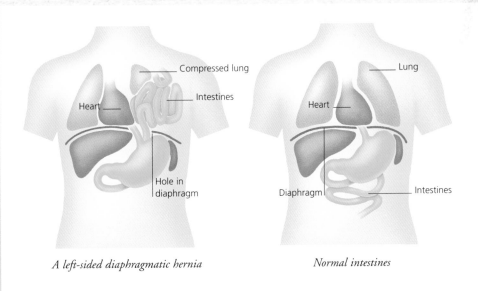

A left-sided diaphragmatic hernia

Normal intestines

closed. In severe cases, however, the lungs are not large enough to allow the baby to survive. There are no reliable ways of predicting which babies have adequate lung growth before birth.

Once a baby has had a successful operation on a hernia, she can expect to have a normal life. Sometimes diaphragmatic hernia is associated with a genetic problem, and a test will be offered to exclude this possibility.

MUSCULOSKELETAL PROBLEMS
Cleft lip or palate
These are among the most common defects affecting babies and may occur singly, or together. The defect occurs when the fetus' upper lip and/ or roof of the mouth does not fuse properly before birth. In many cases, the cause is unknown, although in some the defect may be hereditary. If a baby is severely affected there may be some difficulty in feeding.

How cleft lip and palate are diagnosed
In some units with highly specialized ultrasound equipment, cleft lip or palate can be diagnosed prenatally in a mid-trimester scan. Otherwise it will be seen at birth.

Treatment
A cleft lip is usually repaired surgically by the age of 3 months. A cleft palate is repaired between 6 and 15 months of age. A plate may be fitted into the roof of a baby's mouth before this time if feeding is a problem. Plastic surgery produces good results (see picture, right) and allows speech to develop normally.

Club foot
Some babies are found to have a condition called talipes or "club foot." It affects about 1 in every 1000 babies. It means that one or both feet are turned away from the normal axis. Sometimes babies with this have a genetic condition. More usually it occurs either because the foot has been constricted in the uterus or because the bones of the foot have not developed properly.

How club foot is diagnosed
A routine ultrasound scan usually shows up any limb defects. This will be followed by further scans to check on the baby's development.

Treatment
If the condition is caused by restriction in the uterus all that may be required after birth are physiotherapy exercises to straighten the foot. If the bones of the foot have not developed properly a baby may need surgery in childhood.

Spinal problems
Occasionally one part of a vertebra may be missing or malformed, giving a misalignment of the spine. This can occur in some inherited conditions or where there are chromosomal problems. It is always difficult to judge what the effect will be in the long term.

How spinal problems are diagnosed
Spinal problems can be identified by an ultrasound scan.

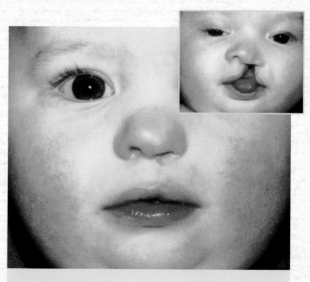

A cleft lip (top right) is usually repaired by surgery (above) when a baby is around 3 months. The outcome is usually very successful.

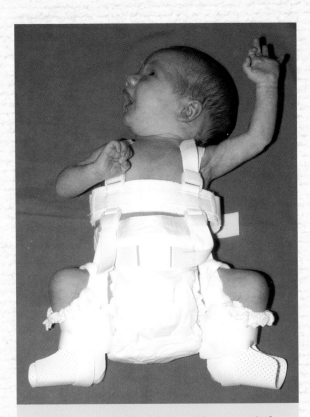

All newborns are checked for hip dislocation and, if found, a Palvick harness is often used to keep the hips in the correct position. The harness is worn for between two and four months and is very effective.

associated with other congenital conditions such as spina bifida or Down syndrome. It is more likely to affect the left hip, although in 25 percent of cases, it is found in both hips.

How congenital hip dislocation is diagnosed
During the standard neonatal pediatric check your baby's hips will be bent and flexed. A click could be a sign of congenital hip dislocation and a further test to confirm the condition is given at 6 weeks. Other symptoms may include asymmetric skin folds on upper legs and the inability to spread legs wide during diaper changes.

Treatment
Early treatment with a special harness (see left) increases the chances of normal hip development. The harness can be removed easily to change the baby's diaper and it does not interfere with feeding, bathing or sleeping. If treatment is needed after 6 months, a plaster cast may be used. Very rarely, surgery is carried out to enlarge the socket. This is usually done before walking begins.

Treatment
Treatment will depend on the severity of the problem. Some children can go on to have quite marked scoliosis (curvature of the spine), which may need surgery.

Congenital hip dislocation
Relatively common, hip dislocation occurs when an incorrectly formed hip joint allows the ball of the femur to slip out of the socket in the pelvic bone. The cause of hip dislocation is unknown; it may be hereditary. Hip dislocation occurs ten times more frequently in girls, and also more frequently in firstborns and breech babies. It is also more likely to occur in twins and may be

THE LOSS OF A BABY

Whether parents lose a baby before the birth or afterward, the loss is devastating. Coming to terms with the death of a much wanted baby and being able to move on can seem an impossibility, but, as many couples have experienced, grieving is an essential part of the healing process.

It's natural to feel shock and denial after losing a baby. Many parents feel as if they're experiencing a bad dream, that what they're going through isn't real and when they wake up, their baby will still be with them.

As reality sets in, feelings of anger and deep sorrow can surface; tearfulness, loss of appetite, and sleeplessness are all part of this process. A woman's feelings are intensified by the massive fall in hormone levels, as her body returns to its pre-pregnancy state.

There's a desperate need to see and hold their baby, and many parents can be wracked with guilt that they didn't do enough for their child. Feelings of anger and the urge to blame the death on someone, anyone—the hospital, the medical staff, each other—can be overwhelming.

As the anger and deep sorrow subside, depression creeps in. What's the point in carrying on when life has been so unfair?

Acceptance is the final stage in the grieving process and will come with time. Acceptance doesn't mean that the pain and anger have disappeared, but that it's time to put the grief away and carry on with life. The death of a baby has changed everything forever, but it's possible to go on and be even stronger in time.

SUPPORT

Every parent's experience of loss is unique. For some, the healing will take a very long time, while others will be anxious to get back to "normal" so that they can try to put the sad event behind them. The important thing is for every parent to experience whatever he or she is feeling, rather than feel that they have to act in the way others think they should.

Losing a baby also can put a huge strain on a relationship. Men have a tendency to internalize their emotions, so while a bereaved father will feel the loss as keenly as his partner he might not be able to express that grief openly. His partner might interpret this reticence as indifference and feel terribly hurt and isolated. The only way through this is for both parents to be as open and honest with each other as they can about the way they are feeling.

It's vital for both parents to accept as much help and support as possible. Most hospitals have support groups for families who have lost a baby and these can be very helpful.

Many parents have derived comfort from having a photograph of their baby or from holding the baby after the birth. Marking the baby's life, no matter how brief, through some sort of service, can also be very healing.

WHY BABIES DIE

Thanks to the advances in medical science, the number of babies who die before labor begins—referred to as stillbirths when the baby is more than 24 weeks gestational age—is exceedingly low, around 1 percent in the United States. It is often not known why a baby dies before birth, but a major cause is abnormal development of the baby or a failing placenta. The mother may notice that something isn't right—the baby has stopped moving—or the healthcare provider is not able to hear the baby's heartbeat. Ultrasound will be used to determine the severity of the baby's problem, and whether a heartbeat can be detected.

If a baby dies in utero, a mother has the difficult choice of going through a normal labor or having a cesarean section.

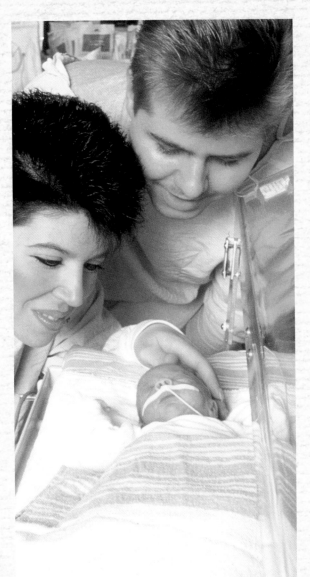

Very rarely, a baby dies during labor—this is called intrapartum death. When this happens, it is most often due to a lack of oxygen. Called fetal distress, there are a variety of reasons for this to occur including placental insufficiency, toxemia of pregnancy, and having the umbilical cord tightly around the neck.

When a newborn dies—neonatal death—it is most often due to breathing difficulties, especially if the baby is premature, or being born late or with serious developmental problems.

Sudden infant death syndrome (SIDS)

Also known as crib death, this is defined as the sudden unexpected death of an infant, under one year of age, that remains unexplained after a thorough case investigation, including an autopsy, examination of the death scene, and review of the clinical history. The causes of SIDS are multifactorial, but since parents have been advised to place babies on their backs rather than on their tummies to sleep (see page 309), the number of deaths attributed to SIDS has plummeted. It is, however, the leading cause of death for Canadian infants between 28 days and one year of age: In 1996, out of 2051 reported infant deaths, 168 (8.2 percent) were attributed to SIDS.

It's not uncommon in a multiple pregnancy for one of the babies not to survive. Losing a twin or triplet can be especially difficult. The parents are torn between grieving for their lost baby, and celebrating the life of the surviving one(s)—an emotional seesaw, which can test the strongest relationship. There's an unfortunate tendency for other people to diminish the loss, thinking that because there's still a living baby, the parents should be thankful. Bereavement doesn't work like that.

INDEX

Incisions, cesarean section 231, 232, 324
Incompetent cervix 279
Incontinence 29, 68, 359
Incubators 373
Indigestion 29, 204
Induction 185, 186, 227–8
Infantile eczema 364, 365
Infections: amniocentesis 244
    food safety 111
    newborn babies 362–4
    postpartum 356
    pre-existing 269
    in pregnancy 256–60
Inherited diseases *see* Genetic diseases
Insects 78, 82
Insomnia 71
Insulin 61, 253, 269, 270
Insurance plans 175, 242
Internal exams 21–23, 214
Intestinal obstruction 378
Intrauterine contraceptive devices 88, 352
Intravenous (IV) lines 214, 227, 228, 230, 324
Invasive tests 241–5
Iodine 108–9
Iron: deficiency 62, 252
    sources of 90, 108–9, 332
    supplements 90, 95, 252
    vegetarian diet 104
Itchiness 66, 273

J

Jaundice, neonatal 365–6
Jealousy 352–3
Joints 145, 211, 260–1

K

Kegel exercises 29, 122, 202, 321, 335, 359
Kick-count sheets 92, 207, 208
Kidneys 239, 259–60, 270, 272, 377
Knotted cord 263

L

Labor: active management of 215
    back labor 251
    birth attendants 177–8
    birth plans 184–5
    complicated 250–1
    emergency births 169
    encouraging 208
    false 212, 213, 250
    fast labor 251
    father's role 166–9, 182–3
    first stage 55, 215–22
    induction 186, 227–8
    length of 215, 228
    monitoring 185, 186–7
    onset of 211–13
    pain 178–81, 217–22
    positions 218, 220–1
    preparation for 201–8
    preterm 244, 250
    second labors 214
    second stage 55–56, 222–5
    signs of 210–14
    slow labor 250–1
    special medical interventions 227–32
    stages of 215–25
    third stage 225
    worries about 159–60
    see also Birth
Lactic acid 218, 219, 338
Lactose 105, 332
Lanugo 36, 45, 50, 283
Large babies 261
Latching on 300, 301
LDRs (birthing rooms) 175, 176
Left-handedness 145–6
Legs: cramps 29, 73
    deep vein thrombosis 252–3, 273, 322
    exercises 118, 337
    swollen 211, 273, 322
    varicose veins 52, 61, 73
Letdown reflex 62, 297–8, 359
Libido 28
Lidocaine 179
Life-saving techniques 371–2

Lifestyle 75–77, 152, 341
Lifting, safety 72, 80
Ligaments 69, 211, 260, 272
Lighting, night-lights 196
Linea nigra 66, 323–5
Lip, cleft 380
Listeriosis 111, 258
Liver 365–6
Lochia 225, 321
Lovemaking *see* Sex
Lunches 104–5, 333
Lungs: baby's 42, 46, 233, 288
    blood clots in 272
    exercise 120, 338
    maturity studies 244
Lupus 264

M

Magnesium 108–9
Malaria 81, 266
Marijuana 75
Mask of pregnancy 131
Massage: baby 296, 306, 346, 361
    breasts 323
    during labor 219
    pain relief 181, 182
    perineal 203
    in pregnancy 126–7, 134, 164–5
Mastitis 358
Masturbation 156, 157–8
Maternal serum alpha-fetoprotein (MSAFP) screen 239–40, 243, 375
Maternity leave 96
Maternity pads 321, 322
Mattresses 196, 197, 310
Meal planners 104–5, 333
Measles 370
Meat 101, 103, 110, 111
Mechanical dilators 228
Meconium 38, 49, 50, 212, 298, 307
Medical history 87, 88
Meditation 127–8
Membranes *see* Amniotic sac
Meningitis 310, 363–4, 370
Menstrual cycle 10–11

Menstruation 10, 14, 19, 275, 326
Midwives 85, 86, 175, 176, 177–8
Milia 285
Milk: bottlefeeding 303–5
    breastfeeding 191, 297–9
    cow's 303, 305
    in diet 102–3
    expressing 302
Milk ducts, blocked 357–8
"Milk rash" 285
Mind, pain control 218
Minerals 107–9, 332
Miscarriage: anxiety about 152
    causes 15, 75, 249, 278–9
    coping with 279
    genetic counseling 247
    invasive tests 241, 242, 244
    later miscarriages 276
    sexual activity and 155
    subsequent pregnancies 96
    ultrasound screening 237
Moisturizers 132, 133, 200, 285
Molar pregnancy 274
Mongolian spots 285
Monitoring 185, 186–7, 208, 217
Monitrices 184
Montgomery's tubercles 28, 63
Mood swings 20, 26, 341
Morning sickness 19, 25, 27, 60, 67, 256
Moro reflex 291
Morphine 179
Morula 14
Movements, baby in uterus 27, 28, 37, 38, 47, 92, 140, 145–7
    kick-count sheets 207, 208
    slowing or absence of 273–4
Mucus, cervical 11, 12
Mucus plug 212, 215
Multifactorial disorders 249
Multiple pregnancies *see* Triplets; Twins
Multiple sclerosis 269
Mumps 370
Muscles: development of 145

see also Body temperature
TENS, pain relief 180–1
Termination of pregnancy 247
Testicles 284, 378
Tests: anxieties about 152
  blood 21, 89–90
  chromosomal 93–94
  HIV 90
  invasive 241–5
  pregnancy 20–21
  screening 236–41
  urine 21, 89, 91
Tetanus 310, 370
Thalassemia 240, 246, 248
Third trimester 23, 44–51,
  52–54
Thirst 274
Thrombophlebitis 253, 273
Thrombosis, deep vein 252–3,
  273, 322
Thrush 259, 299, 308, 358–9,
  364
Thumb-sucking 142
Thyroid disease 270–1, 330
Thyroxine 61
"Tiger in the tree" 346
Tiredness 19–20, 25, 67
Tongue, baby's 142
Touch, sense of 142, 290
Toxoplasmosis 78, 111, 244,
  256, 257–8
Tranquilizers 180
Transition phase 167, 216–17
Translocations, chromosomes
  249
Transvaginal ultrasound 236
Transverse lie 188, 205
Travel 81–82, 197–8, 207,
  318
Trichomoniasis 268
Trimesters 23
Triplets 15, 16, 91
Trisomies 240, 245, 249
Twins: birth 96, 226
  conception 14, 15–16
  identical 14, 16, 96
  monitoring growth 91
  non-identical 16, 96
  placenta 141
  prenatal care 94–96

ultrasound screening 95, 96,
  237–8
in uterus 47, 48, 142

U

Ultrasound scans 28, 87, 92,
  236–9
  biophysical profile 208
  nuchal translucency screen
    238–9
  twin pregnancies 95, 96,
    237–8
Umbilical cord 30, 42, 50
  amniotic fluid problems 262
  at birth 51, 233, 284
  care of the stump 284, 309,
    312
  cutting 223, 225
  emergency births 169
  fetal blood sampling 241,
    245
  functions 141
  prolapse 213, 263
  round baby's neck 262, 263
  small babies 261
Undershirts 200, 317
Underwear 133, 135
Urinary tract infections
  259–60, 270, 273, 322
Urinary tract obstruction 377
Urination: after birth 322
  catheters 179, 231, 322
  during labor 182
  incontinence 29, 68
  infrequent 274
  newborn babies 307
  painful 273
  signs of pregnancy 20
Urine tests 21, 89, 91
Uterus 140–1
  afterpains 320
  baby's position 204–5, 215
  bleeding after delivery 225
  cesarean 231, 232
  delivery of placenta 225
  fibroids 238, 250, 255
  implantation 14–15, 20
  internal exams 23, 214
  placental problems 276–7

prolapse 356–7
rupture 188, 277
ultrasound 238
see also Contractions

V

Vacuum extraction 180, 188,
  229
Vagina: bleeding 274, 275–7
  breech labor 251
  discharges 211, 259, 284
  leaking of fluid 273
  lovemaking 156
  perineal massage 203
  ultrasound 236
Vaginal birth after a cesarean
  (VBAC) 188, 277
Varicose veins 52, 61, 73
Vegetables 101–2, 107
Vegetarian diet 103, 104–5
Veins 52, 61, 73, 252–3, 273,
  322
Vernix 39, 283, 285
Video 185, 192
Vision see Sight
Visitors 327
Visualization 128, 160, 181,
  205
Vitamins 106–9, 331–2
Vitamin A 106, 108–9, 132,
  331
Vitamin B complex 106–7,
  108–9, 332
Vitamin B_{12} 105, 252
Vitamin C 107, 108–9, 332
Vitamin D 61, 107, 108–9,
  332
Vitamin E 107, 108–9, 133
Vitamin K 269, 286
Voice, mother's 143–4
Vomiting 19, 25, 256, 273,
  362

W

Walking reflex 291
Warming up 117, 338
Washing: baby clothes 309
  diapers 308, 316

sponge baths 312–13
Water, drinking 81, 103, 115,
  201, 295, 332
Water birth 175, 176, 181,
  222
Water breaking 212–13
Weight (baby's): after birth
  287, 295, 367–9
  birth weight 283
  prenatal checks 88
  smoking and 75
Weight (mother's): after birth
  323, 333
  during pregnancy 26, 53,
    64–65, 100, 273
Weight training 120–1, 338
Whooping cough 310, 370
Womb see Uterus
Work: announcing pregnancy
  23
  part-time 193
  paternity leave 170
  returning to 158, 193, 350
  safety 79–80

X

X-linked disorders 18, 247–9

Y

Yeast infections 259

Z

Zinc 108–9
Zygote 14

ACKNOWLEDGMENTS

CARROLL & BROWN WOULD LIKE TO THANK:

Additional contributors: Anne Deans, MD, Gavin Evans, Kate Harding, MRCOG, Alison Murdoch

Additional consultants: Lesley Hickin, MD and Michael Janay, Child-Safety Specialist, Child Protection Network, Inc.

Design assistance: Evelyn Bercott and Peggy Sadler

Production Director: Karol Davies

Production Controller: Nigel Reed

Computer Management: Paul Stradling

Picture researcher: Sandra Schneider

Illustration: Peter Sutton, Halli Marie Verrinder, and Amanda Williams

Indexer: Hilary Bird

Proofreader: Geoffrey West

Photographic props: BabyBjörn AB

Models: Jocelyn Best, Michael McEhearney, and George; Frankie Dixon; Donae Hurst and Kyle; Racquel Milan, Jason Moy, and Bella; Alison Potter and Joseph

Make-up: Toka Hombu, Jeseama Owen

Picture credits:
OSF = Oxford Scientific Films
SPL = Science Photo Library
Mother & Baby PL = Mother & Baby Picture Library
Prof. S Campbell = Professor Stuart Campbell, Create Health Clinic
CLAPA = Cleft Lip and Palate Association

Front Jacket LWA-Dann Tardif/Corbis; 6 (top) Powerstock (bottom) Walter Hodges/Corbis; 8 (top) Mother & Baby PL; 10 Francis Leroy, Biocosmos/SPL; 15 Professor P M Motta et al/SPL; 17 Getty Images; 20 BSIP, LA/SPL; 21 (top) Adrian Weimbrecht/Practical Parenting/IPC Syndication; 24 (top) Mother & Baby PL (bottom) Mother & Baby PL/Dan Stevens; 25 (top) Mother & Baby PL/Ian Hooton (bottom) Mother & Baby PL/Dan Stevens; 26 (top) Saturn Stills/SPL (bottom) Mother & Baby PL/Dan Stevens; 27 (top) Mother & Baby PL/Ian Hooton (bottom) Mother & Baby PL/Dan Stevens; 28 (top) Rick Gomez/Corbis (bottom) Mother & Baby PL/Dan Stevens; 29 (top) Mother & Baby PL/Ruth Jenkinson (bottom) Mother & Baby PL/Dan Stevens; 30 Andy Walker, Midland Fertility Services/SPL; 31 (top) Petit Format/Nestle/Photo Researchers, Inc (bottom) Petit Format/Nestle/SPL; 32 (top) OSF/Science Pictures (bottom) Edelmann/SPL; 33 (top) Prof. S Campbell (bottom) SPL; 34 Powerstock; 35 (top) Edelmann/SPL (bottom) Prof. S Campbell; 36 (top) Powerstock (bottom) Edelmann/SPL; 37 (top) Tissuepix/SPL (bottom) James Stevenson/SPL; 38 Edelmann/SPL; 39 (top) Prof. S Campbell (bottom) BSIP DR LR/SPL; 40 OSF/Neil Bromhall; 41 (top) OSF/Dr Derek Bromhall (bottom) Baby Bond; 42 (top) Neil Bromhall/Genesis Films/SPL (bottom) Edelmann/SPL; 43 Prof. S Campbell; 45 Simon Fraser/Royal Victoria Infirmary Newcastle upon Tyne/SPL; 46 (top) Prof. S Campbell (bottom) BSIP, ATL/SPL; 47 (top) Prof. S Campbell (bottom) Innerspace Imaging/SPL; 48 (top) Simon Fraser/SPL (bottom) Edelmann/SPL; 49 (top) Prof. S Campbell (bottom) Simon Fraser/SPL; 52 (top) Mother & Baby PL (bottom) Mother & Baby PL/Dan Stevens; 53 (bottom) Mother & Baby PL/Dan Stevens; 54 (top) Mother & Baby PL/Ian Hooton (bottom) Mother & Baby PL/Dan Stevens; 57 Mother & Baby PL/Ruth Jenkinson; 84 Mother & Baby PL/Ian Hooton; 86 Simon Fraser/SPL; 87 Mother & Baby PL/Ian Hooton; 91 Rick Gomez/Corbis; 110 Imagestate; 120 Getty Images; 135 Jo Jo Maman Bebe; 136 Powerstock; 138 Ariel Shelley/Corbis; 143 Bubbles/Derren Curtis; 144 (top) Retna/Luci Pashley; 152 (top) Camera Press/Ian Boddy; 172 Mother & Baby PL/Ruth Jenkinson; 175 Mother & Baby PL/Moose Azim; 176 Jose Luis Pelaez, Inc/SPL; 178 Getty Images; 179 BSIP, Laurent/SPL; 182–183 Mother & Baby PL/Ruth Jenkinson; 184 Camera Press/Ian Boddy; 190 Getty Images; 191 Getty Images; 193 Mother & Baby PL/Ruth Jenkinson; 195 Powerstock; 199 (bottom) Getty Images; 206 (top) Mother & Baby PL/Ian Hooton (bottom) Powerstock; 210 Mother & Baby PL/Ruth Jenkinson; 213 Juliette Antoine/Oredia/Retna; 214 Mother & Baby PL/Ruth Jenkinson; 217 Ruth Jenkinson/Midirs/SPL; 219 Mother & Baby PL/Indira Flack; 222–223 Mother & Baby PL/Ruth Jenkinson; 224 Walter Hodges/Corbis; 225 James King-Holmes/SPL; 227 Mother & Baby PL/Indira Flack; 230 Michael Donne/SPL; 234 (top) Mehau Kulyk/SPL (center) GJLP/SPL (bottom) BSIP, Veronique Estiot/SPL; 237 Yves Baulieu, Publiphoto Diffusion/SPL; 239 GCa/SPL; 241 Alfred Pasieka/SPL; 242 Saturn Stills/SPL; 245 Colin Cuthbert/SPL; 249 BSIP Vem/SPL; 250 BSIP, Veronique Estiot/SPL; 251 SPL; 253 SPL; 255 GJLP/SPL; 256 Custom Medical Stock Library/SPL; 257 CNRI/SPL; 259 Dr P Marazzi/SPL; 260 Mehau Kulyk/SPL; 262 Mother & Baby PL/Ruth Jenkinson; 264 Damien Lovegrove/SPL; 265 Antonia Reeve/SPL; 267 Dr P Marazzi/SPL; 272 Wellcome Trust Medical Photographic Library; 274 CNRI/SPL; 275 SPL; 280 (top) Powerstock (bottom) BabyBjorn/SPL; 282 Getty Images; 285 (top) SPL (center) Mike Devlin/SPL (bottom) Dr I Williams/SPL; 290 BabyBjorn; 294 Sandra Lousada/Retna; 297 Rick Gomez/Corbis; 303 Juliette Antoine/Oredia/Retna; 320 Getty Images; 323 Powerstock; 325 Getty Images; 327 John Henley/Corbis; 334 Getty Images; 340 Powerstock; 354 (top) BSIP, Chassenet/SPL (center) BSIP Astier/SPL (bottom) Dr P Marazzi/SPL; 358 (left) John Radcliffe Hospital/SPL (right) Dr P Marazzi/SPL; 362 BSIP, Chassenet/SPL; 364 Meningitis Research Foundation (inset) Dr P Marazzi/SPL; 365 Dr I Williams; 366 (inset) Aaron Haupt/SPL (right) BSIP Astier/SPL; 373 Joseph Nettis/SPL; 374 Mediscan; 380 Clapa; 381 Dr P Marazzi/SPL; 383 Hank Morgan/SPL